TRAUMATI BRAIN INJURY

A ROADMAP FOR ACCELERATING PROGRESS

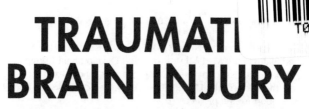

Donald Berwick, Katherine Bowman, and Chanel Matney, *Editors*

Committee on Accelerating Progress in Traumatic Brain Injury Research and Care

Board on Health Sciences Policy

Board on Health Care Services

Health and Medicine Division

A Consensus Study Report of

The National Academies of
SCIENCES · ENGINEERING · MEDICINE

THE NATIONAL ACADEMIES PRESS
Washington, DC
www.nap.edu

THE NATIONAL ACADEMIES PRESS   500 Fifth Street, NW   **Washington, DC 20001**

This activity was supported by Contract No.W81XWH20C0126 between the National Academy of Sciences and the United States Army Medical Research and Development Command of the Department of Defense. Any opinions, findings, conclusions, or recommendations expressed in this publication do not necessarily reflect the views of the United States Army Medical Research and Development Command that provided support for the project.

International Standard Book Number-13: 978-0-309-49043-6
International Standard Book Number-10: 0-309-49043-X
Digital Object Identifier: https://doi.org/10.17226/25394
Library of Congress Catalog Number: 2022933295

Additional copies of this publication are available from the National Academies Press, 500 Fifth Street, NW, Keck 360, Washington, DC 20001; (800) 624-6242 or (202) 334-3313; http://www.nap.edu.

Suggested citation: National Academies of Sciences, Engineering, and Medicine. 2022. *Traumatic brain injury: A roadmap for accelerating progress.* Washington, DC: The National Academies Press. https://doi.org/10.17226/25394.

The National Academies of
SCIENCES · ENGINEERING · MEDICINE

The **National Academy of Sciences** was established in 1863 by an Act of Congress, signed by President Lincoln, as a private, nongovernmental institution to advise the nation on issues related to science and technology. Members are elected by their peers for outstanding contributions to research. Dr. Marcia McNutt is president.

The **National Academy of Engineering** was established in 1964 under the charter of the National Academy of Sciences to bring the practices of engineering to advising the nation. Members are elected by their peers for extraordinary contributions to engineering. Dr. John L. Anderson is president.

The **National Academy of Medicine** (formerly the Institute of Medicine) was established in 1970 under the charter of the National Academy of Sciences to advise the nation on medical and health issues. Members are elected by their peers for distinguished contributions to medicine and health. Dr. Victor J. Dzau is president.

The three Academies work together as the **National Academies of Sciences, Engineering, and Medicine** to provide independent, objective analysis and advice to the nation and conduct other activities to solve complex problems and inform public policy decisions. The National Academies also encourage education and research, recognize outstanding contributions to knowledge, and increase public understanding in matters of science, engineering, and medicine.

Learn more about the National Academies of Sciences, Engineering, and Medicine at **www. nationalacademies.org.**

The National Academies of
SCIENCES · ENGINEERING · MEDICINE

Consensus Study Reports published by the National Academies of Sciences, Engineering, and Medicine document the evidence-based consensus on the study's statement of task by an authoring committee of experts. Reports typically include findings, conclusions, and recommendations based on information gathered by the committee and the committee's deliberations. Each report has been subjected to a rigorous and independent peer-review process and it represents the position of the National Academies on the statement of task.

Proceedings published by the National Academies of Sciences, Engineering, and Medicine chronicle the presentations and discussions at a workshop, symposium, or other event convened by the National Academies. The statements and opinions contained in proceedings are those of the participants and are not endorsed by other participants, the planning committee, or the National Academies.

For information about other products and activities of the National Academies, please visit www.nationalacademies.org/about/whatwedo.

MARTIN SCHREIBER, Chief, Division of Trauma Critical Care and Acute Care Surgery, Professor of Surgery, and Director, Donald D. Trunkey Center for Civilian and Combat Casualty Care, Oregon Health & Science University; and Adjunct Professor of Surgery, Uniformed Services University of the Health Sciences, Bethesda, Maryland
MONICA S. VAVILALA, Professor, Anesthesiology and Pain Medicine and Pediatrics, and Director, Harborview Injury Prevention and Research Center, University of Washington

Study Staff

KATHERINE BOWMAN, Study Director
CLARE STROUD, Senior Program Officer
CHANEL MATNEY, Program Officer
BRIDGET BOREL, Research Associate (*until July 2021*)
EDEN NELEMAN, Senior Program Assistant (*from July 2021*)
CHRISTIE BELL, Finance Business Partner
ANDREW M. POPE, Senior Director, Board on Health Sciences Policy
SHARYL NASS, Senior Director, Board on Health Care Services

National Academy of Medicine Fellow in Osteopathic Medicine

JULIEANNE P. SEES, Pediatric Neuro-Orthopaedic Surgeon and Associate Professor, Departments of Orthopaedic Surgery and Pediatrics, Thomas Jefferson University School of Medicine, Philadelphia, Pennsylvania

Consultants

RONA BRIERE, Senior Editor, Briere Associates, Inc.
ALLIE BOMAN, Editorial Assistant, Briere Associates, Inc.
MARGARET SHANDLING, Editorial Assistant, Briere Associates, Inc.
ANNA NICHOLSON, Science Writer, Doxastic, Inc.
JON WEINISCH, Science Writer, Doxastic, Inc.

Reviewers

This Consensus Study Report was reviewed in draft form by individuals chosen for their diverse perspectives and technical expertise. The purpose of this independent review is to provide candid and critical comments that will assist the National Academies of Sciences, Engineering, and Medicine in making each published report as sound as possible and to ensure that it meets the institutional standards for quality, objectivity, evidence, and responsiveness to the study charge. The review comments and draft manuscript remain confidential to protect the integrity of the deliberative process.

We thank the following individuals for their review of this report:

JANDEL ALLEN-DAVIS, Craig Hospital
JEFFREY BAZARIAN, University of Rochester
DAVID CIFU, Virginia Commonwealth University School of Medicine
SUSAN CONNORS, Brain Injury Association of America
KRISTEN DAMS-O'CONNOR, Icahn School of Medicine at Mount Sinai
JACK EBELER, Health and Medicine Division Committee, National Academies of Sciences, Engineering, and Medicine
JOHN HOLCOMB, The University of Alabama at Birmingham
DAVID OKONKWO, University of Pittsburgh
DAVID WRIGHT, Emory University
JINGZHEN (GINGER) YANG, Nationwide Children's Hospital

Although the reviewers listed above provided many constructive comments and suggestions, they were not asked to endorse the conclusions or recommendations of this report nor did they see the final draft before its release. The review of this report was overseen by **DAN G. BLAZER,** Duke University Medical Center, and **ALAN M. JETTE,** MGH Institute of Health Professions. They were responsible for making certain that an independent examination of this report was carried out in accordance with the standards of the National Academies and that all review comments were carefully considered. Responsibility for the final content rests entirely with the authoring committee and the National Academies.

Acknowledgments

The committee would like to express its gratitude to the many people and families dealing with traumatic brain injury and the scientists and clinicians who generously lent their time and insight to this project. The committee is also grateful for the contributions of Rona Briere, senior editor, and Allie Boman and Margaret Shandling, editorial assistants, Briere Associates, Inc.; Anna Nicholson and Jon Weinisch, science writers, Doxastic, Inc.; Tony Teat and Chantelle Bynum, Masai Interactive; and Christopher Lao-Scott, senior librarian of the National Academies Research Center, for his crucial assistance with fact checking.

Preface

I came to my role as chair of this committee as a newcomer to the topic of traumatic brain injury (TBI). Like any physician—indeed, like any adult—I knew of people whose acute injury from a contact sport, a bicycle accident, or a nursing home fall had led to sidelining for a "concussion," a period of memory loss, or evacuation of a subdural hematoma. "TBI" was for me the name of an unfortunate, usually obvious, accidental episode, occasionally followed by acute intervention. Mild cases resolved, and severe ones led to lifelong functional loss. It was a serious topic, but, in its way, rather simple.

I did not realize how wrong I was. Now, after 15 months of hard work with a superb committee of clinicians, research scholars, and epidemiologists who have devoted their careers to the study and care of TBI, and after eloquent testimony from people living with TBI and their families, I can see the topic more accurately for what it is: complex in texture, massive in scale, full of important research challenges, and largely as unrecognized—or as misunderstood—by the public and most clinicians as it was initially to me. TBI is not the name of an isolated, sometimes dramatic, but largely evanescent event. Instead, TBI is a significant, but remarkably hidden, burden for patients, families, public health, and health care costs throughout the nation, and in every demographic group.

As a longtime student of the deficiencies and opportunities for improvement in chronic disease care and outcomes, I can now recognize in TBI an iconic example of how care as currently designed can fail to reliably meet the needs of people facing chronic, life-changing health care challenges. And, just as for chronic illness broadly, I can see the exciting range of achievable improvements in TBI care, outcomes, and cost if only we set the proper goals and begin to act as an integrated system toward meeting those goals.

From its inception, the members of this committee embraced the value of teamwork and systems thinking in both TBI care and TBI research. They did so in their own work as a committee and in the vision of improvement that they shared for the nation. They rejected, as the clinical community must, the siloing of TBI into specialty channels, and instead noted and celebrated the interdependencies upon which successful TBI care depends: among medical and surgical specialties; among phases of patients' journeys from the point of injury through acute care into timely rehabilitation and, when needed, through lifelong support; between care systems and community systems; and from bench research to bedside application. The committee directly confronted the gaps between current but inadequate conventions of TBI classification (as "mild," "moderate," and "severe") and the more mature understandings of biomarkers, clinical observations, and sequential assessments that support evidence-based management and accurate prognostication. "Mild TBI," they clarified, is often not mild at all in its consequences, and "severe TBI" can have highly favorable outcomes with proper supports. They came to issue a clear call for a new TBI classification system. Much TBI, they concluded, remains undetected, and its behavioral and physical effects misattributed, because too few clinicians and laypeople understand its various forms and masquerades. They came to call, as well, for an end to that ignorance.

The committee agreed early on that clinicians and patients would need a comprehensive set of "bio-psycho-socio-ecological" lenses to see TBI truly in all its dimensions, and that care and concern over time—not just in terms of a bounded episode—were the proper tools for the best possible outcomes and the most responsive and compassionate support. No committee member is likely ever to forget the poignant workshop testimony from patients who described the sense of being "lost" or "forgotten" by a health care system lacking the integration and memory it would have needed to accompany them effectively through their changed lives with their altered needs. The understanding thus gained led the committee to address system design and leadership as inescapably vital resources. TBI, they came to recognize, is a clinical topic largely without a home in American health care, a public health challenge with no identifiable, responsible national or regional owner—no place the buck stops for the design and management of integrated systems of TBI care over time and place. That is not a problem easy to solve in a fragmented health care system, but neither is it one that will go away of its own accord.

I owe a deep debt to the members of the committee I was privileged to chair. Their gracefulness with each other, their shared respect, their willingness to reach across disciplinary boundaries, and their extraordinarily hard work, layered on their busy day (and night) jobs, impressed me at every step. Nothing the National Academies staff and I asked of them seemed too big for them to jump on and carry out quickly and reliably. I have never led a more capable and generous group, and I thank them, each and every one. And as the committee knows, every particle of progress and every positive element of our report traces directly to the skill, resilience, and good humor of the National Academies staff we were blessed to work with: our study director, Katie Bowman, and her Olympic-quality team of Clare Stroud, Chanel Matney, Bridget Borel, and Eden Neleman. They made my role as chair a pleasure and, frankly, for a topic of this size, easy. I am deeply grateful.

Like all chairs of National Academies committees and all committee members and staff, my fondest hope now is that the fate of this ambitious report is not to end up on shelves. It is a working document and a blueprint for action. The lack of a central leadership body for transforming TBI care at either the national or regional level is a real threat to the needed follow-through. Literally millions of people with TBI, present and future, depend now on action to achieve the care and outcomes that science, present and future, can make possible for them. If the buck stops somewhere for systemic redesign of TBI care, as it has not yet done, the gains in life, function, joy, and treasure can be immense. If TBI care as a system remains leaderless and rudderless, immense also will be the continuing human and societal costs.

Donald Berwick, *Chair*
Committee on Accelerating Progress in
Traumatic Brain Injury Research and Care

Contents

Boxes, Figures, and Tables

BOXES

FIGURES

TABLES

Summary[1]

The universe of traumatic brain injury (TBI) is vast, encompassing everyday occurrences such as falls and injuries during recreational activities, as well as motor vehicle crashes, violence, and military armed conflict. TBI affects all segments of society because the circumstances that cause it are common and because a significant brain injury sustained by one family member causes emotional, physical, and often financial disruptions to the family system. Those who live with long-term consequences from TBI may require accommodations to support their fullest possible reintegration into communities in which they live, learn, and work. Individual, family, community, and societal costs from TBI are high.

IMPETUS FOR THE STUDY

Over the past several decades, awareness of the magnitude and consequences of TBI has increased, particularly in sports and among military service members, with new recommendations emerging for screening and management after suspected brain injuries. A 10-year National Research Action Plan for TBI and posttraumatic stress disorder was established in 2012 by executive order among key agencies involved in TBI research. Large translational research initiatives have been undertaken to learn about the pathophysiology of brain injury, patient trajectories, and interventions to support recovery. These efforts from federal agencies, philanthropic organizations, patient and Veterans' advocacy groups, and the clinical care and research communities provide a foundation on which to build as the field looks to the decade ahead.

Despite prior efforts and progress, barriers and challenges remain, including unanswered questions about the most effective preventive, acute, rehabilitative, and long-term

---

[1] This Summary does not include reference citations. References for the information herein are provided in the full report.

care for TBI. Although interventions can prevent further injury and help manage symptoms, research has yet to yield Food and Drug Administration (FDA)-approved therapies for healing TBI. Moreover, not all patients and families have access to the best available care or to integrated follow-up across the care and recovery continuum throughout their lifespan. Box S-1 presents a sampling of statistics that illustrate the magnitude of the TBI problem today.

In this context, the Combat Casualty Care Research Program of the Department of Defense requested that the National Academies of Sciences, Engineering, and Medicine convene an ad hoc committee of experts to examine how progress can be advanced in TBI care and research and to develop a roadmap to help guide the field.

BOX S-1   MAGNITUDE OF THE TBI PROBLEM

TBI is experienced each year by millions of children and adults in the United States and globally.* However, the current system of TBI care does not meet the needs of many patients, families, and communities.

- Annually, as many as 55.9 million people globally are estimated to experience a "mild" TBI, and 5.48 million to experience a "severe" TBI. It is estimated that more than 55 million people—roughly 0.7 percent of the world's population—are living with the effects of a medically treated TBI.
- In the United States, 4.8 million people are evaluated in emergency departments for TBI each year. TBI is diagnosed in approximately 2 percent of total emergency department visits, hospitalizations, and deaths.
- In 2017, 2.5 million U.S. high school students reported experiencing at least one concussion. Modifiable factors, particularly early identification and follow-up with a TBI specialist, are associated with faster recovery and improved outcomes from concussion.
- A year after injury, 53 percent of those experiencing a "mild TBI" report persistent symptoms and functional impairment.
- Only 13–25 percent of people with moderate, severe, or penetrating TBI receive interdisciplinary inpatient rehabilitation.
- TBI is a signature injury of recent wars. Since 2000, more than 439,000 service members have been diagnosed with TBI.
- Half of U.S. Army soldiers report experiencing a TBI prior to enlistment, and one in five report experiencing a TBI during active duty. TBIs are associated with adverse mental health outcomes including posttraumatic stress disorder (PTSD), anxiety, depression, and suicidality.
- Estimates of the lifetime cost of TBI in the United States, including medical care and such indirect costs as lost work, range from approximately $80 million for the roughly 300,000 TBIs resulting in death or hospitalization to more than $750 billion for the more than 2 million total TBIs recorded in 1 year.
- Rural populations have higher TBI incidence and poorer outcomes and often experience longer times to reach care relative to urban populations. Racial and ethnic differences are also linked to disparities and inequities in TBI prevalence, outcomes, and access to care.
- An estimated 2.5 million caregivers are supporting a person with a TBI. Families report substantial emotional and financial burdens from such caregiving.

*Estimates are likely to undercount true rates of TBI. In many cases, data are drawn from health systems and disease classification codes that miss some people who experience TBI.

A ROADMAP FOR ACCELERATING PROGRESS IN TBI CARE AND RESEARCH

The committee's recommendations for actions to advance TBI education, prevention, care, and research toward an optimized system are summarized in Box S-2 and detailed in the text that follows.

The term "traumatic brain injury" evokes an image of a sudden, isolated event; dramatic surgical or medical interventions; and, with good fortune, a cure, as with a broken bone that knits together. According to that image, the injury is clear, the intervention acute, and the episode time-delimited—TBI has a beginning, a treatment, and a predictable outcome. An overarching finding of this committee, however, is that this image is at best incomplete and at worst misleading for many people. Conceiving of TBI as an acute event with a clear endpoint also belies the burden it places on families, communities, and workplaces and its substantial financial and social costs.

It is far more accurate to view TBI through a wider lens encompassing at least four domains that drive the trajectory of recovery—biological, psychological, sociological, and ecological (including economic)—reflecting the mix of personal and social factors that

---

BOX S-2   A ROADMAP FOR ACHIEVING PROGRESS IN TBI CARE AND RESEARCH

To transform TBI care into a learning health system and accelerate improvement in care will require changes in public and professional knowledge about TBI, as well as national goals, care system redesigns, resource allocation, and leadership.

Conclusions

- TBI care in the United States often fails to meet the needs of individuals, families, and communities affected by this condition.
- High-quality care for TBI requires that it be managed as a condition with both acute and long-term phases.
- Public and professional misunderstandings are widespread with respect to the frequency; manifestations; long-term consequences; and proper detection, treatment, and rehabilitation of TBI.
- The United States lacks a comprehensive framework for addressing TBI.

Recommendations

1. Create and implement an updated classification system for TBI.
2. Integrate acute and long-term person- and family-centered management of TBI.
3. Reduce unwarranted variability and gaps in administrative and clinical care guidance to ensure high-quality care for TBI.
4. Enhance awareness and identification of TBI by health care providers and the public.
5. Establish and reinforce local and regional integrated care delivery systems for TBI.
6. Integrate the TBI system of care and TBI research into a learning health care system.
7. Improve the quality and expand the range of TBI studies and study designs.
8. Create and promulgate a national framework and implementation plan for improving TBI care.

affect the experience of and recovery from conditions such as TBI. This "bio-psycho-socio-ecological" lens reveals that for many patients, TBI is more complex and more hidden and imposes a more chronic burden than a simple, event-based model would indicate.

> *Conclusion: TBI care in the United States often fails to meet the needs of individuals, families, and communities affected by this condition. TBI is an ongoing condition that poses significant burdens over time, including substantial financial and social costs. For the most part, the nation has no mechanism in place for long-term follow-up and care of adults or children with TBI. The results of this gap include needless death, squandered human potential, family stress, and soaring social costs. Because of this gap, the true morbidity, mortality, and cost attributable to TBI, though undoubtedly vast, are unknown.*

The following recommendations reflect priorities identified by the committee as necessary for transforming TBI care and research to fill this gap. Achieving each of these priorities will require cooperative action among multiple organizations and communities and investments of substantial time and resources. The committee identified core actors to take each priority forward while emphasizing the critical role of a holistic framework for TBI.

Implement an Evidence-Guided Classification Scheme for Care and Research

The spectrum of initiating circumstances under the rubric of TBI is enormous, magnified by the fact that for many individuals, more than one TBI occurs in a lifetime. Causes range from high-energy kinetic or penetrant injuries to seemingly insignificant events, and result in diverse outcomes ranging from an immediate threat to life to subtle, persistent effects that may not initially be recognized as related to TBI but substantially affect health and function. Across this spectrum, the taxonomic categories of "mild, moderate, and severe," derived from clusters of scores on the Glasgow Coma Scale, are inadequate to capture or guide either proper management of TBI or accurate prognostication of its outcome. The consequences of injuries classified as "mild" can prove, in some instances, to be insidious, and even lifelong in their impact. Conversely, injuries rated as "severe" can vary in long-term outcomes, from devastating disability to high function. Tools are needed to accurately inform clinical decisions, including withdrawal of life-sustaining treatment, a gap that leads to suboptimal care for people across the spectrum of TBI. Clinicians, patients, and payers need a more nuanced, personalized, and evidence-guided taxonomy for TBI, using clinical and biological markers to support more effective assessment, treatment, prognosis, and rehabilitation. Because initial assessment does not reliably predict ultimate outcome, regular reassessment is also essential as a person's condition and needs change.

Recommendation 1. Create and implement an updated classification system for TBI. The current clinical classification scheme for TBI should be updated to be more accurate and informative for care and research:

a. The National Institutes of Health (NIH) should convene a TBI Classification Work-group to review data from recent large-scale clinical studies and determine which elements should be incorporated into a more descriptive, evidence-based, and precise classification system for clinical care and research. In this effort, NIH should engage professional communities that routinely diagnose and classify TBI.

b. Relevant professional societies, including but not limited to those in emergency medicine, trauma care, and rehabilitation, should advise and train clinicians caring for people with TBI to classify patients based on their actual Glasgow Coma Scale (GCS) sum score (e.g., GCS 14) rather than the inaccurate and misleading three-category shorthand mild, moderate, or severe. Optimally, clinicians should also use results from neuroimaging and blood-based biomarkers, when available and clinically indicated, to classify patients. Clinicians should update the TBI classification for each patient as the person's condition evolves.

Progress has been made in identifying markers that can inform TBI assessment, diagnosis, and prognostication since a 2007 National Institute of Neurological Disorders and Stroke (NINDS) workshop on this topic. As one of its initial actions, the Classification Workgroup should evaluate these advances, including the utility of various markers across different TBI populations and injury severities and in different care environments. Data elements that might be considered for incorporation into a revised and updated TBI classification system include advances in neuroimaging, blood-based biomarkers, and other areas.

Manage TBI as Both a Complex Acute and a Chronic Condition

The physical, psychological, and social effects of TBI, along the full range of severity and with time horizons beyond the acute phase of management, have significant impacts on a person's function, relationships, and quality of life. Testimony from experts and people living with TBI conveyed these serious effects and the frequent failures of the health care system to even recognize them, let alone address them adequately. For many people, although thankfully not for all, a TBI is the portal to months, years, or a lifetime of motor, sensory, psychological, behavioral, and cognitive problems. TBI should be understood and managed as a condition with acute and chronic phases and challenges that evolve over time, challenges a truly responsive health care system would anticipate and meet. Instead, evidence suggests that many people with TBI find themselves without continuity of care, integrated professional support, or adequate health insurance downstream from their acute injury. Many TBI patients are lost to follow-up, leaving no mechanism for measuring the long-term effects of this condition.

> **Recommendation 2. Integrate acute and long-term person- and family-centered management of TBI. All people with TBI should have reliable and timely access to integrated, multidisciplinary, and specialized care to address physical, cognitive, and behavioral sequelae of TBI and comorbidities that influence quality of life.**

a. Relevant professional societies should encourage clinicians to recommend that all patients at discharge from inpatient and outpatient acute care settings have an opportunity for follow-up with a clinician experienced in managing TBI. Guidance to clinicians should also emphasize the need to connect patients and family caregivers with care navigation resources as needed.
b. In their intake processes, health care and social services organizations should be aware of lifetime TBI exposure so they can identify those needing accommodations, as well as those at increased risk for TBI-related symptoms or declining trajectories in health and function. These organizations should also give providers guidance on practical strategies and accommodations that can help patients and families cope with TBI-related symptoms, and on resources that can increase reliable and timely access to and appropriateness of care for persons with TBI.

   c. Organizations that oversee or provide long-term care should consider the needs of families and caregivers for education and support as key components of long-term care plans.

Stronger commitment and strategies are needed to ensure quality and continuity of care for all people with TBI. Incorporating family and caregiver needs is also crucial, since many persons with TBI live with family and are dependent upon family members and other caregivers to address their needs, navigate health care and community services, and facilitate community integration.

Ensure Quality and Consistency of Care

   Unwarranted variability and gaps in care guidance need to be addressed, and guidelines and best practices need to be consistently implemented, including to guide reimbursement practices. The evidence to inform TBI care decisions should be based on a range of rigorous methodologies for generating knowledge and include evidence obtained not only from randomized controlled trials but also from observational cohort and other study designs and from expert consensus on best practices.

   Recommendation 3. Reduce unwarranted variability and gaps in administrative and clinical care guidance to ensure high-quality care for TBI. The federal agencies that lead the development of clinical practice guidelines for TBI, including the Department of Veterans Affairs, the Department of Defense, the Agency for Healthcare Research and Quality, and the Centers for Disease Control and Prevention, should convene at regular intervals an expert panel to undertake the actions below in collaboration with clinical and patient community stakeholders. The Centers for Medicare & Medicaid Services (CMS) should be engaged in this effort to ensure alignment of coverage with clinical guidelines:

   a. Survey the landscape of existing clinical care guidelines for all elements of TBI care, during all phases of care, and involving all salient specialties. Synthesize best current clinical practice and evidence to develop consensus-based guidelines where evidence is currently limited, using rigorous methods for such consensus processes. Guidelines should be sensitive to local contexts and potential sources of inequity, such as race/ethnicity, rurality, and limited access to health care resources.
   b. Identify and resolve problems of inconsistency among current clinical care guidelines.
   c. Identify guidelines and practices that are contraindicated by current evidence, and issue guidance on their deimplementation.
   d. Identify common criteria for the inclusion of studies used to inform the development of guidelines and for how topics are covered for which limited evidence from randomized controlled trials or other rigorous study designs is available (see Recommendation 7).
   e. Identify gaps in the evidence base informing current clinical care guidelines, and recommend research to develop the necessary evidence (see also gaps identified in the research agenda presented later).
   f. Develop evidence-guided and consensus-based criteria for identifying patients who should be referred to inpatient and outpatient TBI rehabilitation (see Recommendation 5).
   g. Identify avenues for emerging best practices to guide third-party coverage of care, regardless of payer source and type of medical facility.

Relevant clinical organizations that have been active in TBI guideline development and can be engaged in this effort include the Brain Trauma Foundation, Concussion in Sport Group, American College of Surgeons, American Academy of Neurology, American College of Emergency Physicians, American Congress of Rehabilitation Medicine, Neurocritical Care Society, and others.

Enhance Awareness and Understanding of TBI

Like many neurologic and medical conditions, TBI is sociologically complex. For example, misunderstood, longer-term psychological consequences of TBI may be interpreted as problems of commitment or character rather than as treatable conditions. TBI care and outcomes can be improved with better understanding among clinicians, educators, and the public of the forms and clinical courses of these injuries, and of the medical and community supports needed to help persons living with TBI and their families cope and thrive. Similarly, underinvestment in research on the causes, types, and treatment of TBI may reflect, in part, underestimation by the public and policy makers of the magnitude of the burden TBI imposes on the population and progress that could potentially be made with levels of research support more commensurate with that burden—what quality-of-care researcher John Williamson termed "achievable benefit not achieved."

Recommendation 4. Enhance awareness and identification of TBI by health care providers and the public. Education and awareness are essential for achieving high-quality care and improving outcomes, and are particularly important in the following areas:

a. *Public awareness.* The Centers for Disease Control and Prevention, working with organizations in TBI prevention, care, and rehabilitation and those that work with at-risk groups, should enhance efforts to raise awareness among the public on the context, causes, and long-term effects of TBI; the importance of follow-up; and resources that may be available to the person with TBI.

b. *Professional awareness, education, and training.* Education and training programs for health care professions should include information on the burden, risk factors, and signs and symptoms of TBI and should correct misconceptions about the condition. Materials should emphasize adherence to evidence-based guidelines where they exist to bring greater consistency to TBI care across the United States, while taking into account patient characteristics and preferences in order to provide personalized care. Guidance should also emphasize eliminating practices that are contraindicated by current evidence and reducing inequities in care and outcomes.

c. *Patient and family empowerment.* National- and state-level patient and family organizations should work with clinical communities in primary care, acute care, and rehabilitation to ensure that all TBI patients and families receive anticipatory guidance on expected symptoms and trajectory, steps to decrease the risk of delayed recovery, and available TBI resources.

Groups at particular risk of experiencing a TBI include, but are not limited to, the elderly, those engaged in sports and recreation, and those at risk of experiencing forms of violence. Organizations working closely with these groups should be involved in efforts to develop and disseminate practical information on TBI. Given the prevalence and burden of TBI, multiple health care professionals, including physicians, nurses, emergency medical technicians, psychologists, and rehabilitation professionals, need sufficient training in and guidance on its diagnosis and management. Investigators with complementary expertise in such areas as social sciences, implementation science, and health economics also form part of the roadmap for advancing TBI care (see the research agenda below). Ensuring broad awareness of and education about TBI can help engage these experts and stakeholders in the efforts that make up that roadmap.

Establish an Effective Care System for TBI

TBI and its care are embedded in and affected by the ecology of American communities. As in almost all aspects of U.S. health care access and quality, TBI care and outcomes demonstrate evidence of racial, geographic, and socioeconomic inequity. Achieving high-quality TBI care will require confronting this inequity at its sources and committing to measuring and monitoring progress toward its resolution. Where you live, who you are, and where you receive care should not determine if and how well you live. Yet, with TBI, as with many complex medical conditions, this ambitious goal is not achieved. The reasons are manifold, and overcoming these obstacles will depend on a careful redesign of TBI care as a system, as well as on incorporating into the nation's TBI care the properties of a "learning health care system," as described in National Academies reports of the past decade. Currently the United States has neither an integrated system of care for TBI nor a learning system capable of continual progress toward ideal TBI care everywhere and for everyone.

Individual patients would benefit if clinicians and health care organizations had the capacity and commitment to view the TBI care they provide—and the system's duties—through the lens of the bio-psycho-socio-ecological model, and to do so not just once but continuously and repeatedly through each patient's life journey, adjusting treatments, assessments, and community resources as the patient's status and needs change. Doing so would require a level of continuity and acceptance of responsibility that American health care does not often achieve for chronic illnesses. At present, the majority of people with TBI cannot count on both the acute and longer-term care they need to achieve their full potential of health and well-being. The gap of "achievable benefit not achieved" is enormous.

Efforts by professional and accreditation societies should be leveraged to confront and mitigate the discontinuity of care; government and private philanthropy should invest in developing prototypes of integrated TBI care, including regional system designs; and public and private payers should ensure that benefit structures accord with the evidence for best practice in TBI care across all phases and environments of care.

> **Recommendation 5. Establish and reinforce local and regional integrated care delivery systems for TBI.** The Secretary of Health and Human Services should work to establish geographically based, integrated care delivery systems for TBI, emphasizing the continuum of care across the acute, rehabilitation, and recovery phases and all severities. The effort should build on the nation's success with regional trauma systems and incorporate practices and lessons learned from the Department of Defense (DoD) and the Department of Veterans Affairs (VA). Specifically:
>
> a. The American College of Surgeons (ACS) and other trauma verification systems should incorporate comprehensive standards for TBI care in trauma center verification processes and data systems and as a national trauma system evolves. As part of this effort, ACS should expand efforts to foster communication between acute care and rehabilitation care providers and expand outreach on the signs and management of TBI to the public, first responders, and acute care providers.

b. Settings that provide TBI care across the post-acute rehabilitation continuum should meet standards for integrated, evidence-based, and individualized brain injury care, such as those required by the Commission on Accreditation of Rehabilitation Facilities for the Brain Injury Specialty. The Joint Commission should review and promulgate standards for high-quality TBI care in the broader spectrum of care settings that treat people with TBI, such as primary care, community hospitals, and concussion programs.

c. The Department of Health and Human Services and the Center for Medicare & Medicaid Innovation should support local and regional pilot demonstration projects to create prototype civilian care infrastructures focused on providing continuity of care for follow-up, rehabilitation, and longer-term care and recovery from TBI. The demonstration projects should document best practices and effects on patient outcomes, and identify the components of a chronic care management model that are most effective for persons with TBI. Prototype systems should address the needs of TBI across the spectrum of severity and venues of care, including community-based services.

d. The Centers for Medicare & Medicaid Services (CMS) and commercial health care insurers should align coverage for TBI care with clinical guidelines to ensure equity in access to, affordability of, and quality of care. For example, payers should use criteria identified under Recommendation 3 when authorizing inpatient and outpatient rehabilitation services, including for long-term TBI sequelae. CMS, the VA, and DoD should test alternative benefit structures for TBI rehabilitation care instead of relying on the current time-based metric (e.g., the "3-hour rule") or preset benefits.

Make the TBI Care System into a Learning System

As observed above, TBI care needs to have the properties of a learning health care system. In addition to care and research, such a system encompasses processes for continual quality improvement and education. A full learning system for TBI also will involve public health agencies and community organizations across the phases of prevention, care, and recovery.

Recommendation 6. Integrate the TBI system of care and TBI research into a learning health care system. Reducing the burden of TBI will require a learning system capable of continual improvement. Important elements are thorough surveillance, standardized and longitudinal patient information, and accessibility of data. The Secretary of Health and Human Services (HHS) should therefore work to establish an integrated TBI data system, taking the following actions:

a. *Conduct thorough surveillance.* The Centers for Disease Control and Prevention should expand efforts to track TBI mortality, morbidity, and long-term outcomes more completely and accurately, including by adding validated, standardized TBI questions to population-based and weighted surveys and working to ensure consistency of information across states and surveys. The Agency for Healthcare Research and Quality should modify and expand the Healthcare Cost and Utilization Project to enable improved analysis of TBI care patterns, costs, and outcomes, both acute and long-term.

b. *Standardize the capture of patient-level data.* HHS should work with health care systems and electronic health record vendors to bring data infrastructure into line with the state of the science by investing in and developing the ability to capture high-quality, TBI-relevant data in medical records. This data infrastructure will help in identifying causal factors and longitudinal outcomes, enabling comparative effectiveness, implementation, and translation studies across health care systems.

    c. *Emphasize longitudinal data, and integrate information across the continuum of care.* HHS should work with the owners of national and regional TBI registries and databanks to crosslink patient-level data across sites and through time. In addition, data systems should collect clinical information in alignment with the refined TBI classification system proposed in Recommendation 1.

Organizations in a learning system need access to high-quality data. Relevant databases to involve in these efforts include, for example, the National Highway Traffic Safety Administration's (NHTSA's) National Emergency Medical Services Information System (NEMSIS); the American College of Surgeons' (ACS's) National Trauma Databank and Trauma Quality Improvement Program; state trauma registries; the National Institute on Disability, Independent Living, and Rehabilitation Research's (NIDILRR's) TBI Model Systems database; the DoD Trauma Registry; and VA TBI registries. But a true learning system requires that organizations go further by using the data to drive real-time and iterative improvements in care.

Invest in Continued Research

Despite advances, major gaps remain in scientific understanding of the pathophysiology of TBI and the necessary foundations for novel acute and post-acute treatments that can achieve better outcomes than are achieved today. Compared with many other important conditions, such as cancer and heart disease, biomedical research on TBI has languished, with insufficient investment and no clear institutional ownership. Redesigning and transforming TBI care will require a new level of investment in clinical and basic research commensurate with the enormous burden of TBI. The committee's recommendation for advancing the TBI research enterprise is given below; priority areas for research are detailed in Box S-3.

> **Recommendation 7. Improve the quality and expand the range of TBI studies and study designs.** TBI research and investment by the National Institutes of Health, the Department of Defense, the Department of Veterans Affairs, and private-sector funders should be commensurate with the public health burden of the condition. The research agenda proposed herein identifies eight areas for further progress and additional attention. When identifying research priorities and requests for applications, the above funders should take the following actions:
>
>   a. Significantly expand financial support and research efforts to address the priorities identified in the research agenda.
>
>   b. Establish translational research and implementation science centers to undertake collaborative efforts toward improved standardization and clinical care for TBI throughout the continuum of care. These centers should use insights from implementation science to enable effective translation of study results from the laboratory to clinical trials and from clinical trials to practice.
>
>   c. Encourage multidisciplinary and multistakeholder research efforts to strengthen the evidence base informing care. These efforts should:
>
>   1. Use the TBI classification system called for in Recommendation 1 to better stratify participants in clinical trials of novel interventions for TBI.

BOX S-3	RESEARCH AGENDA TO ACCELERATE THE EXPANSION OF KNOWLEDGE

The following eight areas are among the most urgent priorities for continued and expanded research on TBI:

A. Conduct national and international epidemiological studies to better understand the scope and burden of TBI and inform prevention efforts.
B. Understand the economic impact of TBI both within health care and within the family and broader community.
C. Understand how combinations of injury characteristics, individual factors, and social-environmental variables affect short- and long-term care and outcomes after TBI.
D. Enhance research to understand and reduce disparities in TBI incidence, diagnosis, care, and outcomes.
E. Expand the number and breadth of validated tools for measuring TBI risk factors and improving diagnosis, classification, monitoring, short- to long-term outcome assessment, and prognostication.
F. Develop evidence-guided therapies for treating TBI and improving outcomes.
G. Innovate and disseminate improved designs for coordinated TBI care in organizations and regions, with special attention to patients' and families' long-term needs and follow-up.
H. Expand TBI research in areas with a weak history of TBI focus, including health care quality, health economics, and implementation science research.

2. Engage patient and family voices early in study design by using stakeholder engagement (i.e., community-based participatory research) to identify unmet needs and refine research questions.
3. Recruit diverse study participants to ensure that research is broadly representative of the people who experience TBI.
4. Use all forms of rigorous study designs when appropriate to answer research questions. Study methods should be eclectic and adaptive, and should include not only randomized controlled trials for efficacy but also pragmatic trials, adaptive designs, comparative effectiveness trials, observational studies (including those using statistical control for causal inference), and mixed methods, as appropriate to the research questions.
5. Engage laboratory scientists and clinicians to ensure better research translation, including rigorous parallels across animal and human injury models, therapeutic targets, comorbidities, and study design outcome metrics and endpoints.

Provide Leadership to Drive Collaboration and Change

The actions identified in Recommendations 1 through 7 are needed to advance TBI care and research, link acute and longer-term care, and better align payment models with improved outcomes. But multiple efforts can be uncoordinated or have goals that misalign because so many different agencies, organizations, professional communities, patient groups, and others have roles to play.

Conclusion: The United States lacks a comprehensive framework for addressing TBI. A barrier to dramatic improvement in TBI care and research is the absence of a strategic framework and a lead agency or organization with a systemic view, responsibility for articulating goals and overseeing progress, the capacity to foster change, and the ability to convene the many stakeholders required to address the necessary multiple lines of effort. Absent a leadership entity, no one owns the problem, and major progress is unlikely.

Federal leadership is needed to establish a strategic framework for dramatically improving TBI care. Because this framework will require the efforts of multiple partners as well as investment of substantial resources, it will be essential to develop early on a clear plan for implementation that includes a timeline and metrics of progress and is curated as circumstances change. This coordinated approach will support innovation and improvement in TBI research and care, and will align the expansive range of partners and stakeholders whose efforts are critical to establishing an optimized system that aims to achieve high-quality care and health equity among all groups and across the lifespan.

Recommendation 8. Create and promulgate a national framework and implementation plan for improving TBI care. The Secretary of Health and Human Services (HHS) should, under the aegis of the Assistant Secretary for Health, create, promulgate, and curate a strategic national framework and implementation plan for improving TBI care:

a. To this end, the Secretary of HHS should establish, for a period of 10 years, a national Traumatic Brain Injury Task Force as a successor to the National Research Action Plan. The TBI Task Force should move beyond an emphasis solely on research coordination to encompass a focus on research implementation and application of the evidence in support of better treatment and systems of care delivery, engaging an expanded group of federal, private-sector, and philanthropic partners. It should enlist and help coordinate TBI-related care improvements among HHS components (such as the Centers for Medicare & Medicaid Services, the National Institutes of Health, the Centers for Disease Control and Prevention, the Administration for Community Living, the Agency for Healthcare Research and Quality, and the Health Resources and Services Administration, among others) and should include participation from other relevant departments, such as the Department of Veterans Affairs, the Department of Defense, the Social Security Administration, and the Department of Transportation.

b. The TBI Task Force's first actions should be to develop a strategic framework addressing the issues reflected in the committee's recommendations and within 2 years, to release a specific implementation plan to guide and coordinate efforts within that framework. This plan should be curated and updated over time.

c. The TBI Task Force should engage a multistakeholder public–private coalition to continually advance and accelerate implementation of the national framework and plan. Stakeholders in this coalition should include, but not be limited to, the federal agencies that provide funding for TBI research and clinical care, relevant patient and family advocacy organizations, Veterans service organizations, relevant professional societies, youth and adult sports associations, health payment organizations, philanthropic foundations, and companies developing new tools and treatments for TBI.

FINAL THOUGHTS

Compared with current TBI care management and research, what is needed is not merely improvement, but a transformation of attitudes, understanding, investments, and care systems. Evolutionary changes—such as better national data systems, redesign of insurance coverage for rehabilitation, reconciliation of disparate clinical care guidance, advances in preclinical and clinical research, and a modernized taxonomy for TBI itself—will help. But bringing the best achievable outcomes to persons with TBI and their families will require a wholesale redesign of TBI systems to reflect the timing and many manifestations of the condition, and to guarantee linked and coordinated care across time and sites of care to deliver what matters most to patients and their loved ones.

1

Introduction

D espite significant advances achieved over the past 60 years in addressing the problem of traumatic injury, injury remains today an important cause of death and disability, by one estimate posing a burden of death and disability second only to that of cancer and just slightly greater than that of heart disease (Moses et al., 2015). Reflecting the magnitude of this burden, prior reports of the National Academies of Sciences, Engineering, and Medicine and others have addressed injury prevention and trauma care (see Box 1-1). Yet, funding directed at research on injury is not yet commensurate with the magnitude of the problem (see Figure 1-1).

Traumatic brain injury (TBI), defined in Box 1-2 and the focus of this report, represents only one type of accidental or deliberate injury. However, TBI was diagnosed in approximately 2 percent of the total emergency department (ED) visits, hospitalizations, and deaths in the United States in 2013 (Taylor et al., 2017), and half of military Veterans have reported a lifetime history of experiencing at least one TBI (Shura et al., 2019). TBI has been reported to contribute to 30 percent of injury-related deaths in a U.S. study (Taylor et al., 2017) and to 41 percent of years of life lost to premature death in a study of 16 European countries (Majdan et al., 2017). TBI thus represents a significant component of overall injury, providing an important opportunity to improve health and well-being if prevention, care, and recovery can be advanced.

STUDY CONTEXT

Every community and every segment of the population is affected by TBI. TBI affects civilian and military populations and occurs in both rural and urban settings. Causes as diverse as falls, sports injuries, vehicle collisions, intimate partner violence, and military incidents can result in such injuries across a spectrum of severity and among every age group, from babies and children, to adults, to the elderly.[1] Chapters 2 and 3 present a detailed look at the scope and burden of TBI.

---

[1] Symptoms consistent with experiencing a TBI have also been reported after incidents among U.S. staff in Cuba, China, and other locations, and it has been suggested that these injures may be caused by radiofrequency energy. This report does not focus on such cases. (For a recent assessment, see NASEM, 2020.)

BOX 1-1   PRIOR REPORTS ON INJURY PREVENTION AND TRAUMA CARE

Assessment of the challenges posed by traumatic brain injuries and opportunities for improving care and research to address these challenges builds on a history of engagement in injury prevention and care that stretches back decades (see the figure below).

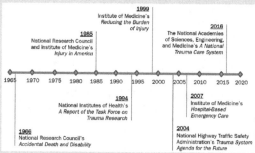

Selected prior reports on injury control and trauma care.

SOURCE: NASEM, 2016.

The 1966 report *Accidental Death and Disability: The Neglected Disease of Modern Society* (NAS and NRC, 1966) called injury a "neglected epidemic" that was "the leading cause of death in the first half of life's span" (NAS and NRC, 1966, p. 5). The committee responsible for that report recommended improved awareness and treatment of trauma and called for establishing trauma registries, expanding support for trauma research, and establishing a national institute of trauma to serve as a coordinated focus of trauma-related activity. The first edition of *Optimal Hospital Resources for Care of the Seriously Injured* was published in 1976 (ACS, 1976) and has since become an important guide for trauma centers. Two decades later, *Injury in America: A Continuing Public Health Problem* (NRC and IOM, 1985) reported that improvements in trauma care had been achieved but that injuries remained the "leading cause of death up to the age of 44 ... [and] cause the loss of more working years of life than all forms of cancer and heart disease combined" (NRC and IOM, 1985, p. 1). The report identified the need for additional research on biomedical mechanisms of injury and on optimal injury management but noted that research on injury and injury control was "disproportionately low and discontinuous, in comparison with that for cancer, heart disease, and other major health problems" (NRC and IOM, 1985, p. 2). The attention to trauma resulting from these and other reports led to a new era of emphasis on the problem in public health, including the establishment of a center at the Centers for Disease Control and Prevention (CDC) focused on injury prevention and control. In 1992, the Defense and Veterans Head Injury Program, now known as the Traumatic Brain Injury Center of Excellence, was established. And in 2005, the Department of Veterans Affairs designated a network for rehabilitation after polytrauma, establishing its Polytrauma System of Care.

A National Trauma Care System: Integrating Military and Civilian Trauma Systems to Achieve Zero Preventable Deaths After Injury (NASEM, 2016) emphasized lessons learned by military and civilian trauma systems and again highlighted the enormous societal burden of traumatic injury, the dramatic contributions it makes to years of life lost before age 75, and its contributions to almost half of all deaths under age 46. The report argued for the value of integrating these two systems to achieve the best possible care, highlighting practices, such as coordinated handoffs, that had contributed to reductions in military trauma deaths. The report stimulated further efforts to strengthen the U.S. trauma care system, including the 2018 launch of the National Trauma Research Action Plan (Bulger et al., 2018).

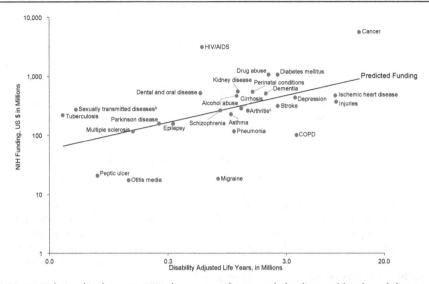

FIGURE 1-1 Relationship between NIH disease-specific research funding and burden of disease for selected conditions. Injury is shown on the right side of the figure and below the line, indicating that it poses a high burden but with less-than-predicted levels of research support.
SOURCE: Moses et al., 2015. Reproduced with permission from the *Journal of the American Medical Association*. © 2015 American Medical Association. All rights reserved.

BOX 1-2   DEFINITION OF TBI USED IN THIS REPORT

As defined by the initiative on Common Data Elements (CDE) for Research on Traumatic Brain Injury and Psychological Health, a traumatic brain injury is "an alteration in brain function, or other evidence of brain pathology, caused by an external force" (Menon et al., 2010, p. 1638). The CDE definition of TBI is both concise and inclusive, encompassing any external force that leads to brain tissue damage of any severity level and resultant disruption in the normal function of the brain. The brain injury can result from an impact, from rotational forces (e.g., angular acceleration or deceleration of the head), or from a pressure wave, and the injury can be blunt or penetrating. Because this study looks broadly across all types of TBI in all military and civilian populations, the CDE definition is the one used as the basis for this report.

It should be noted that different communities addressing TBI have developed operational definitions focused on the signs and symptoms most relevant to their particular foci, including loss of consciousness or alteration of mental state and other postinjury elements. A number of TBI definitions are collected in Appendix B of the report *Evaluation of the Disability Determination Process for Traumatic Brain Injury in Veterans* (NASEM, 2019). Some definitions focus on how individuals experiencing a TBI can be identified, especially at the point of injury (e.g., DoD, 2012, 2015; French et al., 2008; McCrory et al., 2017). Others address injuries for which the injured person can be considered for disability adjudication and compensation (VA, 2015) or for payment of claims against health benefit plans. Still others provide guidance for clinical practice or inclusion criteria for clinical studies (APA, 2013; Giza et al., 2013; Malec et al., 2007). Although this report uses the encompassing CDE definition, such operational definitions remain valuable to the sectors of the TBI field for which they were developed.

Just as the many causes of TBI and the people who experience it are diverse, so, too, are the physiological, cognitive, and behavioral changes that can occur following injury. An impact to the head, brain acceleration and deceleration, and the potential for the brain to shift internally and hit the opposite side of the skull can create bruising, damage the blood–brain barrier and blood vessels, and stretch or shear neurons and other cell types in the brain. These forces can lead to bleeding and swelling, as well as to a host of cellular and molecular events that lead to further damage, including disruption of neurotransmitter and ion flows in brain synapses, alterations in metabolism, and inflammatory responses. Although many people who experience a TBI have minor symptoms that resolve over hours or days, others experience alterations or loss of consciousness and have prolonged symptoms such as headaches, dizziness, vision and speech disturbances, agitation, cognitive dysfunction, and other long-term effects. One study found that even among those who had experienced an injury considered a mild TBI, 53 percent reported continued impairment a year later (Nelson et al., 2019). Headache is one of the most common symptoms after TBI (Lucas, 2015); however, experiencing one or more TBIs has also been connected to increased risk of developing anxiety, anger, depression, substance use disorders, and dementia, and to suicide and reduced life expectancy (Graham and Sharp, 2019; Harrison-Felix et al., 2015; Juengst et al., 2017; Madsen et al., 2018; Neumann et al., 2017; Shura et al., 2019). Table 1-1 lists examples of consequences that may arise after TBI.

The prevalence of TBI and the toll it can exact on those who experience it and their families make it an important area of investigation, although the vast heterogeneity of the condition makes assessment of TBI care and research particularly challenging. TBI is not a single type of injury with a single trajectory. Data from the Department of Defense indicate that more than 80 percent of TBIs are classified as "mild," approximately 10–11 percent as "moderate," and roughly 2 percent as "severe" or resulting from a penetrating head wound.[2] Based on data from the Centers for Disease Control and Prevention (CDC), an unknown percentage of people do not seek or receive initial medical care after a potential TBI (CDC,

---

[2] Information on TBI worldwide totals for the period 2000–2020 Q4, available online at DoD TBI Worldwide Numbers. https://health.mil/About-MHS/OASDHA/Defense-Health-Agency/Research-and-Development/Traumatic-Brain-Injury-Center-of-Excellence/DoD-TBI-Worldwide-Numbers (accessed October 4, 2021).

TABLE 1-1 Examples of Physical, Cognitive, and Behavioral Challenges Experienced After TBI

Physical	Cognitive	Behavioral
Headache	Difficulty concentrating	Depression
Movement problems	Memory problems	Anxiety
Impaired or blurred vision	Reduced attention span	Agitation
Difficulties with speech or swallowing	Difficulty with problem solving	Reduced impulse control
Dizziness and balance problems	Confusion	Increased anger or irritability
Seizures	Increased risk of Alzheimer's disease, Parkinson's disease, and other neurodegenerative disorders	
Fatigue		
Pain		
Sleep problems		

NOTE: This list is intended to illustrate symptoms that can develop after TBI and is not intended to be exhaustive or to represent the experiences of all people who experience such an injury.

2015), while among those seeking care, the CDC data show that 86 percent of those who received initial care were treated and released from the ED (indicating a generally less serious injury), 12 percent were hospitalized and subsequently discharged, and 2 percent died.[3] Chapters 2 and 3 further explore who experiences TBI and what personal and social burdens the condition poses.

Patients with TBIs across the spectrum of severity may enter the medical system through multiple points, ranging from emergency medical services in the field, to presentation to an athletic trainer in a training room, to evaluation in a primary care setting. This breadth of entry points to clinical care for TBI, along with the variety of care providers potentially involved, presents challenges both to the medical system and to patients and families as they navigate care and recovery.

Differing mechanisms and severity of injury may also result in vastly different clinical courses. Adult patients sustaining moderate or severe TBI, such as from a motor vehicle crash, may find themselves transported by emergency medical services to the ED of a trauma center, with subsequent admission to the intensive care unit of the hospital, perhaps after urgent surgical intervention. This may be followed by an inpatient hospital stay and subsequent inpatient and outpatient rehabilitation, potentially over the course of months or even years. In contrast, a pediatric patient sustaining a mild TBI as the result of participation in a sport, such as soccer, may be evaluated immediately by school athletic personnel and referred to a sports medicine physician for evaluation, with management and oversight of return to learning and sports over the course of a few weeks. The many types of TBI and the many types of people who experience it thus contribute to a maze of clinical paths along which TBI patients may travel, making standardization of care for the optimization of outcomes challenging.

Areas for Improvement

Improving TBI care and research will require addressing essential components across the full spectrum of prevention, treatment, and recovery while recognizing and building on patient and community experiences. These components include the following:

- Understanding the scope and causes of TBI and the experiences of those who are faced with or at risk of injury. At the core of any process of improvement in TBI care and research are the needs and participation of those who experience these injuries. Care and research also need to be connected to population-level surveillance to gain insights on the scope of the problem and aid in designing prevention approaches.
- Developing, deploying, and improving prevention strategies. The most effective way to improve outcomes of TBI is to prevent people from experiencing such an injury in the first place. Although primary injury prevention is not the focus of this report, the committee emphasizes its importance in any comprehensive framework for understanding and improving the overall TBI system.
- Identifying everyone who has experienced a TBI and needs care. To this end, accurate and timely screening and diagnosis are required.
- Providing high-quality care to those who have experienced one or more TBIs and facilitating the most successful recovery achievable for that person. Care elements include sufficient access to care and appropriate treatment capacity, provision of the most effective care possible according to current medical understanding and best practices, and delivery of coordinated care. A multidisciplinary response to TBI is

---

[3] See https://www.cohenveteransbioscience.org/traumatic-brain-injury (accessed December 1, 2021).

often required. No single medical specialty or care provider has the clear lead role in TBI.

- Developing a research system capable of supporting improved understanding of TBI and the development of treatments and other interventions that can improve outcomes and address identified gaps and needs for persons with TBI and their families.
- Creating processes for feedback, learning, and improvement within the TBI system. Such processes are part of establishing an interconnected, learning health care system for TBI.

The overall TBI ecosystem also encompasses networks beyond health care and research. It includes the related systems that administer and finance health care, accredit care facilities, and provide regulatory approval and oversight of products and therapies. It also intersects with the wide range of community organizations and institutions in which people return to learning, work, and play after experiencing a TBI, including the education system, work environments, professional and amateur sports associations, the criminal justice system, and others. In short, TBI affects a cross section of society and can touch nearly all health care and community institutions. And it involves more than biomedical factors, encompassing social, psychological, and ecological dimensions that significantly affect care and long-term outcomes (see further discussion in Chapters 2 and 3). The present report cannot delve into these many networks and intersections in detail, but emphasizes that TBI needs to be situated within this bigger picture.

Recent TBI Efforts

Efforts by military and civilian federal agencies, foundations, clinicians and researchers, and patient and family advocacy organizations over decades have focused attention on TBI and raised awareness of the needs and challenges it poses. In 2019, for example, federal agencies provided more than $300 million for TBI research.[4] A variety of efforts to better understand TBI and its management are highlighted in Table 1-2; these and other developments are summarized in Appendix A. Additional efforts and networks address related issues in emergency medical services and trauma care, mental health, and other topics.

These various programs have generated valuable longitudinal data on the recovery trajectories of those who experience TBI, increased researchers' and clinicians' understanding of the pathophysiology of brain injuries, and resulted in such successes as a Food and Drug Administration (FDA)–approved blood-based biomarker to help identify concussion (see FDA, 2018).

Collectively, the knowledge gained represents an important base of information for analyzing both areas of progress and areas in which more widespread implementation of best practices or the acquisition of new knowledge can improve care and outcomes for those who experience TBI. Federal agencies involved in the decade-long National Research Action Plan (NRAP) on posttraumatic stress disorder, mental health conditions, and TBI, established in 2013, are looking ahead to next steps. The Brain Trauma Blueprint is designed to foster public–private collaboration around TBI research needs to advance precision medicine, and the Department of Defense (DoD) is moving forward with its Warfighter Brain Health Strategy. Now is the time to advance military and civilian TBI research and care, and this report is intended to contribute to those strategic planning efforts.

---

[4] Based on a search for traumatic brain injury or TBI in the federal RePORTER database, available at https://federalreporter.nih.gov (accessed August 25, 2021). See also Appendix A for further information on federal support for TBI research.

TABLE 1-2 Selected TBI Research Efforts

Effort	Key Funders	Year(s)	Target Population(s)	Description
Research Consortia, Initiatives, and Networks				
Collaborative European NeuroTrauma Effectiveness Research in TBI (CENTER-TBI)	20 European universities	2013–present	European civilians	Various efforts to study TBI, develop TBI databases, and translate research to policy
Chronic Effects of Neurotrauma Consortium (CENC)	DoD, VA	2013–2019	Military personnel (Veterans)	Study to investigate the long-term effects of mild TBI (mTBI) among military service personnel and Veterans
Collaborative Neuropathology Network Characterizing Outcomes of TBI (CONNECT-TBI)	NINDS, University of Pennsylvania	2020–present	Athletes, military personnel, and civilians	Network to promote the sharing of tissue and datasets
Concussion Assessment, Research and Education Consortium (CARE)	NCAA, DoD	2014–present	Student athletes and cadets	Study to explore concussive injury and recovery
International Initiative for Traumatic Brain Injury Research (InTBIR)	NIH, European Commission, Canadian Institutes of Health Research	2011–2019	Civilians, military personnel, athletes, and pediatric populations	International effort to reduce TBI burden by leveraging and coordinating TBI research
Long-term Impact of Military-relevant Brain Injury Consortium (LIMBIC)	DoD, VA, universities, private research institutions	2019–present	Military (Veterans)	Further research for TBI military personnel and Veterans (newest iteration of CENC)
TBI Endpoint Development Initiative (TED)	DoD, FDA, PPPs	2014–present	Civilians, athletes, military personnel	Efforts to identify/validate measures of TBI and recovery
TBI Model Systems (TBIMS)	NIDILRR, (Administration for Community Living, HHS)	1987–present	Civilian	Longitudinal study of long-term outcomes of individuals with moderate-severe TBI who received inpatient rehabilitation; the network also supports projects aimed at meeting the needs of individuals with TBI
Transforming Research and Clinical Knowledge in TBI (TRACK-TBI)	NIH, DoD, OneMind, NeuroTrauma Sciences LLC, Abbott Laboratories	2009–present	Civilian	Largest-scale initiative to analyze clinical TBI data and TBI outcomes
VA TBMIS Research Program	VA, NIDILRR (HHS)	2008–present	Military service members and Veterans	Longitudinal study of outcomes after inpatient rehabilitation at 5 VA Polytrauma Rehabilitation Centers
Enabling Research Infrastructure				
Common Data Elements (CDE)	NIH, HHS	2010–present		Effort to create data standards for TBI clinical research

continued

TABLE 1-2 Continued

Effort	Key Funders	Year(s)	Target Population(s)	Description
Federal Interagency TBI Research Informatics System (FITBIR)	DoD, VA, NIH	2011–present	Military personnel and civilians	Centralized TBI research database
Research Agenda and Priority Setting				
Brain Trauma Blueprint	Cohen Veterans Bioscience	2019–present	Military personnel and civilians	Framework for identifying gaps and synthesizing information to advance precision diagnostics and therapeutics, building on a 2019 summit
Congressionally Directed Medical Research Program on TBI and Psychological Health	Congress	2007–present	Military personnel	Support for research in TBI prevention, detection, diagnosis, treatment, and rehabilitation
National Research Action Plan on TBI and PTSD (NRAP)	DoD, VA, HHS	2013–present	Military personnel and civilians	Established by a 2012 executive order to address research and care gaps
Education and Awareness				
HEADS UP	CDC	2003–present	Youths and the elderly	Educational initiatives to improve TBI awareness and prevention among youths and the elderly

NOTE: CDC = Centers for Disease Control and Prevention; DoD = Department of Defense; DOE = Department of Energy; FDA = Food and Drug Administration; HHS = Department of Health and Human Services; NCAA = National Collegiate Athletic Association; NFL = National Football League; NIDILRR = National Institute on Disability Independent Living and Rehabilitation Research; NIH = National Institutes of Health; NINDS = National Institute of Neurological Disorders and Stroke; PPP = public–private partnership; TBI = traumatic brain injury; UCSF = University of California, San Francisco; VA = Department of Veterans Affairs.

STUDY PURPOSE, SCOPE, AND APPROACH

Recognizing the importance of and opportunities for improving TBI care and research, DoD's Combat Casualty Care Research Program asked the National Academies to convene an ad hoc committee of experts to consider the challenges entailed in achieving such improvements and recommending steps that can be taken to overcome those challenges. The committee's statement of task is present in Box 1-3. The committee quickly realized that no one study could fully address the many networks and intersections outlined above, and so, while emphasizing the importance of situating TBI within that bigger picture, focused on identifying both gaps in and opportunities to advance TBI care and research. The committee also identified prevention as an essential topic, though not covered explicitly in its statement of task, sitting firmly at the beginning of the chain of care. This report represents the committee's response to its statement of task, documenting its understanding of the many crucial elements that need to form part of an optimized system for TBI care and research and presenting a roadmap for accelerating progress toward achieving that system.

The committee formed to carry out this complex task included 18 members with expertise in basic, translational, and clinical research on TBI; epidemiology; neurotrauma; systems of care for TBI, from acute emergency medicine and trauma care through rehabilitation and community reintegration; neuropsychology and mental health; and health sciences and health care policy. The committee met virtually over the course of the study, holding meetings

---

BOX 1-3   STATEMENT OF TASK

An ad hoc committee under the auspices of the National Academies of Sciences, Engineering, and Medicine will gather input from a wide range of public and private experts and stakeholders; examine the current landscape of basic, translational, and clinical traumatic brain injury (TBI) research; and identify gaps and opportunities to accelerate research progress and improve care for those affected by TBI.

The committee will plan and host a large public workshop that examines the current landscape and explores future opportunities for collaborative action. Workshop attendees will include representatives of federal, state, and local governments; military and Veterans' health stakeholders; the private sector; the academic community; patient advocacy stakeholders; the clinical community; philanthropic organizations; and traditional TBI research funders, as well as other relevant stakeholders involved in related fields aimed at advancing diagnostic tools, therapeutic trials, and systems of care. Presentations and discussions will address the following topics:

- Fostering biomedical research on TBI;
- Accelerating translational and clinical research on TBI;
- Delivering breakthroughs in TBI treatments; and
- Improving TBI systems of clinical care from acute care through rehabilitation.

The study, including the workshop, will address a range of populations affected by TBI and related goals, including improving readiness, retention, return to service, and prevention of long-term sequelae in military populations; and improving return to play and work, and prevention of long-term sequelae in sports participants, older adults who have fallen, individuals affected by traffic/vehicle injuries, and other civilian populations.

Based primarily on the workshop presentations and discussions, supplemented by additional literature review as appropriate, the committee will develop a report, with recommendations, that:

- Identifies major barriers and knowledge gaps that are impeding progress in the field;
- Highlights opportunities for collaborative action (both intergovernmental and public-private) that could accelerate progress in TBI research and care; and
- Provides a roadmap for advancing both research and clinical care that would guide the field over the next decade.

---

approximately monthly to discuss and analyze the evidence and develop the conclusions and recommendations presented in this report. Evidence was gathered through a literature review, as well as a series of public virtual workshop sessions held in March and April 2021 and public webinars held in May and June 2021, with speakers who generously shared their knowledge and experiences with the committee. See Appendix C for further information on how the committee conducted its work and Appendix D for brief biographies of committee members and staff.

ORGANIZATION OF THE REPORT

Chapter 2 of this report describes the extent of the problems posed by TBI and the experiences and burdens reported by patients and families. Chapter 3 describes how biological, psychological, social, and ecological factors affect the experience of and outcomes following TBI, and introduces the care and recovery continuum. Chapter 4 highlights the role of prevention in reducing the numbers of TBIs that occur and explores awareness of and misconceptions about the condition. This information lays the foundation for the committee's identification of actions that can be taken to make progress in improving TBI care and research.

The report then turns to the patient journey and care pathways following a TBI.

Chapter 5 focuses on the acute phase of care, from the point of injury and prehospital assessment through hospital care and transition to rehabilitation. Chapter 6 addresses the post-acute and longer-term phase of care, emphasizing rehabilitation, recovery to the extent possible, and community reintegration. Each of these chapters lays out the goals and main elements of care provided to a person who has experienced a TBI and identifies a number of remaining clinical gaps and needs for that phase of care.

In Chapter 7, the report examines major gaps, challenges, and opportunities for advancing TBI care and research. The opportunities identified include implementing a new clinical classification system for TBI; using emerging biomarkers as part of an expanded TBI toolkit; learning from and building on existing care systems and networks; increasing patient, family, and stakeholder engagement; and employing additional types of study designs.

Finally, Chapter 8 details the essential elements of an optimized system for accelerating progress in the TBI field, emphasizing the need for a coordinated system capable of more effectively connecting current programs and networks and providing a locus for efforts to advance TBI care and research. This chapter provides the committee's recommendations for actions that can be taken to help achieve an optimized TBI system and a research agenda for addressing unanswered questions.

REFERENCES

ACS (American College of Surgeons) Committee on Trauma. 1976. Optimal hospital resources for care of the seriously injured. *Bulletin of the American College of Surgeons* 61(9):15-22.
APA (American Psychiatric Association). 2013. *Diagnostic and statistical manual of mental disorders, fifth edition (DSM-5)*. Arlington, VA: APA.
Bulger, E. M., T. E. Rasmussen, G. J. Jurkovich, T. C. Fabian, R. A. Kozar, R. Coimbra, T. W. Costantini, J. Ficke, A. K. Malhotra, M. A. Price, S. L. Smith, W. G. Cioffi, and R. M. Stewart. 2018. Implementation of a National Trauma Research Action Plan (NTRAP). *Journal of Trauma and Acute Care Surgery* 84(6):1012-1016.
CDC (Centers for Disease Control and Prevention). 2015. *Report to Congress on traumatic brain injury in the United States: Epidemiology and rehabilitation*. National Center for Injury Prevention and Control; Division of Unintentional Injury Prevention: Atlanta, GA.
DoD (Department of Defense). 2012. *Military acute concussion evaluation form*. Defense and Veterans Brain Injury Center. https://health.mil/Reference-Center/Forms/2015/04/30/MACE-2012 (accessed July 31, 2021).
DoD. 2015. *Traumatic brain injury: Updated definition and reporting*. Memorandum for Assistant Secretary of the Army (Manpower and Reserve Affairs), Assistant Secretary of the Navy (Manpower and Reserve Affairs), Assistant Secretary of the Air Force (Manpower and Reserve Affairs), and Director, Joint Staff, from the Assistant Secretary of Defense, April 6, 2015. https://www.health.mil/Reference-Center/Policies/2015/04/06/Traumatic-Brain-Injury-Updated-Definition-and-Reporting (accessed July 31, 2021).
FDA (Food and Drug Administration). 2018. *FDA authorizes marketing of first blood test to aid in the evaluation of concussion in adults*. FDA News Release. https://www.fda.gov/news-events/press-announcements/fda-authorizes-marketing-first-blood-test-aid-evaluation-concussion-adults (accessed July 30, 2021).
French, L., M. McCrea, and M. Baggett. 2008. The Military Acute Concussion Evaluation (MACE). *Journal of Special Operations Medicine* 8(1):68-77.
Giza, C., J. Kutcher, S. Ashwal, J. Barth, T. Getchius, G. Gioia, G. Gronseth, K. Guskiewicz, S. Mandel, G. Manley, D. McKeag, D. Thurman, and R. Zafonte. 2013. Summary of evidence-based guideline update: Evaluation and management of concussion in sports: Report of the Guideline Development Subcommittee of the American Academy of Neurology. *Neurology* 80(24):2250-2257.

Graham, N. S., and D. J. Sharp. 2019. Understanding neurodegeneration after traumatic brain injury: From mechanisms to clinical trials in dementia. *Journal of Neurology, Neurosurgery & Psychiatry* 90:1221-1233.

Harrison-Felix, C., C. Pretz, F. Hammond, J. Cuthbert, J. Bell, J. Corrigan, A. Miller, and J. Haarbauer-Krupa. 2015. Life expectancy after inpatient rehabilitation for traumatic brain injury in the United States. *Journal of Neurotrauma* 32(23):1893-1901.

Juengst, S. B., R. Kumar, and A. K. Wagner. 2017. A narrative literature review of depression following traumatic brain injury: Prevalence, impact, and management challenges. *Psychology Research and Behavior Management* 10:175-186.

Lucas, S. 2015. Posttraumatic headache: Clinical characterization and management. *Current Pain and Headache Reports* 19(10):48. https://doi.org/10.1007/s11916-015-0520-1.

Madsen T, A. Erlangsen, S. Orlovska, R. Mofaddy, M. Nordentoft, and M. E. Benros. 2018. Association between traumatic brain injury and risk of suicide. *Journal of the American Medical Association* 320(6):580-588.

Majdan, M., D. Plancikova, A. Maas, S. Polinder, V. Feigin, A. Theadom, M. Rusnak, A. Brazinova, and J. Haagsma. 2017. Years of life lost due to traumatic brain injury in Europe: A cross-sectional analysis of 16 countries. *PLoS Medicine* 14(7):e1002331. https://doi.org/10.1371/journal.pmed.1002331.

Malec, J. F., A. W. Brown, C. L. Leibson, J. T. Flaada, J. N. Mandrekar, N. N. Diehl, and P. K. Perkins. 2007. The Mayo classification system for traumatic brain injury severity. *Journal of Neurotrauma* 24(9):1417-1424.

McCrory, P., W. Meeuwisse, J. Dvorak, M. Aubry, J. Bailes, S. Broglio, R. C. Cantu, et al. 2017. Consensus statement on concussion in sport—The 5th International Conference on Concussion in Sport held in Berlin, October 2016. *British Journal of Sports Medicine* 51(11):838-847.

Menon, D. K., K. Schwab, D. W. Wright, and A. I. Maas. 2010. Demographics and Clinical Assessment Working Group of the International and Interagency Initiative toward common data elements for research on traumatic brain injury and psychological health. Position statement: Definition of traumatic brain injury. *Archives of Physical Medicine and Rehabilitation* 91(11):1637-1640.

Moses, H., D. Matheson, S. Cairns-Smith, B. P. George, C. Palisch, and E. R. Dorsey. 2015. The anatomy of medical research: US and international comparisons. *Journal of the American Medical Association* 313(2):174-189.

NAS and NRC (National Academy of Sciences and National Research Council). 1966. *Accidental death and disability: The neglected disease of modern society.* Washington, DC: National Academy Press.

NASEM (National Academies of Sciences, Engineering, and Medicine). 2016. *A national trauma care system: Integrating Military and civilian trauma systems to achieve zero preventable deaths after injury.* Washington, DC: The National Academies Press.

NASEM. 2019. *Evaluation of the disability determination process for traumatic brain injury in veterans.* Washington, DC: The National Academies Press.

NASEM. 2020. *An assessment of illness in U.S. government employees and their families at overseas embassies.* Washington, DC: The National Academies Press.

Nelson, L. D., N. Temkin, S. Dikmen, J. Barber, J. Giacino, E. Yuh, H. Levin, et al. 2019. Recovery after mild traumatic brain injury in patients presenting to US level I trauma centers: A Transforming Research and Clinical Knowledge in Traumatic Brain Injury (TRACK-TBI) study. *JAMA Neurology* 76(9):1049-1059.

Neumann, D., J. F. Malec, and F. M. Hammond. 2017. Negative attribution bias and anger after traumatic brain injury. *Journal of Head Trauma Rehabilitation* 32(3):197-204.

NRC and IOM (National Research Council and Institute of Medicine). 1985. *Injury in America: A continuing public health problem.* Washington, DC: National Academy Press.

Shura, R. D., S. Nazem, H. Miskey, T. Hostetter, J. Rowland, L. Brenner, VA Mid-Atlantic Mirecc Workgroup, and K. H. Taber. 2019. Relationship between traumatic brain injury history and recent suicidal ideation in Iraq/Afghanistan-era veterans. *Psychological Services* 16(2):312-320.

Taylor, C., J. M. Bell, M. J. Breiding, and L. Xu. 2017. Traumatic brain injury–related emergency department visits, hospitalizations, and deaths—United States, 2007 and 2013. *Morbidity and Mortality Weekly Report* 66(9):1-16.

VA (Department of Veterans Affairs). 2015. *Fact sheet: Coding guidance for traumatic brain injury (TBI).* http://www.rstce.pitt.edu/va_tbi/documents/11192015/11192015_03.pdf (accessed July 31, 2021).

2

The Scope and Burden of Traumatic Brain Injury

Chapter Highlights

- Traumatic brain injury (TBI) affects millions of Americans annually, with the highest rates of hospitalization and death among the oldest age groups. In the United States in 2017, the leading causes of TBI-related hospitalizations were falls and motor vehicle crashes, while the leading causes of TBI-related deaths were suicide and falls.
- TBI imposes significant health, social, and economic costs. Limitations in current data collection lead to undercounting and underestimates of the true incidence and cost of TBI.

This chapter reviews the scope and burden of traumatic brain injury (TBI), including the frequency of injury among segments of the global and U.S. populations. The chapter examines the economic cost of TBI and the potential for cost savings from improved care and outcomes. Finally, the chapter highlights themes reported by patients and families during the study's information-gathering workshops with respect to the burden imposed by TBI. The data and testimonies summarized in this chapter establish TBI as a significant health challenge.

FREQUENCY OF TRAUMATIC BRAIN INJURY

This section presents epidemiological data on the frequency—incidence and prevalence—of TBI.[1]

---

[1] The incidence of TBI reflects newly diagnosed cases of people with TBI over a specified period, often a year. It provides the rate of TBI—how frequently such injuries are occurring. Prevalence, on the other hand, reflects the total number of cases of people with TBI in a population at a given time. Prevalence is a percentage, representing what proportion of the population is affected by TBI at the measured time.

Limitations in Data and Data Quality

Limitations in TBI surveillance are broadly recognized, and it is widely acknowledged that nearly all TBI estimates are undercounts. These limitations affect estimates of mortality, hospitalization, emergency department (ED) care, and population-level incidence.

The most comprehensive source for mortality data in the United States is the National Vital Statistics System, which collects information from death certificates. Although the death certification process in the United States is very thorough, case identification of deaths due to TBI is challenging. Traumatic deaths disproportionally occur out of hospital, becoming the jurisdiction of a medical examiner's office. If the intent of the death is not in question (e.g., not a homicide)—as in a fall or road traffic injury, both of which are leading causes of TBI—an autopsy is not required, and detailed diagnoses are often not provided on the death certificate. Many deaths of individuals who sustained a TBI are identified as "blunt traumatic injury," and thus are not coded as TBIs in vital statistics data systems. Deaths that occur after an extended period of disability due to TBI may also not be captured, even if the ultimate cause of death is related to the initial injury.

Globally, mortality underestimates are far more problematic. In 2012, the World Health Organization (WHO) examined vital statistics systems and rated only roughly 20 countries, all high-income, as having high-quality death certification systems (WHO, 2014). Many countries use hospital-based death certification systems, yet up to 80 percent of deaths—and disproportionately traumatic deaths—occur outside of health care settings (World Bank/WHO, 2014). WHO estimates that two-thirds of all deaths globally are not counted, with low-income countries the most impacted. Thus, mortality due to TBI may be far greater than is currently known.

The most common source of TBI incidence data is health care records, and sources such as the Healthcare Cost and Utilization Project's (HCUP's) National Inpatient Sample, the National Emergency Department System, the Consumer Product Safety Commission's National Electronic Injury Surveillance System, and the American College of Surgeons' National Trauma Data Bank have all been used to estimate incidence. In each of these sources, cases of people with TBI are ascertained through the *International Classification of Diseases* (ICD) codes (and related Diagnosis Related Group codes)—a detailed listing of individual medical diagnoses. In the Ninth Revision of the ICD (ICD-9), used from the 1990s to 2015, traumatic injury codes were difficult to differentiate from nontrauma and neurologic disease codes. Although the current ICD-10 coding system includes more codes specific to TBI, identification remains challenging. For example, many analyses rely only on the primary diagnosis in a record, defined as the diagnosis requiring the most care. If a patient has multiple injuries and a brain injury is not the most severe of these at the time of admission (e.g., the patient also has an open fracture), the brain injury may be recorded as a secondary code and thus not picked up by case ascertainment algorithms.

Because of differences in the databases available for studying TBI and their coding limitations, TBI incidence estimates vary widely. One study found that the sample population estimates for ED visits in the National Inpatient Survey were 805 percent higher in 2007 and 1,169 percent higher in 2013 than those in the National Trauma Data Bank (Stopa et al., 2020), mainly because the latter source includes primarily large trauma hospitals and so misses many milder brain injuries. Studies have also examined the predictive value of the ICD-10 system in detecting cases of people with TBI by comparing those data against the corresponding full medical records. One study focused on intracranial injury and skull fracture. Because these are severe injuries with very specific ICD-10 codes, the authors hypothesized that the codes would have very high predictive value (i.e., ability to catch all cases). They found, however, that the predictive value for intracranial injury ranged from 82 percent to 92 percent and for skull fracture from 57 percent to 61 percent (Gabella et al., 2021). A study in New Zealand designed to prospectively identify people with TBI found that the medical records of only 312 (18.6 percent) of 1,369 identified TBI cases contained one of the TBI ICD-10 diagnostic codes (Barker-Collo et al., 2016). And an analysis of Department of Veterans Affairs (VA) data comparing three ICD algorithms for capturing TBI found only partial sensitivity (Carlson et al., 2013).

Estimating the incidence of people with cases on the milder end of the TBI spectrum poses even more substantial challenges relative to TBIs causing death or requiring acute care. Because many individuals with less severe injury do not seek acute care, no secondary data sources are available with which to enumerate them, and acute care for some such cases may be provided in outpatient or sports medicine clinics, for which nationally weighted data are not collected. Studies have found that a large proportion of people with TBI do not seek medical care at all. For example, in the New Zealand prospective study referenced above, 64 percent of people with TBI went to a hospital, 8 percent saw a family doctor, and 28 percent were identified through other sources (Feigin et al., 2013). Studies of medical sources show that 75–80 percent of TBI is in the mild category (Bruns and Hauser, 2003; CDC, 2003; Sosin et al., 1996), and the impact of undercounting such a prevalent outcome results in vastly underestimating the burden of TBI. The recognized limitations in data from such sources as medical coding, insurance claims, and death certificates also highlight the complementary role of self-reporting using structured and validated screening tools, including questionnaires and interviews, in helping to better understand the prevalence and burden of TBI.

Finally, it should be noted that data on race, ethnicity, and rates of TBI are difficult to interpret. One challenge is that race/ethnicity categories between TBI sources and population data often do not align, with different categories, different options for identifying multiple races, and different formats for differentiating race and ethnicity. Ongoing discussions with agencies that collect data to study race/ethnicity as a health determinant, such as the National Center for Health Statistics, to identify more uniform coding protocols will be valuable in improving the capture and presentation of race/ethnicity health data.

Global TBI Incidence and Prevalence

According to the most comprehensive study to date on the estimated global incidence of TBI, more than 27 million new cases of people with medically treated TBI occurred in 2016, for an age-standardized incidence of 369 per 100,000 world population (James et al., 2019). This study estimated global TBI prevalence at more than 55 million, indicating that about 0.7 percent of the world's population was living with a medically treated brain injury. These estimates are from the

> This estimate of the global incidence of TBI in 2016 is equal to the number of people that would be involved if 148 jumbo jets (Boeing 747-8) crashed every day.

Global Burden of Disease study and literature review, however, and the authors acknowledge many limitations in their TBI estimation. For example, these estimates include only hospital-treated TBI, which excludes deaths occurring prior to hospital arrival (at-scene), injuries treated in nonhospital settings or not treated at all, and individuals seeking treatment for symptoms after their original injury.

Several studies have extrapolated global TBI estimates from more focused studies. The BIONIC study in New Zealand estimated population-level TBI incidence (Barker-Collo and Feigin, 2009; Feigin et al., 2013; Theadom et al., 2012) using multiple-source prospective case ascertainment of TBIs of all severity, regardless of medical treatment. The authors of this study estimated a TBI incidence of 790 per 100,000, which extrapolates globally to more than 50 million TBIs occurring each year, with approximately 30 percent of these individuals not seeking acute medical care (Feigin et al., 2013). Dewan and colleagues (2019) estimated the global incidence of TBIs of all severity, regardless of medical care, based on the proportion of TBIs in road traffic injuries (such as motor vehicle crashes) and incidence ratios in more than 240 published studies (Dewan et al., 2019). They estimated a TBI incidence of 939 per 100,000 population, which included 55.9 million mild and 5.48 million severe TBIs annually. These estimates are far higher than any other global estimates, yet are unlikely to include falsely identified cases of people with TBI, and therefore provide some idea of the extent of TBI undercounting.

Comparing rates of TBI across countries and over time is highly problematic because of underreporting and difficulty in ascertaining cases. The Lancet Neurology Commission on TBI reported that estimates from region-specific population studies range from 200 to 600 TBIs per 100,000 people, with variance based on such factors as case definition and ascertainment, the qualities of data systems, and methodological differences (Johnson and Griswold, 2017). Based on data from the Global Burden of Disease consortium, TBI rates were highest in central and eastern Europe and central Asia (James et al., 2019). Dewan and colleagues (2019) concluded that although their measured per capita TBI rates were highest in high-income countries, low- and low-middle income countries experienced nearly three times more total TBIs. Access to trauma care is an important factor in considering global estimates of TBI. Indeed, by one estimate, approximately 2 million lives could be saved if trauma care available in high-income countries were available in lower- and middle-income countries (Mock et al., 2012).

Studies generally find that TBI is increasing globally. From 1990 to 2016, the incidence and prevalence of medically treated TBI rose globally by 3.6 percent and 8.4 percent, respectively (James et al., 2019). These increases were driven mainly by increases in fall-related TBI among older adults, particularly in high-income countries, as well as by road traffic injuries and violence, which rose particularly rapidly in low- and middle-income countries.

Measures that reflect disproportionately high TBI rates among the young and account for the high rates of disability among survivors are important for understanding the true population-level burden of TBI. However, very few studies have estimated such measures as premature loss of life or years lived with disability. One study of 16 European countries found that TBI contributed more than 1.3 million years of potential life lost (YPLL) in 2013, which accounted for 41 percent of overall YPLL among all injuries (Majdan et al., 2017). The Global Burden of Disease TBI consortium estimated that TBI was responsible for 8.1 million years lived with disability, with a global disability rate of 111 per 100,000 population (James et al., 2019).

TBI Incidence in the U.S. Civilian Population

The Centers for Disease Control and Prevention (CDC) initiated efforts to create a system for national surveillance for TBI by launching the multistate Traumatic Brain Injury Surveillance Program in 1989 (Thurman et al., 1999). The program began by funding 4 states to collect population-based incidence data and by 1997 had grown to include 15 states. In the first official report from this program, it was estimated that each year, a TBI was sustained by 1.5 million Americans, 50,000 of whom died; 230,000 of whom were hospitalized; and 90,000 of whom experienced long-term disability, with an estimated prevalence of 5.3 million people living with a permanent TBI-related disability. In addition to generating among the first population-based TBI incidence estimates, CDC's TBI Surveillance Program initiated efforts to standardize data definitions and reporting. For example, *Guidelines for Surveillance of Central Nervous System Injury* was published in 1995 to support the collection of valid, comparable data (Thurman et al., 1995).

CDC's National Center for Injury Prevention and Control continues to report TBI incidence data for the United States but now relies on death certificates and weighted national samples of health data, enabled by improvements in electronic medical records. The center's most recent report provides information on TBI mortality in 2017, including an estimated 61,131 TBI deaths (Daugherty et al., 2019).[2] TBI-related death rates remained steady at about 17.5 per 100,000 from 2000 through 2005, decreased to 16.3 in 2014, and increased back to 17.5 in 2017. Throughout this period, TBI death rates were significantly higher for males than for females and were higher for American Indian/Alaska Native people than for other reported racial/ethnic groups. The leading causes of TBI death included motor vehicle crashes, falls, suicide, and homicide. Suicide became the leading cause of TBI-related death, increasing by 32 percent over this period, with the highest increase among non-Hispanic White people.

The most recent report on the incidence of nonfatal TBI provides data for 2016–2017 (CDC, 2021). This report, as well as prior reports for 2014 (CDC, 2019) and 2007 and 2013 (Taylor et al., 2017), use data from the Health Resources and Services Administration's (HRSA's) HCUP Nationwide Emergency Department Sample and National Inpatient Sample. Prior studies, from 2003 (Rutland-Brown et al., 2006) and 2002 to 2006 (Faul et al., 2010), used data from the National Hospital Discharge Survey and National Hospital Ambulatory Medical Care Survey. All of the above sources represent nationally weighted samples of electronic medical records.

According to the CDC (2021) report, in 2017 there were almost 224,000 TBI-related hospitalizations, with the rates highest among those over age 75 (320.8 per 100,000), those aged 65–74 (102.7), and those aged 55–64 (67.5). The leading causes of TBI hospitalization were falls (49.1 percent) and motor vehicle crashes (24.5 percent). An estimated 61,000 deaths were attributed to TBI in 2017, with mortality rates highest among those over age 75 (77.0 per 100,000), those aged 65–74 (24.3 per 100,000), and those aged 55–64 (19.5 per 100,000). See Figure 2-1 and Table 2-1 for rates of hospitalizations and deaths by age group.

---

[2] Note that this number represents an undercount of cases of people with TBI because it requires an ICD-10 TBI code and uses new methodology that requires the presence of a cause-of-injury code.

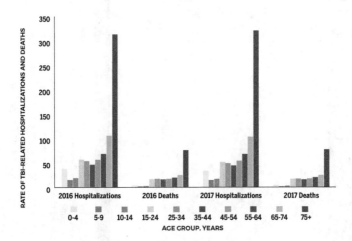

FIGURE 2-1 Estimated rates of TBI-related hospitalizations and deaths in the United States, by age group. The data show trends by age range among those who were hospitalized or died during 2016 and 2017.
SOURCE: CDC, 2021.

TABLE 2-1 Estimated Rate of TBI-Related Hospitalizations and Deaths by Age Group in the United States (2014, 2016, and 2017)

Age Group (years)	Hospitalization Rate per 100,000 Population (95% CI)			Death Rate per 100,000 Population (95% CI)		
	2014	2016[a]	2017[a]	2014	2016	2017
0–17	31.4 (27.6–35.1)	26.5 (23.3–29.7)	23.9 (21.0–26.9)	3.4 (3.3–3.6)	3.7 (3.5–3.8)	3.8 (3.7–4.0)
0–4	45.1 (38.5–51.7)	37.1 (31.4–42.8)	32.7 (27.2–38.1)	3.6 (3.4–3.9)	3.6 (3.3–3.8)	3.8 (3.5–4.0)
5–9	—	14.4 (12.1–16.8)	14.1 (11.9–16.3)	—	1.5 (1.3–1.7)	1.3 (1.2–1.5)
10–14	—	18.5 (15.8–21.3)	16.7 (14.2–19.2)	—	2.5 (2.2–2.7)	2.5 (2.3–2.7)
5–14	20.0 (17.1–22.9)	—	—	1.9 (1.7–2.0)	—	—
15–24	60.1 (55.3–64.9)	55.9 (51.3–60.5)	51.0 (47.0–55.0)	14.4 (14.0–14.7)	15.9 (15.5–16.3)	16.3 (15.9–16.7)
25–34	58.6 (54.1–63.2)	53.0 (48.7–57.3)	48.5 (44.6–52.4)	14.7 (14.3–15.0)	16.8 (16.4–17.1)	16.7 (16.3–17.1)
35–44	51.8 (48.1–55.4)	45.6 (42.0–49.1)	43.4 (40.0–46.8)	13.7 (13.3–14.1)	15.2 (14.8–15.6)	15.1 (14.7–15.5)
45–54	70.8 (66.4–75.2)	55.6 (51.6–59.6)	53.6 (49.8–57.4)	16.9 (16.5–17.3)	16.5 (16.2–16.9)	17.0 (16.6–17.4)
55–64	89.5 (84.8–94.2)	67.7 (63.3–72.1)	67.5 (63.5–71.6)	19.1 (18.7–19.5)	19.1 (18.7–19.5)	19.5 (19.1–19.9)
65–74	145.5 (139.2–151.8)	104.8 (99.2–110.4)	102.7 (97.3–108.1)	24.7 (24.1–25.3)	24.2 (23.6–24.7)	24.3 (23.7–24.9)
75+	470.6 (452.8–488.5)	313.4 (298.5–328.4)	320.8 (305.8–335.7)	78.5 (77.2–79.7)	75.5 (74.3–76.7)	77.0 (75.8–78.1)
Total[b]	90.5 (86.5–94.6)	70.3 (66.5–74.1)	68.8 (65.2–72.4)	17.8 (17.7–18.0)	18.4 (18.3–18.6)	18.8 (18.7–19.0)[c]
Adjusted[d]	86.1 (84.3–88.0)	65.7 (64.3–67.2)	63.6 (62.3–65.0)	17.0 (16.9–17.2)	17.3 (17.1–17.4)	17.5 (17.4–17.7)

NOTES: In 2016, the TBI surveillance definition was updated to reflect the transition from the use of the *International Classification of Diseases, Ninth Revision* (ICD-9) to ICD-10 diagnostic codes. Differences in the definitions used before and after 2016 mean that the 2014 numbers are not directly comparable to those for 2016 and 2017. See CDC, 2021 for an explanation. CI = confidence interval.

[a] In-hospital deaths and patients who transferred from another hospital were excluded.
[b] Cases with missing age were included. Numbers subject to rounding error.
[c] Rate significantly different compared with 2016; t-tests p-value <0.05.
[d] For 2014 rates: age-adjusted to the 2000 U.S. standard population. For 2016 and 2017 rates: cases with missing age were excluded; rates age-adjusted to National Center for Health Statistics (NCHS) 2000 U.S. standard population.

SOURCES: CDC, 2019, 2021.

In 2017, the leading causes of TBI death were suicide (34.7 percent) and falls (28 percent) (CDC, 2021). Differences in rates by age and mechanism indicate differing levels of severity by mechanism (for example, suicide is more likely to cause death than is being struck by/against an object) and reduced resiliency/increased severity among older individuals, who have much higher rates of hospitalization and death by falls compared with younger age groups.

In 2014, approximately 2.5 million TBIs were treated in EDs. Rates for ED treatment were highest for those over age 75 (1,682 per 100,000) and aged 0–17 (1,104 per 100,000). The leading mechanisms for TBI in ED patients were falls (47.9 percent); being struck by/against an object, which is a common mechanism for sports injuries (17.1 percent); and road traffic injuries (13.2 percent) (CDC, 2019). According to CDC, between 2006 and 2014, TBI ED visits increased substantially for all leading mechanisms, including road traffic injuries (24 percent increase), falls (80 percent), being struck by/against an object (58 percent), self-harm (60 percent), and assault (18 percent). During this period, however, the TBI-related hospitalization rate decreased 8 percent, primarily as the result of a 34 percent decrease in road traffic–related hospitalizations. A similar decrease of 6 percent was noted for TBI deaths. These estimates are similar to those provided through the Global Burden of Disease study, which reported a 2016 U.S. TBI incidence of 333 per 100,000, with a 3.3 percent decrease between 1990 and 2016 (James et al., 2019).

CDC does not report such measures as YPLL or disability-adjusted life years (DALYs).[3] However, Rosenbaum and colleagues (2014) estimated YPLL among hospitalized patients using the National Inpatient Sample, the same hospitalization source as that used by CDC (Rosenbaum et al., 2014). They estimated more than 25.5 million years of potential life lost for all ICD-9 neurologic disease categories between 1988 and 2011, with the highest contribution from the codes of intracerebral hemorrhage and cerebral ischemia. Two other studies have included estimates of YPLL. The first, conducted using TBIs in 1985, yielded an estimate of 1.4 million YPLL and 2.6 million life years lost as a result of temporary and permanent disability (Max et al., 1991). The second study used TBIs from 2012 and estimated DALYs among survivors to be 117,000 lifetimes of quality lost (Lawrence et al., 2018). These estimates are difficult to compare because they are based on different TBI case inclusion criteria, as well as different analytic methods.

TBI incidence rates in the United States have been estimated in a number of studies the majority of which have focused on those who are hospitalized (Bruns and Hauser, 2003; Fife, 1987; Guerrero et al., 2000; Jager et al., 2000; Sosin et al., 1996; Thurman and Guerrero, 1999). These studies have yielded varying rates, generally ranging from 180 to 250 hospitalizations per 100,000 population, 392 to 444 ED visits per 100,000, and 600 to more than 800 total TBIs per 100,000. This variance is attributable to multiple definitions of TBI (e.g., many early studies did not include skull fracture), sampling frames, and data sources (Bruns and Hauser, 2003). Most of these estimates are now outdated, moreover, because of the shift from ICD-9 to ICD-10 codes in the third quarter of 2015, which makes analysis of data from that year particularly difficult. This change improved TBI case ascertainment because the ICD-10 codes are more specific to trauma, and the TBI codes are more detailed. One consistent finding, however, is that the number of TBI-related ED visits is far higher than the hospitalization rate; further, when estimated, the number of people who experience a potential TBI but do not seek medical attention is high.

These studies provide a foundation for increased focus in recent years on what has been considered "mild" TBI. In addition, recognition has grown that "mild" TBI can cause long-

---

[3] DALYs are a measure of the health burden of a condition, and reflect an estimation of the number of years of life lost due to premature death and the number of years of life lived with illness or disability.

term effects in some people. A burst of research activity over the past decade has sought to advance understanding of TBI, its diagnosis and management, and influences on the trajectories of recovery. Yet despite the resulting advances in knowledge, gaps remain with regard to understanding of the breadth of the burden of disease; objective tools with which to diagnose milder forms of TBI, such as concussion; and treatments to improve outcomes. And the advances in understanding that have been achieved are tempered by substantial gaps in implementation that continue to exist, preventing the potential of these research advances from reaching those adult and pediatric patients who would most benefit (Haarbauer-Krupa et al., 2017).

Pediatric TBI

TBI represents a substantial burden in childhood, resulting in the United States in more than 2,000 deaths and more than 17,500 hospitalizations in 2017 and more than 812,000 ED visits in 2014 (CDC, 2019, 2021). According to CDC's 2021 Surveillance Report on TBI in the United States,[4] children and adolescents aged <18 accounted for roughly 8 percent of TBI-related hospitalizations and about 4.5 percent of TBI-related deaths in 2016 and 2017 (CDC, 2021). Among that age group, falls and motor vehicle crashes were the most common principal mechanisms of injury for hospitalization related to TBI.

The vast majority (>70 percent) of all TBIs, including those in pediatric populations, are defined as mild (Dewan et al., 2016), and more than 70 percent of pediatric patients with mild TBI recover within 1–3 months (Lumba-Brown et al., 2018). Pediatric TBI, including concussion, can result from participation in sports or recreation or from other mechanisms of injury, such as motor vehicle crashes or falls (CDC 2003, 2021). These statistics also likely represent a substantial undercount of the burden of TBI, as many children either do not seek care or seek care with their primary care physician for milder injures (Arbogast et al., 2016), numbers not easily captured in estimates that typically use ED and hospitalization data. In fact, according to the 2017 National Youth Risk Behavior Survey, 2.5 million high school students reported at least one concussion within the prior year (DePadilla et al., 2018). In light of these data, it is clear that TBIs, especially mild TBIs, including concussions, have a wide-ranging impact on children in the United States.

As noted above, there is increasing awareness that the effects of TBI can be experienced not merely acutely, at the time of injury, but also long-term, even throughout the lifespan, and even for injuries classified as mild. This potential for lifetime impact is particularly important for children, for whom TBI can affect both current function and future potential. More than 62 percent of children with moderate-to-severe TBI, and even 14 percent of those with mild TBI, experience ongoing disability, requiring specialized medical services and educational support (Rivara et al., 2012).

TBI Among Older Adults

The distribution of TBI is bimodal with respect to age: the incidence of TBI is highest among the youngest and oldest age groups, which are more susceptible to TBI caused by particular kinds of injuries, including falls and motor vehicle crashes (Haarbauer-Krupa et al., 2021). The majority of TBIs in older adults involve falls, and a single fall is a risk factor for later falls (Faul et al., 2010; Narapareddy et al., 2019). In 2016 and 2017, roughly half of

---

[4] The report does not include TBIs from VA, military, or federal hospitals; patients who sought care outside of a hospital setting; or those who did not seek care.

TBI-related hospitalizations due to unintentional falls in the United States occurred among adults aged ≥75 (CDC, 2021).

In 2016 and 2017, adults aged ≥55 had the highest rate of TBI-related hospitalization in the United States (CDC, 2021). The rate among adults aged ≥75 (2016: 313.4/100,000; 2017: 320.8/100,000) far exceeded that among those aged 65–74 (2016: 104.8/100,000; 2017: 102.7/100,000) and those aged 55–64 (2016: 67.7/100,000; 2017: 67.5/100,000). During this same period in the United States, the most recently reported CDC data indicate that the rates of TBI-related death were highest in adults aged ≥75 (2016: 75.5/100,000; 2017: 77.0/100,000), followed by those aged 65–74 (2016: 24.2/100,000; 2017: 24.3/100,000) and those aged 55–64 (2016: 19.1/100,000; 2017: 19.5/100,000) (CDC, 2021). In 2017, these figures translated to more than 67,000 hospitalizations and more than 16,000 deaths among adults aged 75 and older (CDC, 2021).

Another study evaluated age group-specific trends in rates of TBI using U.S. census data and data from the National Trauma Data Bank. The investigators found a 20–25 percent increase in trauma center admissions for TBI among those aged 75 and over between 2007 and 2010 (Dams-O'Connor et al., 2013). They noted the tendency for older adults (aged ≥65) with TBI to be White females who had suffered injury from a fall.

A review of the literature on TBI sustained in older adulthood found that the highest incidence of TBI-related ED visits, hospitalizations, and deaths occurred in older adults (Gardner et al., 2018). Another study of TBI in older adults found that TBI was responsible for more than 80,000 ED visits per year among persons aged 65 and older; furthermore, three-quarters of these visits resulted in hospitalization (Thompson et al., 2006). Similarly, a population-based descriptive epidemiological study of TBI-related ED visits in the United States between 2006 and 2010 found that children younger than 3 years and adults older than 60 had the largest increase in TBI rates during that period (Marin et al., 2014).

In addition to exhibiting among the highest rates of TBI-related hospitalization and death, persons 65 years of age and over face especially poor TBI outcomes.

Gender Differences in TBI Incidence

TBI incidence in the United States is significantly higher among males (388 per 100,000) than females (195 per 100,000) (Haarbauer-Krupa et al., 2021). Data indicate that females, who account for just over 50 percent of the U.S. population, account for approximately half of all TBI-related ED visits, 41 percent of TBI-related hospitalizations, and 27 percent of TBI-related deaths (Haarbauer-Krupa et al., 2021). As with other rates of TBI, these may be underestimates, as brain injury often is not reported or detected, particularly in cases of mild injury. There are also no national prevalence estimates for TBI caused by intimate partner violence, although an estimated 30–74 percent of women who experience intimate partner violence have a history of TBI (Haarbauer-Krupa et al., 2021).

Compared with females, males had significantly higher age-adjusted rates of principal mechanisms of injury contributing to TBI-related hospitalization and death in the United States between 2016 and 2017 (CDC, 2021). The most common injuries precipitating hospitalization were unintentional falls, motor vehicle crashes, unintentionally being struck by an object, intentional self-harm, and assault; the latter was more than four-fold higher among men than women (see Figure 2-2 and Table 2-2). Unintentional falls, motor vehicle crashes, suicide, and homicide were the most common injuries contributing to TBI-related death. Additionally, males have higher rates of concussion in certain contact sports, such as football; however, females have higher rates of concussion in gender-comparable sports, such as soccer (Haarbauer-Krupa et al., 2021). An analysis of sex differences in injury rates and recovery

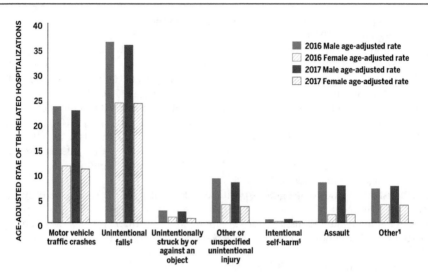

FIGURE 2-2 Estimated age-adjusted rate of TBI-related hospitalizations, by sex and mechanism of injury, United States (2016 and 2017).
SOURCE: CDC, 2021.

times among National Collegiate Athletic Association (NCAA) athletes who experienced TBI found that females had higher concussion rates than males in baseball/softball, basketball, ice hockey, and soccer; females also took longer than males to recover (longer to return to nonrestricted participation) in almost all sports (Covassin et al., 2016).

TBI Incidence in the U.S. Military Population

TBI incidence is higher among military than civilian populations, in part because of the physical demands of military service and the potentially dangerous activities associated with military operations and training (Haarbauer-Krupa et al., 2021). Notably, military personnel are at greater risk of exposure to explosions that can lead to blast overpressure injuries, and

TABLE 2-2 Age-Adjusted Rates of Males and Females Among Major Unintentional and Intentional Principal Mechanisms That Contributed to a TBI-Related Hospitalization in the United States (2016 and 2017)

TBI Principal Mechanism	Rate (per 100,000 population)			
	Males (2016)	Females (2016)	Males (2017)	Females (2017)
Unintentional falls	36.2	24.0	35.6	23.9
Motor vehicle crashes	23.3	11.4	22.5	10.8
Unintentionally being stuck by or against an object	2.5	1.2	2.3	0.9
Intentional self-harm	0.7	0.3	0.8	0.3
Assault	8.1	1.7	7.5	1.7

SOURCE: CDC, 2021.

penetrating brain injuries from fragments and bullets are an important concern for them as well. Among the U.S. armed services, the incidence of TBI is highest among those in the Army, and is generally higher among those on versus not on active duty. Data from the largest study to date on mental health risk, resilience, and pathophysiology in army service members (Army STARRS), however, found that nearly half of those entering the service reported experiencing a concussion or mild TBI prior to enlistment (Naifeh et al., 2019; Stein et al., 2012), highlighting the prevalence of brain injury in the civilian population. By comparison, according to unpublished data from this same study, approximately 20 percent reported having been "knocked out" or "dazed" at some time while in or after joining the service.[5] Although preenlistment TBIs are common, however, deployment-acquired TBIs are more strongly associated with elevated risk for posttraumatic stress disorder (PTSD), generalized anxiety disorder, major depressive episodes, and suicidality (Naifeh et al., 2019; Stein et al., 2019).

The Department of Defense (DoD) provides publicly available information about the number of service members who have sustained a mild, moderate, penetrating, or severe TBI since 2000 (see Table 2-3). TBIs are identified based on billing codes from insurance claims for inpatient or outpatient TBI medical encounters defined by the appropriate ICD coding guidelines.[6] These statistics include TBIs sustained by service members during military training, military deployment, and day-to-day activities. Of note, among service members having sustained more than one TBI, the reporting counts only a single TBI; if a service member has sustained multiple TBIs of different types, the injury with the highest severity is reported. Of more than 434,000 TBIs reported since 2000, the majority (82.3 percent) were classified as mild (for example, concussion).

The VA's Traumatic Brain Injury Veterans Health Registry captures data about TBIs experienced by Veterans who seek care or benefits from the VA and who served in Operation Enduring Freedom (OEF), Operation Iraqi Freedom (OIF), or Operation New Dawn (OND). Data in the registry are drawn from such sources as the VA TBI Screen, administered when

---

[5] Communication from Ronald C. Kessler, Ph.D., McNeil Family Professor, Department of Health Care Policy, Harvard Medical School, regarding data from Army STARRS program to Eric Schoomaker, M.D., Ph.D. September 13, 2021. Similar findings are reported in Stein et al., 2015.

[6] According to the DoD website, "The International Classification of Diseases, 10th edition, Clinical Modification (ICD-10-CM) took effect Oct. 1, 2015, replacing the ICD-9-CM coding guidelines. Military treatment facilities code medical encounters using ICD-10-CM and other DOD specific codes" https://www.health.mil/Military-Health-Topics/Centers-of-Excellence/Traumatic-Brain-Injury-Center-of-Excellence/DOD-TBI-Worldwide-Numbers (accessed October 4, 2021).

TABLE 2-3 Department of Defense Numbers for TBI Among Service Members Worldwide

TBI Severity	2014	2016	2017	2020	2000–2021 Q1
Penetrating	174	92	73	70	5,544
Severe	173	184	134	100	4,545
Moderate	2,335	2,633	2,559	2,503	46,716
Mild	20,837	15,420	15,042	13,802	361,848
Not Classifiable	1,549	13	33	1	20,956
Total	25,068	18,342	17,841	16,476	439,609

NOTE: Q1 = Quarter 1.
SOURCE: https://www.health.mil/Military-Health-Topics/Centers-of-Excellence/Traumatic-Brain-Injury-Center-of-Excellence/DOD-TBI-Worldwide-Numbers (accessed October 8, 2021).

Veterans seek health care from the VA, as well as information from diagnostic codes in electronic medical records and the VA's disability benefit file. Between 2001 and 2013, a total of 221,895 Veterans were included in the registry, most of whom (185,437, or 84 percent) were identified using the TBI screen (Whiteneck et al., 2015). Veterans identified through their positive responses on the screen are offered a clinical evaluation to confirm the TBI diagnosis, as well as a plan of care. Those with clinically confirmed TBI commonly report blast injuries (77 percent), loss of consciousness (52 percent), and posttraumatic amnesia (40 percent). Most of the cases of people with TBI in the registry are classified as mild (81 percent), followed by moderate (9 percent) and severe (6 percent).

ECONOMIC COSTS

The economic costs associated with injury, in general, are high. In 2019, for example, CDC estimated that "the economic cost of injury was $4.2 trillion, including $327 billion in medical care, $69 billion in work loss, and $3.8 trillion in value of statistical life and quality of life losses" (Peterson et al., 2021, p. 1656). TBI represents only one condition that can result from an injury, and the report does not break down economic costs by such types, but notes among its limitations that the costs derived for nonfatal injuries are based on the year following injury, and thus do not account for costs of potential long-term consequences that may also be significant.

The first TBI cost study estimated the direct costs (medical care) and indirect costs (nonmedical costs, such as lost work) accrued over the lifetime of individuals who experienced a TBI in 1985 that led to hospitalization or death (Max et al., 1991). The lifetime accrual of costs for an annual cohort of injuries is a common estimation used by health economists, but is one of the most misinterpreted findings in cost studies because the total lifetime cost is often interpreted as an annual cost. Max and colleagues (1991) estimated that the 327,907 head injuries sustained in 1985 that resulted in death or hospitalization incurred $37.8 billion in total lifetime costs. The per-person lifetime cost was $115,300 averaged across minor, moderate, severe, and fatal injuries. Direct costs were estimated as $4.5 billion and accounted for 12 percent of total lifetime costs; indirect morbidity costs (e.g., lost work) were $20.6 billion and accounted for 54 percent; and the costs associated with premature death from TBI accounted for the remaining 34 percent.

Lawrence and colleagues (2018) conducted a study on lifetime cost estimation for TBIs that occurred in 2012. For the 2,123,120 TBIs recorded in that year, the estimated lifetime costs totaled $758 billion. To compare, the Max et al. (1991) estimate in 2012 dollars would be $80.51 billion,[7] making the Lawrence et al. estimate nearly 9.5 times higher. Lawrence and colleagues derived these higher estimates by including nonhospitalized cases of people with TBI, both civilian and military, and also more categories of indirect costs, illustrating that cost estimates are greatly influenced by such factors as case inclusion, valuation of premature life lost, wage valuation, and categories and values of costs that are included in quality-of-life estimates. Lawrence and colleagues (2018) further estimated that of the $758 billion in total lifetime costs, $250 billion could be attributed to fatal, $335 billion to nonfatal hospitalized, and $173 billion to nonhospitalized TBIs. Medical costs were estimated to account for $26 billion of the $758 billion total, which the authors note represents 1 percent of total U.S. personal health care spending. Of the total lifetime costs, they estimated that 2.4 percent was direct costs, 13.3 percent was for work loss, and 83.3 percent ($631 billion) was for quality of life lost.

Using a claims database for 2016, authors of a recent study estimated the direct costs per year of nonfatal TBI care, including inpatient and outpatient care and prescription drugs

---

[7] Converted based on the Consumer Price Index and inflation.

(Miller et al., 2021). Costs were determined over the year following diagnosis and totaled approximately $40 billion, with approximately $10 billion coming from private insurance and $22.5 billion from Medicare. The majority of cases in the database were classified as "head injury unspecified." However, "total estimated annual healthcare costs attributable to low severity TBIs were substantially higher than total estimated annual healthcare costs attributable to middle and high severity TBIs" (Miller et al., 2021).

In a study of the Rochester Epidemiology Project, the authors found that costs for moderate and severe TBI were generally incurred in the first 6 months after injury, whereas costs for mild TBI began to increase above comparison control levels at 1 year, and overall accounted for a large proportion of incremental costs above comparison controls (Leibson et al., 2012). These costs may also represent an underestimate, failing to account for additional indirect costs, such as travel for appointments, tutoring for academic difficulties, and lost time from work (Graves et al., 2020).

Several other studies and reviews have examined the costs of TBI. Humphreys and colleagues (2013) summarize findings from 10 studies published between 2010 and 2012, 8 of which are from the United States. These 10 studies examine direct and lifetime costs and include cost/benefit analyses, mainly of rehabilitation care. Van Dijck and colleagues (2019) review 25 studies published before 2018 that measure annual costs for hospital treatment, reporting a range of in-hospital treatment costs of $2,130 to $401,808 per patient. The authors of both of these reviews conclude that TBI cost estimates are rare; generally have weaker designs (van Dijck and colleagues assigned an overall low quality score of 71 percent); do not adequately describe methods; and have large inconsistencies in their inclusion criteria, definitions, and analytic approaches.

Cost of Pediatric TBI

The cost of pediatric TBI has been estimated to be as high as $1.0–$2.56 billion based on data from the Pediatric Health Information System and the HCUP Kids' Inpatient Database. The data show 15- to 17-year-olds shouldering most of the burden with the highest rates of inpatient hospitalization for pediatric TBI, and with motor vehicle crashes and falls causing most of the injuries (Robertson et al., 2013; Schneier et al., 2006; Shi et al., 2009). Estimates of the costs for hospitalized pediatric patients are greater than $1 billion a year, excluding ongoing costs incurred after discharge, including rehabilitation and other support necessary after a life-changing injury (Schneier et al., 2006).

Pediatric mild TBI or concussion is often overlooked in cost estimation as it is treated primarily in the ambulatory outpatient setting and generally incurs less cost per case relative to moderate or severe TBI, the latter cases entailing emergency diagnostic imaging; procedures; inpatient hospitalization, sometimes in the intensive care setting; and longer-term rehabilitation care, both inpatient and outpatient. However, the vast majority of pediatric TBI is classified as mild, and it is increasingly recognized that these cases can have both lingering and longer-term impacts on function and quality of life and benefit from treatment with rehabilitation, often requiring short- to medium-term academic accommodations as children return to school. Therefore, analyses of the costs associated with these cases have been undertaken, and have found that the costs of pediatric mild TBI may actually exceed those of moderate and severe TBI (Graves et al., 2015). Estimates of the costs associated with pediatric mild TBI or concussion range from $277–$284 per pediatric visit to the ED (Hardesty et al., 2019) to greater than $3,500 per child for those with persisting postconcussion symptoms (Corwin et al., 2020), estimated to be 30 percent of all children sustaining concussion (Zemek et al., 2016). The analysis by Corwin and colleagues includes estimates of direct outpatient costs for specialist appointments, rehabilitation therapies, medications, and education-related support, but does not include indirect costs of lost wages due to parental time spent accompanying the child to medical treatment or address important issues related to quality of life. Based on the sheer numbers of children sustaining concussion or mild TBI, then, the overwhelming proportion of the costs of pediatric TBI is attributable to injuries on the milder end of the spectrum of severity.

Cost-Effectiveness and Cost Savings

Research suggests that providing optimal care for TBI is cost-effective and yields cost savings. A study evaluating the use of Brain Trauma Foundation guidelines for those with severe TBI found that routine use of the guidelines helped achieve substantial cost savings; furthermore, the net savings were associated with improved TBI outcomes and decreased burden on social support systems (Faul et al., 2007). A multicenter cohort analysis of prospectively collated clinical data from the UK Rehabilitation Outcomes Collaborative national database found that specialist rehabilitation was highly cost-effective for TBI patients who were severely disabled, despite their reduced lifespan (Turner-Stokes et al., 2019). The authors found that specialist rehabilitation could potentially generate savings of more than £4 billion in the cost of ongoing care for the 8-year cohort. Another study used a decision-analytical model to compare the costs, outcomes, and cost-effectiveness of three strategies for treating patients with severe TBI (Whitmore et al., 2012). The authors found aggressive treatment for severe TBI to be a cost-effective option even for older patients. Furthermore, they found an association between the provision of comfort care and poorer outcomes and higher costs. A scoping literature review investigating economic evaluations of inpatient and outpatient neuropsychological rehabilitation in individuals with acquired brain injury found that the majority documented cost savings (Stolwyk et al., 2021). However, the review acknowledged methodologic limitations in many of the cost evaluations reviewed, making it difficult to eliminate potential confounding effects or to capture a full picture of indirect and societal costs and savings and highlighting a role for further economic analyses addressing TBI. Another literature review concluded that little research has been published on the economic impacts of mild and moderate TBI on families, caregivers, and society. The authors of that study called for more research on this issue, emphasizing the need to estimate the economic burden of mild and moderate TBI on health care providers and social services (Humphreys et al., 2013).

Overall, the number and breadth of studies estimating cost, cost-effectiveness, and cost/benefit for TBI are lacking, with a dearth of evidence for either the most or the least promising strategies. This lack of evidence hinders the ability to identify state-of-the-art treatment and translate it into practice.

Burden of TBI on Patients and Families

In addition to economic costs, TBI imposes a tremendous burden on individuals, families, and communities. To better understand the perspectives of individuals and families recovering from TBI, the committee made patient and family voices an important component of its information-gathering workshop. The participating patients and family members expressed seven illustrative themes that help provide a more comprehensive understanding of the challenges faced following a TBI.[8]

---

[8] The content of this section was drawn from the committee's discussions during sessions of the public workshop held on March 16, 2021. See Appendix B for additional information on the workshop topics and speakers.

1. Overwhelmingly, speakers were grateful for the care they had received and for the providers who listened to their concerns and needs. Having one provider with whom they had a strong connection was vital to recovery, and one essential quality was the provider's ability to hear their concerns and help with the total experience of the individual and family. One parent reported the following experience based on participation in a research study:

> What transpired after that [referral because of research] was just really a very careful coordinated plan for [her son]. And it was really the first time as a parent or a patient that I've ever experienced a doctor really listening and wanting to collaborate with other fields.
>
> General health care practitioners, including mental health therapists and primary care physicians, often serve people with TBI and their caregivers, but may not have the knowledge of their unique needs and how to assist them.

2. Families wanted comprehensive information about what to do, what to expect, and how to negotiate the many life changes involved in accommodating ongoing TBI symptoms. The information they received was not coordinated and often had gaps in addressing their concerns and situations.

> When I graduated [from rehab], there was no guidance on the best recovery process going forward, what would be good to do and what I shouldn't be doing.... Bad is that no doctor was officially on my case post-acute rehab.
>
> And, you know, work issues and stuff like that kept coming up. There was no support on that aspect to where, you know, I could comfortably tell people what was wrong with me.
>
> A second challenge is a lack of information and training for families.... Wouldn't it be great if case managers and discharge planners were paid based on patient and family satisfaction?
>
> [After four months in the hospital], I was discharged home to my parents without much care after that. And my parents had no idea really about what to do, what to do with me and I had no idea. And I was, I had a lack of insight and I was very impulsive.
>
> I was faced in 2013, when my husband shared with me that he would rather take his life than to face that daily burden of, putting the burdens on not only myself but our family and loved ones, Nobody understood the pain he was going through. And so from that moment on, I knew that this was something very serious and we needed to find out what was happening.
>
> As a family, the impacts on my children have been so severe that my oldest son was suicidal at times because the impacts of caregiving on him was too much.

3. Many speakers reported that care felt far less comprehensive and cohesive after hospital discharge, and there was little or no real support after treatment was over, even though symptoms often persist and impact the patient's life.

> I don't have follow up. I go see the doctor once a year for my annual checkup. But I don't get the opportunity to really be diagnosed or re-diagnosed.
>
> I was discharged from a neurological intensive care unit directly from the ICU to

home with no follow up. Zero follow up. I just had to hunt down all the various other doctors I needed to see to take care of my problems.

Everyone who has a severe TBI should have some doctor assigned who calls them and who they can call with questions, issues, I think.

4. Speakers identified a disconnect between the symptoms on which doctors were focused and the symptoms that had the most impact on patients and their families.

    I feel I did not get enough information about my recovery and perhaps the doctors didn't know it.... You know, practical things like when could I actually drive again. I mean, how do you know when you're to the point when you know you recovered sufficiently to be able to drive.

    [I brought up my headaches] over and over and over and over again. And I honestly, every time, like I said, I'm constantly told there's nothing wrong with me.

5. Speakers identified the need for patients to have advocates to help ask questions and seek resources. Several speakers mentioned that they had advocates or served in the advocate role, and they worried about patients and families who did not have this support.

    It's almost impossible to advocate for yourself. So you need another person to advocate on your behalf, whether it's a family member or friend. And unfortunately some people don't have those advocates and they really suffer.

    It became just this dark process of trying to figure out what can we do to treat this next symptom that's popping up.... It just became a trial and error for us. And I mean, fortunately for my husband. I am an advocate. I am a go getter. I'm a pusher and ... [what do people without this do]?

6. Speakers mentioned that insurance was challenging with respect to what was and was not covered and the process of negotiating coverage.

    I just wanted to reiterate my experience of having to really fight.... [Insurance company] was going to put me in a nursing home because it's a lot cheaper. To me it's just criminal that so many victims of TBI are just forced by insurance companies into bed rest, which is just killing their chances of a good recovery.

    Many people actually max out their benefits at that point [inpatient rehab]. And so then when they are home they have problems and they don't have any insurance funds to help with those.

7. A wide range of research needs was identified—in particular, research integrating patient and family experiences.

    The research that documents negative impact on family caregivers has not been matched with research funding to develop and systematically disseminate interventions and programs that can assist them.... There also appears to be a disconnect between existing research evidence and clinical practice.

8. Some patients and families reported that clinical research programs helped make them aware of and gain access to specialty TBI care.

> *We were lucky enough to be at [school] that was partnering ... for some research on pediatric concussions. [Son] had already completed baseline testing as part of the program and was immediately referred [to provider] for evaluation. And what transpired after that was just really a very careful, coordinated plan for him. They said hey, we have a study that's going on [at university] and you should probably sign up and see what happens, and I finally did, and it worked. Some things finally came to fruition. Things started making sense*

These themes and quotations were instrumental in guiding this report to focus on a holistic approach to TBI treatment and care, integrating individuals within their families and support structures and acknowledging the many systems (including health care, work, school, social, and recreational) with which patients interact.

CONCLUSIONS

The committee identified a clear need to better document TBI's incidence, burden, and vulnerable populations through improved data collection and analysis systems and further research. Obtaining high-quality data, at the population level and from patient care, is an integral component of a learning health care system, in which data are used to inform research and improve care, among other features (see Chapter 8). Despite significant gaps in measurement of the incidence and prevalence of TBI at all levels of severity, existing data create a compelling picture that TBI is a prevalent health issue with increasing incidence in the civilian and military U.S. populations, as well as globally. A similar dearth of evidence is available for measuring the full burden of TBI, including monetary costs, but again, existing data indicate that TBI imposes a high burden on individuals, families, and communities, as well as the nation as a whole. Despite the data limitations, moreover, the information that does exist supports the need to disseminate and implement best practices that can improve the lives of all TBI patients and their families. Reducing the burden of TBI will require developing not only treatments and interventions for those who experience it, but also prevention policies and programs to reduce the frequency with which it occurs.

REFERENCES

Arbogast, K. B., A. E. Curry, M. R. Pfeiffer, M. R. Zonfrillo, J. Haarbauer-Krupa, M. J. Breiding, V. G. Coronado, and C. L. Master. 2016. Point of health care entry for youth with concussion within a large pediatric care network. *JAMA Pediatrics* 170(7):e160294.

Barker-Collo, S. L., and V. L. Feigin. 2009. Capturing the spectrum: Suggested standards for conducting population-based traumatic brain injury incidence studies. *Neuroepidemiology* 32(1):1-3.

Barker-Collo, S., Theadom, A., Jones, K., Feigin, V. L., and M. Kahan. 2016. Accuracy of an International Classification of Diseases Code surveillance system in the identification of traumatic brain injury. *Neuroepidemiology* 47(1):46-52.

Bruns, J., Jr., and W. A. Hauser. 2003. The epidemiology of traumatic brain injury: A review. *Epilepsia* 44(s10):2-10.

Carlson, K. F., J. E. Barnes, E. M. Hagel, B. C. Taylor, D. X. Cifu, and N. A. Sayer. 2013. Sensitivity and specificity of traumatic brain injury diagnosis codes in United States Department of Veterans Affairs administrative data. *Brain Injury* 27(6):640-650.

CDC (Centers for Disease Control and Prevention). 2003. *Report to Congress on mild traumatic brain injury in the United States: Steps to prevent a serious public health problem*. National Center for Injury Prevention and Control. Atlanta, GA: Centers for Disease Control and Prevention.

CDC. 2019. *Surveillance report of traumatic brain injury-related emergency department visits, hospitalizations, and deaths—United States, 2014*. Atlanta, GA: Department of Health and Human Services.

CDC. 2021. *Surveillance report of traumatic brain injury-related hospitalizations and deaths by age group, sex, and mechanism of injury—United States, 2016 and 2017*. Atlanta, GA: Department of Health and Human Services.

Corwin, D. J., C. L. Master, M. F. Grady, and M. R. Zonfrillo. 2020. The economic burden of pediatric postconcussive syndrome. *Clinical Journal of Sport Medicine* 30(5):e154-e155.

Covassin, T., R. Moran, and R. J. Elbin. 2016. Sex differences in reported concussion injury rates and time loss from participation: An update of the national collegiate athletic association injury surveillance program from 2004-2005 through 2008-2009. *Journal of Athletic Training* 51(3):189-194.

Dams-O'Connor, K., J. P. Cuthbert, J. Whyte, J. D. Corrigan, M. Faul, and C. Harrison-Felix. 2013. Traumatic brain injury among older adults at level I and II trauma centers. *Journal of Neurotrauma* 30(24):2001-2013.

Daugherty, J., D. Waltzman, K. Sarmiento, and L. Xu. 2019. Traumatic brain injury-related deaths by race/ethnicity, sex, intent, and mechanism of injury—United States, 2000–2017. *Morbidity and Mortality Weekly Report* 68(46):1050-1056.

DePadilla, L., G. F. Miller, S. E. Jones, A. B. Peterson, and M. J. Breiding. 2018. Self-reported concussions from playing a sport or being physically active among high school students—United States, 2017. *Morbidity and Mortality Weekly Report* 67(24):682-685.

Dewan, M. C., N. Mummareddy, J. C. Wellons 3rd., and C. M. Bonfield. 2016. Epidemiology of global pediatric traumatic brain injury: Qualitative review. *World Neurosurgery* 91:497-509.

Dewan, M. C., A. Rattani, S. Gupta, R. E. Baticulon, Y. C. Hung, M. Punchak, A. Agrawal, A. O. Adeleye, M. G. Shrime, A. M. Rubiano, J. V. Rosenfeld, and K. B. Park. 2019. Estimating the global incidence of traumatic brain injury. *Journal of Neurosurgery* 130:1080-1097.

Faul, M., M. M. Wald, W. Rutland-Brown, E. E. Sullivent, and R. W. Sattin. 2007. Using a cost-benefit analysis to estimate outcomes of a clinical treatment guideline: Testing the Brain Trauma Foundation guidelines for the treatment of severe traumatic brain injury. *Journal of Trauma* 63(6):1271-1278.

Faul, M., M. M. Wald, L. Xu, and V. G. Coronado. 2010. *Traumatic brain injury in the United States: Emergency department visits, hospitalizations, and deaths, 2002–2006*. Atlanta, GA: Centers for Disease Control and Prevention.

Feigin, V. L., A. Theadom, S. Barker-Collo, N. J. Starkey, K. McPherson, M. Kahan, A. Dowell, P. Brown, V. Parag, R. Kydd, K. Jones, A. Jones, S. Ameratunga, and B. S. Group. 2013. Incidence of traumatic brain injury in New Zealand: A population-based study. *Lancet Neurology* 12(1):53-64.

Fife, D. 1987. Head injury with and without hospital admission: Comparisons of incidence and short-term disability. *American Journal of Public Health* 77(7):810-812.

Gabella, B. A., J. E. Hathaway, B. Hume, J. Johnson, J. F. Costich, S. Slavova, and A. Y. Liu. 2021. Multisite medical record review of emergency department visits for traumatic brain injury. *Injury Prevention* 27(S1):i42-i48.

Gardner, R. C., K. Dams-O'Connor, M. R. Morrissey, and G. T. Manley. 2018. Geriatric traumatic brain injury: Epidemiology, outcomes, knowledge gaps, and future directions. *Journal of Neurotrauma* 35(7):889-906.

Graves, J. M., F. P. Rivara, and M. S. Vavilala. 2015. Health care costs 1 year after pediatric traumatic brain injury. *American Journal of Public Health* 105(10):e35-41.

Graves, J. M., M. Moore, L. Kehoe, M. Li, A. Chan, K. Conrick, W. Williams-Gilbert, and M. S. Vavilala. 2020. Family hardship following youth concussion: Beyond the medical bills. *Journal of Pediatric Nursing* 51:15-20.

Guerrero, J. L., D. J. Thurman, and J. E. Sniezek. 2000. Emergency department visits associated with traumatic brain injury: United States, 1995-1996. *Brain Injury* 14(2):181-186.

Haarbauer-Krupa, J., A. Ciccia, J. Dodd, D. Ettel, B. Kurowski, A. Lumba-Brown, and S. Suskauer. 2017. Service delivery in the healthcare and educational systems for children following traumatic brain injury: Gaps in care. *Journal of Head Trauma Rehabilitation* 32(6):367-377.

Haarbauer-Krupa, J., M. J. Pugh, E. M. Prager, N. Harmon, J. Wolfe, and K. C. Yaffe. 2021. Epidemiology of chronic effects of traumatic brain injury. *Journal of Neurotrauma*. https://doi.org/10.1089/neu.2021.0062.

Hardesty, W., B. Singichetti, H. Yi, J. C. Leonard, and J. Yang. 2019. Characteristics and costs of pediatric emergency department visits for sports- and recreation-related concussions, 2006–2014. *Journal of Emergency Medicine* 56(5):571-579.

Humphreys, I., R. L. Wood, C. J. Phillips, and S. Macey. 2013. The costs of traumatic brain injury: A literature review. *ClinicoEconomics and Outcomes Research* 5:281-287.

Jager, T. E., H. B. Weiss, J. H. Coben, and P. E. Pepe. 2000. Traumatic brain injuries evaluated in us emergency departments, 1992–1994. *Academic Emergency Medicine* 7(2):134-140.

James, S. L., A. Theadom, R. G. Ellenbogen, M. S. Bannick, W. Montjoy-Venning, L. R. Lucchesi, N. Abbasi, et al. 2019. Global, regional, and national burden of traumatic brain injury and spinal cord injury, 1990-2016: A systematic analysis for the Global Burden of Disease study 2016. *Lancet Neurology* 18(1):56-87.

Johnson, W. D., and D. P. Griswold. 2017. Traumatic brain injury: A global challenge. *Lancet Neurology* 16(12):949-950.

Lawrence B. A., J. A. Orman, T. R. Miller, R. S. Spicer, and D. Hendrie. 2018. Ch. 32. Cost of traumatic brain injuries in the United States and the return on helmet investments. In *Neurotrauma and critical care of the brain*, 2nd ed., edited by J. Jallo and C. M. Loftus. New York: Thieme Medical Publishers, Inc.

Leibson, C. L., A. W. Brown, K. Hall Long, J. E. Ransom, J. Mandrekar, T. M. Osler, and J. F. Malec. 2012. Medical care costs associated with traumatic brain injury over the full spectrum of disease: A controlled population-based study. *Journal of Neurotrauma* 29(11):2038-2049.

Lumba-Brown A., K. O. Yeates, K. Sarmiento, M. J. Breiding, T. M. Haegerich, G. A. Gioia, M. Turner, E. C. Benzel, S. J. Suskauer, C. C. Giza, M. Joseph, C. Broomand, B. Weissman, W. Gordon, D. W. Wright, R. S. Moser, K. McAvoy, L. Ewing-Cobbs, A. C. Duhaime, M. Putukian, B. Holshouser, D. Pauk, S. Wade, S. Herring, M. Halstead, H. Keenan, M. Choe, C. Christian, K. Guskiewicz, P. Raskin, A. Gregory, A. Mucha, H. Taylor, J. Callahan, J. Dewitt, M. Collins, M. Kirkwood, J. Ragheb, R. Ellenbogen, T. Spinks, T. Ganiats, L. Sabelhaus, K. Altenhofen, R. Hoffman, T. Getchius, G. Gronseth, Z. Donnell, R. O'Connor, and S. Timmons. 2018. Centers for Disease Control and Prevention guideline on the diagnosis and management of mild traumatic brain injury among children. *JAMA Pediatrics* 172(11):e182853.

Majdan, M., D. Plancikova, A. Maas, S. Polinder, V. Feigin, A. Theadom, M. Rusnak, A. Brazinova, and J. Haagsma. 2017. Years of life lost due to traumatic brain injury in Europe: A cross-sectional analysis of 16 countries. *PLoS Medicine* 14(7):e1002331.

Marin, J. R., M. D. Weaver, D. M. Yealy, and R. C. Mannix. 2014. Trends in visits for traumatic brain injury to emergency departments in the United States. *Journal of the American Medical Association* 311(18):1917-1919.

Max, W., E. J. MacKenzie, and D. P. Rice. 1991. Head injuries: Costs and consequences. *Journal of Head Trauma Rehabilitation* 6(2):76-91.

Miller, G. F., L. DePadilla, and L. Xu. 2021. Costs of nonfatal traumatic brain injury in the United States, 2016. *Medical Care* 59(5):451-455.

Mock, C., Joshipura, M., Arreola-Risa, C., and R. Quansah. 2012. An estimate of the number of lives that could be saved through improvements in trauma care globally. *World Journal of Surgery* 36(5):959-963.

Naifeh, J. A., Mash, H., Stein, M. B., Fullerton, C. S., Kessler, R. C., and R. J. Ursano. 2019. The Army Study to Assess Risk and Resilience in Servicemembers (Army STARRS): Progress toward understanding suicide among soldiers. *Molecular Psychiatry* 24:34-48.

Narapareddy, B., L. Richey, and M. Peters. 2019. *The growing epidemic of TBI in older patients.* NeurologyLive. https://www.neurologylive.com/view/growing-epidemic-tbi-older-patients (accessed November 10, 2021).

Peterson, C., G. F. Miller, S. Barnett, and C. Florence. 2021. Economic cost of injury—United States, 2019. *Morbidity and Mortality Weekly Report* 70(48):1655–1659.

Rivara, F. P., T. D. Koepsell, J. Wang, N. Temkin, A. Dorsch, M. S. Vavilala, D. Durbin, and K. M. Jaffe. 2012. Incidence of disability among children 12 months after traumatic brain injury. *American Journal of Public Health* 102(11):2074-2079.

Robertson, B. D., C. E. McConnel, and S. Green. 2013. Charges associated with pediatric head injuries: A five year retrospective review of 41 pediatric hospitals in the US. *Journal of Injury & Violence Research* 5(1):51-60.

Rosenbaum, B. P., M. L. Kelly, V. R. Kshettry, and R. J. Weil. 2014. Neurologic disorders, in-hospital deaths, and years of potential life lost in the USA, 1988–2011. *Journal of Clinical Neuroscience* 21(11):1874-1880.

Rutland-Brown, W., J. A. Langlois, K. E. Thomas, and Y. L. Xi. 2006. Incidence of traumatic brain injury in the United States, 2003. *Journal of Head Trauma Rehabilitation* 21(6):544-548.

Schneier, A. J., B. J. Shields, S. G. Hostetler, H. Xiang, and G. A. Smith. 2006. Incidence of pediatric traumatic brain injury and associated hospital resource utilization in the United States. *Pediatrics* 118(2):483-492.

Shi, J., H. Xiang, K. Wheeler, G. A. Smith, L. Stallones, J. Groner, and Z. Wang. 2009. Costs, mortality likelihood and outcomes of hospitalized us children with traumatic brain injuries. *Brain Injury* 23(7):602-611.

Sosin, D. M., J. E. Sniezek, and D. J. Thurman. 1996. Incidence of mild and moderate brain injury in the United States, 1991. *Brain Injury* 10(1):47-54.

Stein, M. B., R. J. Ursano, N. A. Sampson, and R. C. Kessler. 2012. *Suicide and traumatic brain injury.* Annual Meeting of the American College of Neuropsychopharmacology. Hollywood, Florida.

Stein, M. B., R. C. Kessler, S. G. Heeringa, S. Jain, L. Campbell-Sills, C. Colpe, C. Fullerton, M. Nock, N. Sampson, M. Schoenbaum, X. Sun, M. Thomas, R. Ursano, and Army STARRS collaborators. 2015. Prospective longitudinal evaluation of the effect of deployment-acquired traumatic brain injury on posttraumatic stress and related disorders: Results from the Army Study to Assess Risk and Resilience in Servicemembers (Army STARRS). *American Journal of Psychiatry* 172:1101-1111.

Stein, M. B., S. Jain, J. T. Giacino, H. Levin, S, Dikmen, L. D. Nelson, M. J. Vassar, D. O. Okonkwo, R. Diaz-Arrastia, C. S. Robertson, P. Mukherjee, M. McCrea, C. L. Mac Donald, J. K. Yue, E. Yuh, X. Sun, L. Campbell-Sills, N. Temkin, G. T. Manley, TRACK-TBI Investigators, ... and R. Zafonte. 2019. Risk of posttraumatic stress disorder and major depression in civilian patients after mild traumatic brain injury: A TRACK-TBI study. *JAMA Psychiatry* 76(3):249-258.

Stolwyk, R. J., J. R. Gooden, J. Kim, and D. A. Cadilhac. 2021. What is known about the cost-effectiveness of neuropsychological interventions for individuals with acquired brain injury? A scoping review. *Neuropsychology Rehabilitation* 31(2):316-344.

Stopa, B. M., M. Harary, R. Jhun, A. Job, S. Izzy, T. R. Smith, and W. B. Gormley. 2020. Divergence in the epide-miological estimates of traumatic brain injury in the United States: Comparison of two national databases. *Journal of Neurosurgery.* Online ahead of print.

Taylor, C. A., J. M. Bell, M. J. Breiding, and L. Xu. 2017. Traumatic brain injury-related emergency department visits, hospitalizations, and deaths—United States, 2007 and 2013. *Morbidity and Mortality Weekly Report Surveillance Summaries* 66(9):1-16.

Theadom, A., S. Barker-Collo, V. L. Feigin, N. J. Starkey, K. Jones, A. Jones, S. Ameratunga, P. A. Barber, and B. R. Group. 2012. The spectrum captured: A methodological approach to studying incidence and outcomes of traumatic brain injury on a population level. *Neuroepidemiology* 38(1):18-29.

Thompson, H. J., W. C. McCormick, and S. H. Kagan. 2006. Traumatic brain injury in older adults: Epidemiology, outcomes, and future implications. *Journal of the American Geriatrics Society* 54(10):1590-1595.

Thurman, D., and J. Guerrero. 1999. Trends in hospitalization associated with traumatic brain injury. *Journal of the American Medical Association* 282(10):954-957.

Thurman, D. J., J. E. Sniezek, D. Johnson, A. Greenspan, and S. M. Smith. 1995. *Guidelines for surveillance of central nervous system injury.* Atlanta, GA: National Center for Injury Prevention and Control, Centers for Disease Control and Prevention.

Thurman, D. J., C. Alverson, D. Browne, K. Dunn, J. Guerrero, R. Johnson, V. Johnson, J. Langlois, D. Pilkey, J. Sniezek, and S. Toal. 1999. *Traumatic brain injury in the United States: A report to Congress.* Atlanta, GA: National Center for Injury Prevention and Control, Centers for Disease Control and Prevention. https://www.cdc.gov/traumaticbraininjury/pdf/TBI_in_the_US.pdf (accessed December 1, 2021).

Turner-Stokes, L., M. Dzingina, R. Shavelle, A. Bill, H. Williams, and K. Sephton. 2019. Estimated life-time savings in the cost of ongoing care following specialist rehabilitation for severe traumatic brain injury in the United Kingdom. *Journal of Head Trauma Rehabilitation* 34(4):205-214.

van Dijck, J., M. D. Dijkman, R. H. Ophuis, G. C. W. de Ruiter, W. C. Peul, and S. Polinder. 2019. In-hospital costs after severe traumatic brain injury: A systematic review and quality assessment. *PLoS One* 14(5):e0216743.

Whiteneck, G. G., J. Cuthbert, and D. Mellick. 2015. *VA Traumatic brain injury veterans health registry report.* Washington, DC: Department of Veterans Affairs.

Whitmore, R. G., J. P. Thawani, M. S. Grady, J. M. Levine, M. R. Sanborn, and S. C. Stein. 2012. Is aggressive treatment of traumatic brain injury cost-effective? *Journal of Neurosurgery* 116(5):1106-1113.

WHO (World Health Organization). 2014. *Improving mortality statistics through civil registration and vital statistics systems: Strategies for country and partner support.* Geneva, Switzerland: World Health Organization.

World Bank/WHO. 2014. *Global civil registration and vital statistics: Scaling up investment plan, 2015—2024.* https://www.worldbank.org/en/topic/health/publication/global-civil-registration-vital-statistics-scaling-up-investment (accessed November 11, 2021).

Zemek, R., N. Barrowman, S. B. Freedman, J. Gravel, I. Gagnon, C. McGahern, M. Aglipay, G. Sangha, K. Boutis, D. Beer, W. Craig, E. Burns, K. J. Farion, A. Mikrogianakis, K. Barlow, A. S. Dubrovsky, W. Meeuwisse, G. Gioia, W. P. Meehan, 3rd, M. H. Beauchamp, Y. Kamil, A. M. Grool, B. Hoshizaki, P. Anderson, B. L. Brooks, K. O. Yeates, M. Vassilyadi, T. Klassen, M. Keightley, L. Richer, C. DeMatteo, M. H. Osmond, and the Pediatric Emergency Research Canada Concussion Team. 2016. Clinical risk score for persistent postconcussion symptoms among children with acute concussion in the ED. *Journal of the American Medical Association* 315(10):1014-1025.

3

Understanding Patients with Traumatic Brain Injury

Chapter Highlights

- Traumatic brain injury (TBI) needs to be viewed and managed as a condition, not a one-time event, and it needs to be viewed through a framework that considers multiple factors. The bio-psycho-socio-ecological model recognizes that injury and recovery are influenced by an interplay among many elements—physical and medical, psychological and behavioral, and social and economic, among others. This framework enables a more complete understanding of complex conditions such as TBI.
- Multiple factors affect a person's access to care and an increased likelihood of negative outcomes after TBI, including age, preinjury status, presence of comorbidities, and propensity for resilience, as well as social and environmental factors related to sex/gender, race, ethnicity, socioeconomic status, insurance status, employment status, geographic location, and social and family support. Although studies have identified these factors, the ways in which these varied factors interact to cause the reported effects remain largely unknown.
- The health care system needs to function as a lens to direct or redirect the trajectory of a person's care and recovery after TBI toward an optimal path. People who experience TBI may encounter the health care system at multiple points as their symptoms arise, abate, or change or as they experience more than one TBI.

One of the essential features of quality health care is patient- or person-centeredness (IOM, 2001), a key feature of the optimized traumatic brain injury (TBI) system described in Chapter 8. To achieve a patient-centered system, it is necessary first to understand those who experience TBI: their journeys and the multiple dimensions—biological, psychological, social, and ecological (contextual)—that feed into and help shape their experiences; the complex, dynamic interactions among these dimensions; and the associated inequities in access to care and in long-term outcomes.

THE PATIENT JOURNEY AND TBI PREVENTION, CARE, AND RECOVERY

The pathway toward addressing TBI starts with *prevention* (see Chapter 4). Although not the focus of this report, the committee emphasizes that the identification and implementation of effective strategies for reducing the numbers and severity of brain injuries that occur is the most effective way to reduce the burden of TBI.

Despite efforts at prevention, however, brain injuries will inevitably occur. Figure 3-1 depicts an overarching and generalized view of a person's pathway from recognition of a potential injury through care; recovery; and return to community, work, and school environments. TBI is a complex condition with many unknowns. Some people completely recover over time, while in other people TBI becomes a chronic and often disabling disease.

The care journey for a person who experiences a TBI can involve different elements and care providers depending on the nature of the injury and the recovery process. Acute and longer-term elements may include the following:

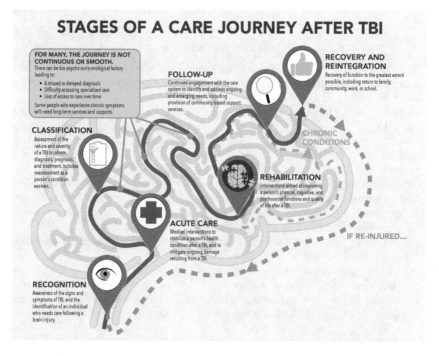

FIGURE 3-1 Illustrative stages of a person's journey through recognition of, treatment for, and recovery after TBI. After a TBI, stages of care may include recognition of the injury, acute care, classification, rehabilitation care, further follow-up, and recovery to the greatest extent possible. This care journey is not always continuous or smooth, and a person may experience chronic symptoms that necessitate ongoing care, or may be reinjured and experience another TBI.
SOURCE: Graphic developed by Masai Interactive.

- *Recognition and provision of early care or aid*: In the context of a sports-related TBI, an athletic trainer or team physician on the field may make an initial assessment to guide a return-to-play decision. In the case of an event such as a vehicle crash, emergency aid may need to be provided at the scene until emergency medical services (EMS) personnel arrive. In a military context, a soldier or medic on the battlefield may provide early aid to an injured comrade.

- *Prehospital EMS care to stabilize vital functions*: In the civilian context, EMS personnel may be called on to stabilize the vital functions of a person who has experienced a TBI and transport them to a higher level of medical care, such as a local hospital emergency department (ED) or a trauma center. In the military trauma system, care may be provided by a forward surgical team or in a combat hospital. A person who experiences a suspected TBI that appears to be minor may receive no hospital-based care beyond an initial evaluation, perhaps coupled with guidance to rest and to seek follow-up should symptoms develop.

- *Acute hospital care to address injuries*: For someone who has experienced a TBI or concomitant injuries of a serious nature, this stage of care includes medical interventions provided in a hospital ED or intensive care unit, aimed at saving the person's life and preventing further negative consequences of the injury. In the military, a person may be evacuated to a regional or U.S.-based military hospital able to provide more advanced levels of care.

- *Rehabilitation and longer-term follow-up to minimize disability*: Rehabilitation and longer-term follow-up can take many pathways and forms, depending on the nature of the injuries sustained. Rehabilitation interventions aim to improve a person's function and quality of life after TBI. Delivery of this care may occur in both military and civilian and both inpatient and outpatient settings. In the military, post-acute rehabilitation therapies are provided through the Department of Veterans Affairs (VA).

- *Recovery and reintegration into society and the workforce to the extent possible*: The goal after TBI is for the person to return to independent living in their home or community and to work or school to the extent possible. A person who experiences a less serious TBI may recover fully, while someone who experiences a more severe injury may deal with ongoing, long-term symptoms and impairments, including a need to receive continued follow-up and rehabilitation care, as well as community-based patient and caregiver support services. In some cases, a person may experience another TBI, potentially starting the journey again.

A FRAMEWORK FOR UNDERSTANDING TBI: THE BIO-PSYCHO-SOCIO-ECOLOGICAL MODEL

Understanding the medical course of TBI is important, but to fully address effective TBI prevention and care requires a framework that is broader than a medical model of injury, given the multiple personal and social/environmental factors that affect the experience of and recovery from such an injury. Models that recognize the interactions among such factors have been applied to a variety of prevention and disease contexts and are required to understand TBI.

The Unique Array of Factors Brought by Each Individual to an Injury

Experienced clinicians, patients and patient advocates, and rehabilitation specialists know that a variety of preexisting and current attributes of the patient, including physiological, interpersonal, and other critical factors, as well as family and community relationships, play key roles in how significant a TBI will be for the patient. In many cases, the role played by these attributes in determining the trajectory of immediate recovery; rehabilitation; and long-term physical, emotional, intellectual, spiritual, and social outcomes is as important as the nature of the injury itself.

Biomedical Aspects of a TBI

Biomedical aspects of a TBI include the nature of the forces and stresses acting on a person's brain, the potential occurrence of traumatic hemorrhage and swelling, and the existence of co-occurring injuries. A person's own physiological responses to the injury are also important in the context of their genetics and endocrine, metabolic, and immune systems. As described in Chapter 2, a majority of TBIs result in what have been termed "mild" injuries with less severe damage to the brain and lesser threats to long-term cognitive, motor, sensory, social, and psychological functions. A smaller number of TBIs have more consequential traumatic impacts and far-ranging effects.

Psychosocial and Ecological Aspects of a TBI

The role of factors beyond the nature of the physical injury lies within a construct that examines the "whole person" in relation to intersecting domains of physical and nonphysical personal characteristics, interpersonal family and immediate community relationships, and socioeconomic factors within the individual's living environment. This construct was first formally described by Engel as the biopsychosocial model (Engel, 1977). Systems theory, including related socioecological models, similarly view health conditions through a framework that considers interactions among individual characteristics, interpersonal relationships, community settings, and wider societal policies, applying the model to prevention, public health, and clinical settings (see, e.g., Karriker-Jaffe et al., 2020; Register-Mihalik and Callahan, 2020; van Erp et al., 2019, and the Centers for Disease Control and Prevention's [CDC's] violence prevention efforts[1]). In the context of TBI, an expanded bio-psycho-socio-ecological (BPSE) model includes the wide and complex array of qualitative and quantitative elements of the living and inanimate network within which each human lives and flourishes. The ecological dimensions of TBI also encompass economic forces, recognizing that challenges in U.S. health care and social systems, such as a scarcity of rehabilitation venues and limited insurance coverage, can limit a person's access to care.

TBIs are not the only illnesses or injuries whose management and outcomes of care are influenced by various elements of a BPSE model. Chronic pain, diabetes, asthma, cardiovascular disease, various cancers, stroke, and Alzheimer's disease and other dementias are among the many chronic health conditions that share this range of influence. In fact, one could argue that no significant survivable injury, illness, or combat-related wound is free of the influence of BPSE factors. For all of these conditions, biological, psychological, social, and human ecological factors play significant roles in the patient's degree of suffering, extent of functional capacity, and even length of survival, and must be assessed and addressed if these illnesses and injuries are to be managed optimally. Improvement in the patient's condition depends on more than a short-term medical-surgical model of treatment, even in

---

[1] See The Social-Ecological Model: A Framework for Prevention at https://www.cdc.gov/violenceprevention/about/social-ecologicalmodel.html (accessed September 27, 2021).

the hands of the most talented clinicians employing the most advanced, state-of-the-art and science modalities.

The prism in Figure 3-2 represents these BPSE factors. The array of BPSE factors unique to each patient can "refract" that person's trajectory after TBI, in some cases leading to outcomes that are better than initially anticipated and in some cases to outcomes that are worse. Collectively, these factors affect the process of recovery and the level of function ultimately achieved for an individual person. The BPSE construct is always present, but the balance of factors and their interactions can change over time for any one patient.

This multifactorial model of human health and well-being is increasingly being recognized as having a major effect at the population level. Direct clinical care may contribute only 20 percent of the overall well-being of a nation's citizenry (Hood et al., 2016), with lifestyle and behavioral factors and social and physical determinants of health playing a more dominant role (NRC and IOM, 2013). Life expectancy, maternal–child health, and a variety of other objective measures of population health are strongly related to these factors, although no one factor plays a more dominant role than others in the U.S. population as a whole.

How the BPSE Framework Describes the Course of a Person's Trajectory After TBI

A TBI can represent the start of a potentially lifelong experience with the long-term consequences of a brain injury, and one cannot predict with certainty at the time of the initial injury what the long-term effects of any one TBI might be for a given person. As reported by providers across the continuum of care, as well as patients and family members, the prism of the BPSE model plays an essential role in affecting outcomes and long-term function. An initial classification of a TBI in a range from less to more severe can be refracted into an array of outcomes, from very poor to very favorable. Illustrating this point, a person's chances of immediate survival from the initial injury have been summarized by the comment, "Where you live actually can determine if you live."[2]

Beyond immediate survival, people who live in rural communities or are injured in remote sites with austere resources for emergency response, evacuation to definitive care,

---

[2] Robinson, J. 2021. TBI Care Gaps and Opportunities: Provider Perspectives on the Acute-Stage Continuum of Care. Panel discussion during virtual workshop for the Committee on Accelerating Progress in Traumatic Brain Injury Research and Care, March 18, 2021.

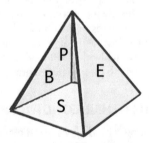

FIGURE 3-2 The BPSE prism. The prism represents the multiple dimensions—biological, psychological, sociological, and ecological—that interact with and influence a condition such as TBI. These dimensions encompass an individual's biological and personal history; people's relationships and the community settings in which they live, work, and play; and broader sociocultural environments and policies.

and access to intensive care treatment, as well as those who live in some urban communities where social determinants of health[3] can affect well-being, are less likely to receive prompt, comprehensive, long-term care and rehabilitation after TBI relative to people without these impediments. Factors in American social and political life that have existed for the duration of the republic's history and have contributed to institutional racism and stratification of educational, economic, employment, residential, and other opportunities have had a serious impact on the optimal management of TBI among disenfranchised groups, including people of color and Native Americans, the poor, and those living in rural areas.

How the Influence of the BPSE Prism and Engagement with an Effective Health Care System Affect a Person's Experiences with TBI Across the Lifespan

After a TBI has been sustained, an "ideal" or optimal treatment and rehabilitation pathway represents what is achievable for that person under the best of conditions. Any deviation from that ideal pathway results in an outcome that is less than optimal. The BPSE prism can steer a person's recovery trajectory away from the ideal pathway, reflecting how the biological nature of the injury, psychological enablers or disablers, social influences (family, race, ethnicity, political, community, faith group, etc.), and the wider ecological environment all impact prospects for short-term survival and longer-term function and potential disability (see Figure 3-3).

In Figure 3-3, an effective health care system provides the lens that refocuses a person's pathway back toward the best possible recovery trajectory. This health care lens encompasses diagnosis, treatment, rehabilitation, and reintegration. Ideally, the lens is able to recognize a deviation, identify requirements for achieving improved care and outcomes, and adjust a person's course accordingly. A person with TBI may need to engage with the health care system multiple times over the course of their lifespan as post-TBI recovery evolves.

While BPSE factors play a role in all phases of TBI management and in the ultimate outcome for each patient, success in incorporating a full understanding of these factors into a patient's clinical course and functional end state has been limited. Any fundamental advances in understanding TBI and in improving prevention, diagnosis, treatment, rehabilitation, and recovery will require integrating BPSE factors into the management scheme and research agenda for TBI, and engaging not only the medical system but also research, financial, educational, community support, and other key elements.

As explored in subsequent chapters, however, the current system for understanding and managing TBI does not function optimally for everyone. Challenges include the heterogeneity of TBI; the need for further research; gaps in the handoffs and transitions that occur along the continuum of care; the need for involvement of multiple types of care providers; the variety of data and payment systems involved in TBI care and research; and the diversity of organizations and communities in which people live, learn, work, and play.

INTERSECTION OF TBI WITH OTHER CONDITIONS

Confounding both acute and long-term diagnosis and management of TBI is the frequent coexistence of posttraumatic stress disorder (PTSD) and pain, especially chronic pain. This

---

[3] Social determinants of health are "conditions in the places where people live, learn, work, and play that affect a wide range of health risks and outcomes," including aspects of health care access and quality, education access and quality, social and community context, economic stability, and neighborhood and built environment (https://www.cdc.gov/socialdeterminants/about.html [accessed March 2, 2022]).

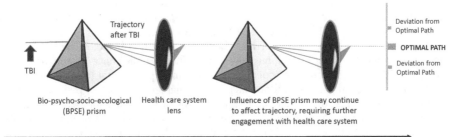

FIGURE 3-3 Conceptual depiction of how BPSE elements can affect the trajectory after a TBI and the role of an effective health care system. The optimal treatment and recovery pathway for a person after experiencing a TBI represents the best outcome that is achievable (center red line). The elements in the BPSE prism can distort or refract the pathway to make it less than ideal. An effective care system serves as a lens for refocusing a person's recovery by recognizing these disablers and providing appropriate interventions and support. A person with TBI may require ongoing follow-up and interactions with a care system to maintain an optimal recovery trajectory, including after the occurrence of any future TBIs.

constellation, often termed the "polytrauma triad" (Cifu et al., 2013), occurs frequently in military service members who are injured or wounded in combat (Hoge et al., 2008). These comorbidities undoubtedly contribute as well to the difficulty of making an accurate diagnosis and designing optimal management for civilian victims of terrorist attacks, natural disasters, violent crimes, and motor vehicle crashes. Much work and controversy surround the attribution of symptoms of TBI and PTSD in the military setting. The principal symptoms of the two conditions overlap substantially in the absence of a penetrating head wound or severe crush injury, with headache alone being one of the few symptoms that accompany TBI but not PTSD. Large population studies have documented marked overlap between and among several comorbid conditions—notably TBI, PTSD, chronic pain, depression, and drug and alcohol abuse—in Veterans of military service (Cifu et al., 2013). Less severe forms of TBI, PTSD, and chronic pain are all clinical diagnoses largely, if not exclusively, reliant upon patient-reported subjective symptoms. This fact injects a level of uncertainty into these diagnoses and often complicates optimal management of the conditions, especially when adjudication of disability or health insurance benefits necessitates attribution for the symptoms involved.

Disparities and Inequities in TBI Outcomes and Access to Care

Equity and TBI

To realize a vision of optimal treatment for and recovery from TBI for all military and civilian populations, it will be necessary to understand and overcome inequities that exist in the current state of TBI treatment, support, and research. Broadly, health inequity arises from the confluence of (1) the interpersonal and systemic mechanisms that organize the distribution of power and resources differentially by individual and group identity, and (2) unequal allocation of power and resources, which is manifested in unequal social, economic, and environmental conditions—that is, the social determinants of health (NASEM, 2017).

Systemic inequities exist in the risk of sustaining a brain injury; access to timely and definitive treatment and recovery; and access to work, family, and community infrastructures that support long-term quality of life. As Chapter 2 documents, being male is associated with higher rates of TBI than is being female. Other studies have identified greater risks of experiencing TBI associated with living in rural or high-poverty areas (Brown et al., 2019; Karb et al., 2016), or have identified higher rates of lifetime TBI among homeless or incarcerated populations, for example (Ferguson et al., 2012; Stubbs et al., 2020).

Inequities in outcomes after TBI have been associated with factors including race, ethnicity, biological sex, socioeconomic status, and others. Studies have documented inequities after TBI in access across the spectrum of care, from prehospital to rehabilitation, as evidenced by the examples that follow later in this chapter. A subset of patients with TBI experience a delayed recovery that can last for months or years after the injury, often with persistent functional impairments that can undermine their emotional health and quality of life (Haarbauer-Krupa et al., 2021). A host of factors have been linked to an increased likelihood of negative TBI-related outcomes, including the patient's age, preinjury status (e.g., mental health, previous head injuries), presence of comorbidities, and propensity for resilience, as well as social and environmental factors related to gender and biological sex, race, ethnicity, socioeconomic status, insurance status, employment status, education status, and geographic location (Haarbauer-Krupa et al., 2021). The cognitive impairment that can result from TBI also presents barriers to self-advocacy and participation in and access to care (Dams-O'Connor et al., 2018).

All of these factors can interact to compound and exacerbate inequities in outcomes and access to care across different populations of TBI patients. However, although many of the causal factors leading to these disparities have been identified, those factors and the ways in which they interact are not yet fully understood. For example, Piatt (2021) identifies injury severity as the major contributing factor in a higher TBI mortality rate among Black relative to White children, with insurance status making only a small contribution. Lack of attention to social drivers—including structural racism, inequities, and bias—plays a role in poor access to quality TBI care and in particular, to rehabilitation and longer-term follow-up across the lifespan (Moore et al., 2019; NASEM, 2017). Access to rehabilitation services after acute care for a TBI is influenced as well by the individual patient's characteristics, the behavior of the health care providers involved, processes of referral, and the broader context of the health care system (Foster and Tilse, 2003). Making progress toward mitigating the inequities detailed above will require considering all of these factors.

There are limited systematic, evidence-based, culturally resonant, and patient-centered interventions in the TBI realm. Research agendas need to address various types of inequities directly; help identify the affected populations; and, more important, build the evidence base for overcoming these inequities. Building this evidence base will require research of all types. Laboratory research is needed to ensure that animal and cell lines are representative of the diverse human populations suffering from TBI. Epidemiological research can identify populations suffering from inequities and evaluate approaches for overcoming them, while implementation and translational research can measure the impacts of intervention approaches. And policy research is needed to ensure that approaches found to be effective reach all populations affected by TBI.

Gender and Sex Differences in TBI Outcomes and Access to Care

Civilian Population

Although it has been established that women with TBI tend to experience worse outcomes than men, gender and sex differences in TBI outcomes have not yet been well characterized (Fabricius et al., 2020). This is largely because women have long been excluded from or greatly underrepresented in TBI preclinical studies and clinical trials, and many studies that do include women are not stratified by sex (NINDS, 2017). Prevalence data are particularly lacking on TBI caused by intimate partner violence, often in the form of repetitive injuries and strangulation (NINDS, 2017). In 2019, PINK Concussions launched the Partner-Inflicted Brain Injury Task Force[4] to foster collaboration between brain injury professionals and domestic violence/intimate partner violence professionals. In addition to the Pink Concussions effort, the Enhancing Neuroimaging Genetics through Meta-Analysis (ENIGMA) Consortium Intimate Partner Violence Working Group is a global collaboration working to collect data on this issue, advance understanding of the neurobehavioral and neurobiological effects, and characterize how TBIs related to intimate partner violence affect long-term health (Esopenko et al., 2021).

New avenues of research demonstrate differences in TBI by sex related to neuroanatomy, neural mechanisms, gonadal hormones, immunity response, and symptoms, underscoring the need for further research (NINDS, 2017). For instance, in women with TBI, hormonal factors can affect recovery outcomes (Haarbauer-Krupa et al., 2021). Social factors also shape the experiences of women who sustain a TBI or provide care for a TBI patient. A qualitative study exploring the lived experience of women with mild and moderate-to-severe TBIs found that their experiences during recovery and caregiving were highly shaped by their gender and gender expectations (Fabricius et al., 2020). In addition, there is evidence that, despite biological sex differences, extrinsic factors that, importantly, are modifiable by policy change or enhanced funding or both can improve outcomes for women, at least in the arena of sports-related concussion (Master et al., 2021).

Military Population

TBI has been called a signature injury of the wars in Iraq and Afghanistan (Tanielian et al., 2008). Although female service members tend to experience a lower rate of TBI compared with their male counterparts, they are more likely to report certain neurobehavioral symptoms after mild TBI (Bouldin et al., 2021; Gray et al., 2020; Haarbauer-Krupa et al., 2021; Kim et al., 2018). For instance, a study of Veterans of the conflicts in Afghanistan and Iraq (Operation Enduring Freedom and Operation Iraqi Freedom, respectively) who experienced TBI during deployment found that PTSD was the most commonly reported condition for both men and women, but that women were more likely to be diagnosed with depression, non-PTSD anxiety disorders, and PTSD with comorbid depression (Iverson et al., 2011). Other studies have yielded similar findings that female Veterans with mild TBI are likely to report neurobehavioral symptoms, are more frequently diagnosed with depression relative to their male counterparts, and are more likely to experience long-term postconcussion syndrome and to opt for non-VA health services (Cogan et al., 2020; Kim et al., 2018). It has been posited that female Veterans may experience more neurobehavioral symptoms in part because they are more likely to experience TBI secondary to interpersonal violence or sexual trauma, as well as because they are more likely to be screened for TBI than are men (Haarbauer-Krupa et al., 2021; Pugh et al., 2019). However, more research is needed on gender differences in the neurobehavioral sequelae of TBI, as female Veterans are not well represented in the existing literature. These issues are being explored in the Women Warriors Initiative, which was launched by the nonprofit Wounded Warrior Project.[5]

---

[4] More information about the PINK Concussions Partner-Inflicted Brain Injury Task Force is available at https://www.pinkconcussions.com/violence (accessed August 3, 2021).
[5] More information about the Women Warriors Initiative is available at https://www.woundedwarriorproject.org/media/tt0ftq4a/wwp-women-warriors-initiative-report-2021.pdf (accessed August 3, 2021).

Age Differences in TBI Outcomes and Access to Care

Children

Individual outcomes among children who experience TBI are shaped by a range of variables, including the type of injury, parenting style, intellectual ability, and socioeconomic factors (Haarbauer-Krupa et al., 2021). One study found higher lifetime prevalence of TBI among U.S. children in states with higher rates of private insurance and insurance adequacy, suggesting that children with less access to care are undercounted in TBI prevalence statistics (Haarbauer-Krupa et al., 2018). The authors also found a significant amount of variability in treatments for pediatric TBI. The experience of TBI can change the social and emotional life of adolescents; for instance, they may need to create new identities for themselves if they can no longer participate in athletics.[6] Coordination between health systems and school systems is critical to ensuring that children continue to meet educational requirements during the TBI recovery process. However, parents of TBI patients are often overwhelmed and do not know how to help their children, as that information may not be readily available and may be difficult for parents to find (Haarbauer-Krupa et al., 2017).

Older Adults

Older adults (generally aged 65 and above) experience the highest rates of TBI-related hospitalization and death, as well as poor functional outcomes (Dams-O'Connor et al., 2013a). Older adults account for 10 percent of all patients with TBI, but 50 percent of deaths attributed to TBI (Stippler et al., 2012). An analysis of TBI trends in United States between 2007 and 2010 found that trauma center admissions increased by about 20–25 percent among adults aged ≥75 compared with the general population (Dams-O'Connor et al., 2013a). During that period, adults aged ≥65 with TBI tended to be White females with severe fall-related injuries. Compared with their younger adult counterparts, older adults tended to require more in-hospital procedures, longer hospital stays, and continued medical care. Older age also increased the likelihood of death in the hospital. Other studies have found that older compared with younger TBI patients tend to have worse functional outcomes (Marquez de la Plata et al., 2008), a greater likelihood of reinjury (Dams-O'Connor et al., 2013b), and more ED visits (Albrecht et al., 2016). Older adults with TBI do worse than younger adults even after mild TBI (Albrecht et al., 2016), and older age predicts worse functional trajectories after TBI post-inpatient rehabilitation (Howrey et al., 2017). Differences in outcome begin to appear even in patients aged 45–59 (Livingston et al., 2005; MRC CRASH Trial Collaborators et al., 2008). Additionally, a history of TBI may accelerate age at onset of cognitive impairment (Li et al., 2016).

Although older age has been clearly established as a strong risk factor for morbidity and mortality after TBI, the factors underlying these outcomes are not well understood. Clearly, however, the observation underscores the need to conceptualize TBI as a long-term condition in which pathophysiological processes interact with age-related changes (Griesbach et al., 2018). Some studies suggest that age moderates the relationship between injury severity and health outcomes, indicating that the effect of injury severity on functioning depends on the patient's age at the time of injury. For instance, the fact that older patients with TBI have higher rates of mortality and worse functional outcomes compared with younger patients holds true despite their tendency to have apparently less severe head injuries (Susman et al., 2002). In

---

[6] Patient Experiences with TBI Systems of Care. Panel discussion during virtual workshop for the Committee on Accelerating Progress in Traumatic Brain Injury Research and Care, March 16, 2021.

Marquez de la Plata and colleagues' (2008) study of age and long-term recovery from TBI, older patients, despite having less severe TBI upon admission, had poorer functional status at discharge and less improvement at 1 year. Livingston and colleagues (2005) found that older TBI patients had poorer functional status at discharge and less improvement at 1 year compared with all other patients, despite less severe TBI upon admission (Livingston et al., 2005).

Given that TBI among older adults remains understudied, predicting outcomes and developing more effective treatment protocols for TBI in older adults will remain problematic in the absence of sufficient clinical data (Thompson et al., 2006). Age and TBI severity are inadequate prognostic markers, as many older adults can respond well to management and rehabilitative treatment (Gardner et al., 2018). However, there are no geriatric-specific TBI guidelines, and the performance of TBI prognostic models for geriatric patients is suboptimal (Dams-O'Connor et al., 2013a; Gardner et al., 2018). Moreover, older adults with TBI may be "misdiagnosed as having dementia and deemed not candidates for intensive rehabilitation."[7] There is clearly a need to develop geriatric-specific prognostic models and evidence-based geriatric TBI treatment and management guidelines.

Rural and Urban Differences in TBI Outcomes and Access to Care

As noted earlier, the care received by individual TBI patients may vary depending on where they live or receive care. For instance, one study evaluated differences in TBI mortality across urban and rural areas in the United States and found that the TBI fatality rate was 13 deaths per 100,000 persons higher in the most rural compared with the most urban areas (Brown et al., 2019). The median fatality rate from all causes of TBI was 23 percent higher in rural than in urban areas, with the greatest differences at the ends of the spectrum of metropolitan and nonmetropolitan counties (Brown et al., 2019).[8] Yue and colleagues (2020) found that the burden of TBI in terms of injury severity, outcomes, and survival is worse in rural than nonrural areas. Underlying factors include reduced or variable access to prehospital care, trauma centers, neurosurgical interventions, and rehabilitative services (Haarbauer-Krupa et al., 2021). Rural populations tend to experience longer delays in reaching care relative to urban populations, which affects long-term outcomes (Tiesman et al., 2007).

Individuals living in rural areas face unique challenges in accessing TBI care and achieving optimal outcomes. Rural areas are home to fewer people with access to fewer public resources compared with those living in nonrural areas. Thus, people in rural areas frequently rely on volunteer emergency response workforces and service providers. Furthermore, injuries occurring in rural areas often are sustained in remote settings with even more limited access to care. This remoteness is associated with greater delays in access to care, greater variability in hospital care capabilities, and the challenge of transporting patients to specialized trauma care when needed, as well as other economic and demographic challenges. For example, people living in remote areas may be older, less able to travel, or less able to afford travel for acute and post-acute care (Tiesman et al., 2007).

The term "rural" can be defined using various indices or criteria, but rural populations, however defined, frequently must contend with conditions of environmental austerity, such as geographic remoteness, isolation, and severe weather conditions. The similarities between

---

[7] Connors, S. 2021. Family Impacts from TBI and Engagement in TBI Care. Panel discussion during virtual workshop for the Committee on Accelerating Progress in Traumatic Brain Injury Research and Care, March 16, 2021.

[8] See Figure 3 from Brown and colleagues (2019), which compares TBI fatality rates per 100,000 persons in the United States by urban influence code. Garcia and colleagues (2017, p. 5) similarity report that "during 1999-2014, the age-adjusted death rates for unintentional injuries were approximately 50% higher in rural areas than urban areas."

these challenges faced by rural populations and those faced by the armed forces may present an opportunity for collaboration among rural providers, special operations medical staff, and wilderness organizations to develop best practices for trauma care in austere conditions.

In terms of health systems and the experiences of rural and urban health care providers, urban providers practice in higher-resource settings where patients are typically closer to the point of care, and these providers have relatively frequent opportunities to practice and maintain skills in providing critical care. In contrast, rural providers practice in lower-resource settings where patients are often injured in remote settings far from the point of care, and these providers therefore have fewer opportunities to practice and maintain critical care skills. Moreover, there are very few neurosurgeons located in rural areas. Most trauma experts working in so-called rural settings in fact work in urban Level I or Level II trauma centers, that is, urban hubs that serve surrounding rural areas. Unfortunately, these providers often lack a comprehensive understanding of how trauma care is provided in truly rural settings or the experiences of providers in those settings. During 2020, for example, the committee learned that no members of the American College of Surgeons' Rural Trauma Committee worked in a rural center. Similarly, the report *A National Trauma Care System: Integrating Military and Civilian Trauma Systems to Achieve Zero Preventable Deaths* (NASEM, 2016a) mentions the term "rural" fewer than ten times, exemplifying the insufficient focus on rural trauma care systems.[9]

In fact, the typical conditions for highly rural trauma care are austere and often comparable to the conditions faced by deployed military personnel. Many medical centers in rural areas have fewer than 25 beds, and half of these centers are at least 75 miles from a Level I or II trauma center. Providers working in these rural settings have variable capability to treat severely injured patients, and data are sparse regarding the transfer of patients from rural settings to more capable trauma centers.[10] Rural populations are doubly impacted by the lack of access to specialized trauma care. The current understanding of how best to treat TBI patients in rural settings is insufficient, and because these settings have reduced access to effective treatments, patients often do not receive the standard of care that is known to be effective in other settings.

In addition to the challenges associated with acute TBI care, access to post-acute and rehabilitative services is even more limited in rural areas. Comparing vocational rehabilitation outcomes between TBI survivors from rural versus urban settings, Johnstone and colleagues (2003) found that despite similar injury severity, neuropsychological test scores, and demographic characteristics, survivors residing in urban areas received significantly greater funds for basic needs required for full participation in the vocational rehabilitation program, as well as significantly more transportation assistance and on-the-job training.

The substantial burden of rural trauma highlights the need for additional study to evaluate the mechanisms of and possible solutions for the disparity between rural and urban trauma care and outcomes (Brown et al., 2019). Such studies might also have implications for trauma care in low- and middle-income countries.

A systematic approach to improved access to acute care for traumatic injuries in rural areas has been proposed.[11] The starting point for such a system could be a notification system that, upon the reporting of an injury, would transmit SMS notifications to a dispatch center that would have up-to-date status and capacity information for all nearby hospitals.

---

[9] Sidwell, R. 2021. Traumatic Brain Injury in the Rural Environment. Presentations and panel discussion during virtual workshop on Accelerating Progress in Traumatic Brain Injury Research and Care, March 16, 2021.
[10] Ibid.
[11] Ibid.

Patients could then be directed to the nearest appropriate center capable of delivering optimal care for a given patient.

Racial and Ethnic Differences in TBI Outcomes and Access to Care

Racial and ethnic differences have been linked to disparities and inequities in TBI prevalence, outcomes, and access to care. Many of the leading causes of TBI, such as road traffic crashes and violence, occur more frequently among populations of color relative to their White counterparts. Illustrating this point, the ED admission rate for the White population was 66 per 1,000 in 2019, compared with 74 per 1,000 for the non-White population (WISQARS, 2019 query).[12] A retrospective cohort study of adults presenting to California EDs between 2005 and 2014, for example, found a 58 percent increase in TBI ED visits and a 34 percent decrease in the proportion of patients admitted to the hospital. Patients who were older adults, Black, and publicly insured had the highest visit rates (Hsia et al., 2018). Assaults, a leading cause of brain injury, occurred three times more often in Black people (10.7/1000) than in White people (3/1000) (WISQARS, 2019 query). Referral to inpatient posthospital care was lower for non-White patients and those without private insurance (Kane et al., 2014). Racial, ethnic, and socioeconomic disparities have also been identified among children who experience TBI. According to a 2006 study, among children under 10 in the United States who experienced a TBI related to a motor vehicle crash between 1995 and 2001, Black children experienced significantly higher rates of death and hospitalization compared with their White peers (Langlois et al., 2005).

A comprehensive literature review explored racial differences in post-TBI outcomes, as well as the potential causes of racial and ethnic disparities in TBI rehabilitation and post-acute services (Gary et al., 2009). The review found that compared with their White counterparts, Black and Hispanic patients who experienced a TBI tended to have worse functional outcomes, were less integrated into their communities, were less likely to receive treatment, and were less likely to be employed. Black and Hispanic caregivers for people with TBI also reported experiencing greater burden, having more unmet needs, and using different types of coping strategies relative to White caregivers. The authors highlight emerging research that suggests racial and ethnic differences in TBI with respect to marital stability, emotional and neurobiological sequelae, and quality-of-life outcomes, although more research is needed to explore these associations.

Numerous studies have identified relationships of race and ethnicity to rehabilitation outcomes after TBI, including utilization of posthospital care, access to rehabilitation, functional status, community reintegration, and employment. This research has shown that survivors from racial and ethnic minority groups are significantly less likely to utilize posthospital health care after brain injury (Gao et al., 2018; Odonkor et al., 2021). For example, a study using data from the National Trauma Databank (NTDB) between 2012 and 2015 on more than 100,000 TBI survivors found that only 16.1 percent of Black patients and 12.5 percent of Hispanic patients with TBI had been discharged from acute care to inpatient rehabilitation, compared with 23.3 percent of White patients (Haines et al., 2019). Black survivors with TBI were more likely to be discharged from acute care to home and less likely to utilize outpatient physical medicine and rehabilitation (PM&R) services (Schiraldi et al., 2015). Compared with White TBI survivors, Hispanic survivors also experienced a lower likelihood of discharge to rehabilitation (Asemota et al., 2013;

---

[12] WISQARS is CDC's Web-based Injury Statistics Query and Reporting Systems, available at https://www.cdc.gov/injury/wisqars/index.html (accessed March 2, 2022).

Budnick et al., 2017; McQuistion et al., 2016) or posthospital care (Kane et al., 2014) and lower odds of discharge to high-level rehabilitation services despite similar insurance coverage (Meagher et al., 2015). Moreover, Black and Hispanic versus White survivors had poorer disability ratings, functional independence scores, and community reintegration (Arango-Lasprilla et al., 2007a,b; Hart et al., 2005), while Hispanic survivors were less likely to obtain employment or to receive on-the-job supports compared with European Americans (da Silva Cardoso et al., 2007).

Demographic data at the local and national levels are currently too limited to enable a full understanding of the needs of many minority communities. During the committee's information-gathering workshop, for instance, Megan Moore from the University of Washington reported that there have been more than 400 studies on the impacts of structural inequities by race and ethnicity, but far fewer studies based on other facets of inequity.[13] She noted that the literature on racial and ethnic differences in TBI often describes disparities in outcomes without adequately identifying the drivers of those disparities, and that even fewer address solutions. Research on these disparities is impeded by the pooling of many racial and ethnic groups in the TBI literature, resulting in gaps in personal/identity-related data. Moore stressed that more data are needed to support the research needed to fully understand these disparities by race and ethnicity, taking into account that not all disparities are differentially negative.[14]

To mitigate the underlying inequities that contribute to these disparate outcomes, it will be necessary to design interventions targeting post-acute care that are specifically tailored to these groups (Gary et al., 2009). At the patient and family level, interventions need to be shaped by an awareness of sociocultural conditions and traditions, as well as the impact of preinjury resilience on outcomes. At the provider level, interventions need to include cultural competency assessments and training that are specific to the needs of a diverse population of TBI patients. At the level of the health care system, strategies are needed for increasing the proportion of Black, Indigenous, and people of color (BIPOC) health care professionals who are part of multidisciplinary teams. To support these efforts, research will be needed to explore the foundational factors driving these disparities, such as discrimination and cultural incongruence (Moore et al., 2015).

Finally, resources for Black and Hispanic families facing TBI are limited, and it is often difficult to reach these communities, in part because they are not well represented in the TBI community. Information about TBI also needs to be made more broadly accessible by addressing language barriers, for example.

Examples of Other Factors Associated with Disparities After TBI

A variety of other pre- and postinjury social determinants of health, including unemployment, housing insecurity, and lack of health insurance, have been associated with disparities in TBI care and outcomes. Other factors, such as criminal history or substance abuse, may be stigmatized and can serve as additional barriers to TBI care and rehabilitation.

Unemployment

Preinjury unemployment among persons with mild TBI has been associated with decreases in functional outcomes and increases in postconcussion symptom reporting, psy-

---

[13] Moore, M. 2021. Reducing disparities in traumatic brain injury. Presentation and panel discussion during virtual workshop on Accelerating Progress in Traumatic Brain Injury Research and Care, March 16, 2021.
[14] Ibid.

chiatric symptoms, and PTSD 6 months after injury (Yue et al., 2018), while unemployment in survivors of severe TBI has been associated with lower 1-year outcome scores and more severe 8-year dysexecutive problems (Ruet et al., 2019). Several studies have also explored the intersection of employment status with racial and ethnic differences. In a sample of 3,468 White and 1,761 Black, Hispanic, Asian, and Native American persons with moderate to severe TBI, odds of unemployment at 1-year follow-up were twice as high among non-White versus White persons (Arango-Lasprilla et al., 2008). Another study found that, after controlling for preinjury status, age, education, injury mechanism, rehabilitation length of stay, and disability rating at discharge, non-White compared with White persons had 3.59 times greater odds of being unemployed than stably employed, 1.91 times greater odds of being unstably employed than stably employed, and 1.88 times greater odds of being unemployed than unstably employed (Arango-Lasprilla et al., 2009).

Housing Insecurity

TBI is often an unrecognized condition in persons experiencing housing insecurity. A systematic review and meta-analysis by Stubbs and colleagues (2020) found that the lifetime prevalence of TBI of any severity in homeless and marginally housed individuals was approximately 53 percent.

Lack of Health Insurance

A recent review of disparities in health insurance coverage and utilization of health services among U.S. TBI survivors (Gao et al., 2018) found that lack of insurance was associated with decreased use of posthospital care. Concerns about losing eligibility or coverage for disability benefits or care provided through such programs as Medicaid may also serve as disincentives for people with TBI to return to work. A meta-analysis of the U.S. labor market from 1990 to 2018 found that expanded eligibility for disability benefits was associated with reduced employment (McHale et al., 2020).

Lessons and Recommendations from Recent National Academies Reports Addressing Equity in Health Care

Several recent National Academies studies and workshops have explored strategies for advancing equity in health care systems (NASEM, 2016b, 2019a,b,c, 2021a,b). Although not directed specifically at TBI, many of the reflections and recommendations emerging from these sources are potentially applicable to efforts to increase equity in systems of care for TBI and may be worthy of consideration by the TBI community. These reflections and recommendations span a range of areas, including improving workforce education and performance monitoring, building interdisciplinary care teams, increasing access to care, forging institutional partnerships beyond health systems, reforming payment systems, and leveraging digital health technology and implementation science (see Box 3-1).

In 2017, the National Quality Forum published *A Roadmap for Promoting Health Equity and Eliminating Disparities,* highlighting four pillars: (1) identify priority disparity areas, (2) implement evidence-based interventions to reduce disparity, (3) invest in health equity performance measures, and (4) incentivize the reduction of disparities (NQF, 2017). These four pillars can also serve as a guiding structure for the design and implementation of strategies for reducing the impact of structural barriers and providing more equitable access to TBI care for those populations currently underserved. Adopting an equity lens to shape such efforts

BOX 3-1 **ADVANCING EQUITY IN HEALTH CARE SYSTEMS: APPLYING REFLECTIONS AND RECOMMENDATIONS FROM NATIONAL ACADEMIES CONSENSUS STUDIES AND WORKSHOPS TO TBI**

The examples below reflect how selected recommendations from recent reports may be relevant to efforts to improve TBI care and research. Further multistakeholder efforts would be needed to explore or adapt these ideas further.

Improve Workforce Education and Performance Monitoring

- Educate TBI care providers on the impacts of diversity, equity, and inclusion on health care outcomes for their TBI patients, including the distinctions between equality and equity and privilege and oppression.[a]
- Provide cultural competency training for health care workers seeing TBI patients, including training in communication processes that reduce implicit bias.[b]
- Train providers to acknowledge the historical and current experiences of vulnerable populations that impact patient care[b] and to advocate for patients who need to address obstacles outside of health care that impact their health.[b]
- Train TBI clinicians in community settings (such as schools, workplaces, prisons, home health care, and public clinics) alongside nonphysician care providers.[c]
- Use diverse, team-based approaches to leadership development that include community health workers.[d]
- Establish incentives for TBI clinicians to receive training in how to communicate about serious conditions, such as TBI, to patients.[b]
- Teach and implement trauma-informed care practices so that TBI clinicians can address individual-, family-, and community-level trauma underlying disparities in risk factors for TBI and in health outcomes for TBI survivors.[b]
- Train TBI clinicians to deliver care that is consistent with patient preferences.[b]
- Stratify clinical performance measures by such factors as race/ethnicity, socioeconomic status, disability status, and serious illness status.[b]
- Conduct performance monitoring and quality improvement based on updated content of care.[d]
- Address organizational culture when implementing measures to improve care equity.[b]

Build Interdisciplinary Care Teams

- Promote integrated care systems, interdisciplinary care, whole-person care, family-centered care, and team-based care for people with TBI along with their caregivers and families.[b,d]
- Include nontraditional health care workers, such as community health workers and peer navigators, in health care teams. These individuals can serve as cultural bridges and advocates to help people with TBI navigate a complex health care system across the course of treatment.[b]
- Empower nurses and other nonphysician members of care teams to be bridge builders, collaborators, connectors, care coordinators, and patient/community advocates.[e]

Increase Access to Care

- Expand access to health care for people with TBI across the lifespan, including access to patient/family-centered care and preventive services.[b,d]
- Increase access points to make TBI care available closer to where people live, work, and enjoy recreation.[f]
- Encourage community health workers and places of worship to support advance care planning for people with TBI, a process that considers how a person's personal values, life goals, and preferences inform their medical care preferences.[b]

BOX 3-1 CONTINUED

- Recognize that clinical environments may feel uncomfortable or unsafe for TBI patients who have experienced trauma or had negative encounters with institutions and authorities (e.g., foster care, intimate partner violence, incarceration).[b]
- Ensure that people with TBI and with low English proficiency can communicate with providers.[b]
- Provide information on the relevant social services and public benefits for people with TBI in resource directories.[f]
- Expand transportation services and mobility, especially for people with disabilities.[f]

Forge Institutional Partnerships Beyond Health Systems

- Connect health care delivery systems to partners outside of health care, including government, civil society organizations, and implementation organizations.
- Connect health care delivery systems to expertise in other domains that contribute to health inequity, such as housing, employment, and education.[b,d,f]
- Partner with the people and institutions in the community where patients have daily interactions outside of health care systems.[b]
- Institutionalize equity in the infrastructure of organizations and their community partnerships.[d]

Reform Payment Systems

- Where appropriate, consider alternatives to the standard fee-for-service payment model in favor of performance-based payment models that reward clinicians for better patient outcomes.[d]
- Consider payment models that give health care organizations the flexibility to address patients' social needs and social determinants of health.[c]
- Address payment structures and incentives as an essential component of advancing equity; seek input from severely affected and vulnerable populations.[b]
- Design funding mechanisms to sustain data-driven equity programs that are working.[b]

Leverage Digital Health Technology and Implementation Science

- Expand the use of digital health technology,[c] electronic health records,[c] telehealth,[e] and virtual health assistants in TBI care. For example, these tools could be used to refer TBI patients to social services and public benefits via a technology platform that was two-way and integrated electronic health records.[f] Leverage implementation science when rolling out new interventions for TBI in health systems.[b]

[a] NASEM, 2016b.
[b] NASEM, 2019b.
[c] NASEM, 2021a.
[d] NASEM, 2019c.
[e] NASEM, 2021b.
[f] NASEM, 2019a.

will require awareness of assumptions that constrain the way people perceive, understand, and feel the world (NASEM, 2016b), ingrained viewpoints and expectations that must be changed to achieve a more inclusive perspective. In some contexts, health care inequity can be framed most effectively as a systemic and unsustainable issue of moral justice that affects all of society, not just particular minority groups, improvements in which will yield benefits for all. In other scenarios, it may be more appropriate to leverage a value-proposition argument for improving diversity, equity, and inclusion.

Lessons from Care Systems That Minimize Disparities

The early phases of assessment and acute management of TBI for military personnel and athletes on sports teams, such as those in the National Football League (NFL) and selected other professional sports leagues, provide lessons for minimizing the effect of disparities on immediate management at the site of injury, as well as on the quality and location of definitive emergency care.

Injuries to some of these individuals occur in the most dangerous, remote, and inaccessible places in the world. In battle zones where military service members are wounded, priority is given to mitigating the limitations of available health care capacity with evidence-based TBI protocols, extensive medical and nonmedical training, and timely evacuation and definitive care. Assessment, reporting, and rest protocols are an important component of early phases of TBI management for active duty service members.[15] TBI is considered a potential risk for all service members deployed to war zones, engaged in training, or participating in sports programs, as well as for athletes in high-risk professional and university sports programs.[16] As a consequence, potential TBIs in combat or on the playing field are treated aggressively, particularly given the attention to TBI resulting from the past two decades of war in Southwest Asia and increased focus on the long-term effects of concussions in athletics.

After acute TBI care, mid- and long-term management of the consequences of TBI is affected by access to and the nature of specialty care and institutional, community, and educational rehabilitation. In the management of sports-related concussion, such modifiable factors as early identification and follow-up with a specialist experienced in TBI are associated with faster recovery and improved outcomes (Desai et al., 2019; Kontos et al., 2020; Master et al., 2020). For military service members, a Transition and Care Management Program for Veterans who have served since the terrorist attacks of 9/11 extends comprehensive care into their transition to civilian life. The Department of Defense's (DoD's) military care system and the facilities and programs of the VA strive to ensure the availability of a system of care that encompasses prevention, early recognition and treatment of a potential TBI, and access to long-term rehabilitation.

Testimony during the committee's information-gathering sessions included examples

---

[15] DoD Instruction 6490.11, enacted in 2012 (DoD, 2019), provides policy guidance on management of concussion or "mild" TBI among deployed service members, and includes requirements for reporting, conduct of medical evaluations, and mandatory rest. For example, all service members must be assessed for a potential concussion after such circumstances as vehicle collisions or rollovers, exposure within 50 meters of an explosion, a blow to the head, or loss of consciousness. The military has also developed the Military Acute Concussion Evaluation-2 (MACE-2) screening tool (https://health.mil/Reference-Center/Publications/2020/07/30/Military-Acute-Concussion-Evaluation-MACE-2 [accessed August 24, 2021]).

[16] The consensus statement of the Concussion in Sport Group recommends that "In all suspected cases of concussion, the individual should be removed from the playing field and assessed by a physician or licensed healthcare provider" (CISG, 2017, p. 839). The group has developed a standardized Sport Concussion Assessment Tool, now in its fifth edition, to aid in rapid evaluation (https://bjsm.bmj.com/content/bjsports/early/2017/04/26/bjsports-2017-097506SCAT5.full.pdf [accessed August 24, 2021]).

of optimal management of health challenges with lifelong impacts. Optimal management of stroke, for example, relies on prompt recognition of its occurrence, rapid transport to a facility capable of performing appropriate brain imaging studies, and thrombolytic/hemostatic intervention (Powers et al., 2019). Failure to take these steps may result in early death or prolonged disability. Recovery and rehabilitation after stroke requires a multidisciplinary approach with active family and patient support and community engagement to achieve optimal function for the patient. BPSE factors also play important roles in achieving an optimal management scheme for pain care, and a comprehensive national program is currently under way aimed at combining the efforts of basic and clinical researchers, clinicians, community health and health care organizations, patient advocacy groups, and public and private funding sources to reduce the impact of these factors.[17]

Similarly, optimal management of Alzheimer's disease relies on prompt identification and multidisciplinary engagement (Bradley et al., 2015). These efforts may forestall the full impact of neurodegeneration and promote patient function, reduce family and community suffering, and lessen individual financial impacts and community economic costs as the disease progresses. As with stroke management, a multidisciplinary approach with active family and patient support, as well as community engagement, is needed to achieve optimal function for the patient and reduce long-term secondary and tertiary effects. The access of individual patients and their supportive families and friends to these collective services is a function of BPSE factors that are being addressed on a national scale.[18]

CONCLUSIONS

TBI needs to be viewed through the lens of a BPSE model. Outcomes from TBI are affected by factors beyond medical care, and TBI interacts strongly with other physical, psychological, and social conditions. Factors associated with disparities in TBI care and outcomes include geographic location, race and ethnicity, age, and gender, and current care and research systems do not function ideally for many patients and their families. A life-course approach to understanding and managing TBI is also required. A person who experiences TBI, of whatever initial severity, needs to be able to reengage with the health care system if new symptoms emerge or as needs change. These engagement points represent potential opportunities for intervention to refocus a patient's post-TBI pathway toward more optimal recovery and outcomes.

REFERENCES

Albrecht, J. S., J. M. Hirshon, M. McCunn, K. T. Bechtold, V. Rao, L. Simoni-Wastila, and G. S. Smith. 2016. Increased rates of mild traumatic brain injury among older adults in US emergency departments, 2009-2010. *Journal of Head Trauma Rehabilitation* 31(5):E1-E7.
Arango-Lasprilla, J. C., M. Rosenthal, J. Deluca, E. Komaroff, M. Sherer, D. Cifu, and R. Hanks. 2007a. Traumatic brain injury and functional outcomes: Does minority status matter? *Brain Injury* 21(7):701-708.

---

[17] See the VA program of team-based pain care, which draws on a biopsychosocial model of pain and uses a Stepped Care Model linking elements from self-care to care at specialized centers (https://www.va.gov/PAIN MANAGEMENT/Providers/IntegratedTeambasedPainCare.asp [accessed August 25, 2021]). In addition, the National Institutes of Health (NIH)-DoD-VA Pain Management Collaboratory involves multiple workgroups conducting 11 multisite pragmatic clinical trials (https://painmanagementcollaboratory.org [accessed August 24, 2021]).
[18] See, for example, the CDC website for information on the intersections of social determinants of health with Alzheimer's' disease (https://www.cdc.gov/aging/disparities/social-determinants-alzheimers.html [accessed August 24, 2021]). See also the Department of Health and Human Services' Healthy People 2030 initiative to improve health and well-being (https://health.gov/healthypeople [accessed August 24, 2021]).

Arango-Lasprilla, J. C., M. Rosenthal, J. DeLuca, D. Cifu, R. Hanks, and E. Komaroff. 2007b. Functional outcomes from inpatient rehabilitation after traumatic brain injury: How do Hispanics fare? *Archives of Physical Medicine and Rehabilitation* 88(1):1-18.

Arango-Lasprilla, J. C., J. Ketchum, K. Williams, J. Kreutzer, C. Marquez de la Plata, T. O'Neil-Pirozzi, and P. Wehman. 2008. Racial differences in employment outcomes after traumatic brain injury. *Archives of Phsyical Medicine and Rehabilitation* 89(5):988-995.

Arango-Lasprilla, J. C., J. Ketchum, K. Gary, J. Kreutzer, T. O'Neil-Pirozzi, P. Wehman, C. Marquez de la Plata, and A. Jha. 2009. The influence of minority status on job stability after traumatic brain injury. *Physical Medicine and Rehabilitation* 1(1):41-49.

Asemota, A., B. George, C. Cumpsty-Fowler, A. Haider, and E. Schneider. 2013. Race and insurance disparities in discharge to rehabilitation for patients with traumatic brain injury. *Journal of Neurotrauma* 30(24):2057-2065.

Bouldin, E. D., A. A. Swan, R. S. Norman, D. F. Tate, C. Tumminello, M. E. Amuan, B. C. Eapen, C. P. Wang, A. Trevino, and M. J. Pugh. 2021. Health phenotypes and neurobehavioral symptom severity among post-9/11 veterans with mild traumatic brain injury: A chronic effects of neurotrauma consortium study. *Journal of Head Trauma Rehabilitation* 36(1):10-19.

Bradley, P., R. Akehurst, C. Ballard, S. Banerjee, K. Blennow, J. Bremner, K. Broich, J. Cummings, K. Dening, B. Dubois, W. Klipper, C. Leibman, V. Mantua, J. L. Molinuevo, S. Morgan, L. A. Muscolo, F. Nicolas, L. Pani, L. Robinson, P. Siviero, J. van Dam, J. Van Emelen, A. Wimo, M. Wortmann, and L. Goh. (2015). Taking stock: A multistakeholder perspective on improving the delivery of care and the development of treatments for Alzheimer's disease. *Alzheimer's & Dementia* 11(4):455-461.

Brown, J. B., M. Kheng, N. A. Carney, A. M. Rubiano, and J. C. Puyana. 2019. Geographical disparity and traumatic brain injury in America: Rural areas suffer poorer outcomes. *Journal of Neurosciences in Rural Practice* 10(1):10-15.

Budnick, H., A. Tyroch, and S. Milan. 2017. Ethnic disparities in traumatic brain injury care referral in a Hispanic-majority population. *Journal of Surgical Research* 215:231-238.

Cifu, D. X., B. C. Taylor, W. Carne, D. Bidelspach, N. Sayer, J. Scholten, and E. Campbell. 2013. Traumatic brain injury, posttraumatic stress disorder, and pain diagnoses in OIF/OEF/OND veterans. *Journal of Rehabilitation Research and Development* 50(9):1169-1176.

CISG (Concussion in Sport Group). 2017. Consensus statement on concussion in sport—The 5th international conference on concussion in sport held in Berlin, October 2016. *British Journal of Sports Medicine* 51:838-847.

Cogan, A. M., V. K. McCaughey, and J. Scholten. 2020. Gender differences in outcomes after traumatic brain injury among service members and veterans. *PM&R: The Journal of Injury, Function, and Rehabilitation* 12(3):301-314.

da Silva Cardoso, E., M. Romero, F. Chan, A. Dutta, and M. Rahimi. 2007. Disparities in vocational rehabilitation services and outcomes for Hispanic clients with traumatic brain injury: Do they exist? *Journal of Head Trauma Rehabilitation* 22(2):85-94.

Dams-O'Connor, K., J. P. Cuthbert, J. Whyte, J. D. Corrigan, M. Faul, and C. Harrison-Felix. 2013a. Traumatic brain injury among older adults at level I and II trauma centers. *Journal of Neurotrauma* 30(24):2001-2013.

Dams-O'Connor, K., L. E. Gibbons, J. D. Bowen, S. M. McCurry, E. B. Larson, and P. K. Crane. 2013b. Risk for late-life re-injury, dementia and death among individuals with traumatic brain injury: A population-based study. *Journal of Neurology, Neurosurgery and Psychiatry* 84(2):177-182.

Dams-O'Connor, K., A. Landau, J. Hoffman, and J. St De Lore. 2018. Patient perspectives on quality and access to healthcare after brain injury. *Brain Injury* 32(4):431-441.

Daugherty, J., D. Waltzman, K. Sarmiento, and L. Xu. 2019. Traumatic brain injury-related deaths by race/ethnicity, sex, intent, and mechanism of injury—United States, 2000–2017. *Morbidity and Mortality Weekly Report* 68(46):1050-1056.

Desai, N., D. J. Wiebe, D. Corwin, J. Lockyer, M. Grady, and C. L. Master. 2019. Factors affecting recovery trajectories in pediatric female concussion. *Clinical Journal of Sport Medicine* 29(5):361-367.

DoD (Department of Defense). 2019. Instruction 6490.11. *DoD policy guidance for management of mild traumatic brain injury/concussion in the deployed setting.* September 8, 2012. Incorporating Change 2, effective November 26, 2019.

Engel, G. 1977. The need for a new medical model: a challenge for biomedicine. *Science* 196 (4286):129-136.

Esopenko, C., J. Meyer, E. Wilde, A. Marshall, D. Tate, A. Lin, I. Koerte, K., et al. 2021. A global collaboration to study intimate partner violence-related head trauma: The ENIGMA consortium IPV working group. *Brain Imaging and Behavior* 15(2):475-503.

Fabricius, A. M., A. D'Souza, V. Amodio, A. Colantonio, and T. Mollayeva. 2020. Women's gendered experiences of traumatic brain injury. *Qualitative Health Research* 30(7):1033-1044.

Ferguson, P. L., E. E. Pickelsimer, J. D. Corrigan, J. A. Bogner, and M. Wald. 2012. Prevalence of traumatic brain injury among prisoners in South Carolina. Journal of Head Trauma Rehabilitation 27(3):E11-E20.

Foster, M., and C. Tilse. 2003. Referral to rehabilitation following traumatic brain injury: A model for understanding inequities in access. *Social Science & Medicine* 56(10):2201-2210.

Gao, S., R. Kumar, S. Wisniewski, and A. Fabio. 2018. Disparities in health care utilization of adults with traumatic brain injuries are related to insurance, race and ethnicity: A systematic review. *Journal of Head Trauma Rehabilitation* 33(3):e40-e50.

Garcia, M. C., M. Faul, M., Massetti, G., Thomas, C. C., Hong, Y., Bauer, U. E., and M. F. Iademarco. 2017. Reducing potentially excess deaths from the five leading causes of death in the rural United States. *Morbidity and Mortality Weekly Report Surveillance Summaries* 66(2):1-7.

Gardner, R. C., K. Dams-O'Connor, M. R. Morrissey, and G. T. Manley. 2018. Geriatric traumatic brain injury: Epidemiology, outcomes, knowledge gaps, and future directions. *Journal of Neurotrauma* 35(7):889-906.

Gary, K. W., J. C. Arango-Lasprilla, and L. F. Stevens. 2009. Do racial/ethnic differences exist in post-injury outcomes after TBI? A comprehensive review of the literature. *Brain Injury* 23(10):775-789.

Gray, M., M. M. Adamson, R. C. Thompson, K. I. Kapphahn, S. Han, J. S. Chung, and O. A. Harris. 2020. Sex differences in symptom presentation and functional outcomes: a pilot study in a matched sample of veterans with mild TBI. *Brain Injury* 34(4):535-547.

Griesbach, G. S., B. E. Masel, R. E. Helvie, and M. J. Ashley. 2018. The impact of traumatic brain injury on later life: Effects on normal aging and neurodegenerative diseases. *Journal of Neurotrauma* 35(1):17-24.

Haarbauer-Krupa, J., A. Ciccia, J. Dodd, D. Ettel, B. Kurowski, A. Lumba-Brown, and S. Suskauer. 2017. Service delivery in the healthcare and educational systems for children following traumatic brain injury: Gaps in care. *Journal of Head Trauma Rehabilitation* 32(6):367-377.

Haarbauer-Krupa, J., A. H. Lee, R. H. Bitsko, X. Zhang, and M. J. Kresnow-Sedacca. 2018. Prevalence of parent-reported traumatic brain injury in children and associated health conditions. *JAMA Pediatrics* 172(11):1078-1086.

Haarbauer-Krupa, J., M. J. Pugh, E. M. Prager, N. Harmon, J. Wolfe, and K. C. Yaffe. 2021. Epidemiology of chronic effects of traumatic brain injury. *Journal of Neurotrauma* 8(23):3235-3247.

Haines, K., B. Nguyen, C. Vatsaas, A. Alger, K. Brooks, and S. Agarwal. 2019. Socioeconomic status affects outcomes after severity-stratified traumatic brain injury. *Journal of Surgical Research* 235:131-140.

Hart, T., J. Whyte, M. Polansky, G. Kersey-Matusiak, and R. Fidler-Sheppard. 2005. Community outcomes following traumatic brain injury: Impact of race and preinjury status. *Journal of Head Trauma Rehabilitation* 20(3):158-172.

Hoge, C. W., D. McGurk, J. Thomas, A. Cox, C. Engel, and C. Castro. 2008. Mild traumatic brain injury in U.S. Soldiers returning from Iraq. *New England Journal of Medicine* 358(5):453-463.

Hood, C. M., K. Gennuso, G. Swain, and B. Catlin. 2016. County health rankings: Relationships between determinant factors and health outcomes. *American Journal of Preventive Medicine* 50(2):129-135.

Howrey, B. T., J. E. Graham, M. R. Pappadis, C. V. Granger, and K. J. Ottenbacher. 2017. Trajectories of functional change after inpatient rehabilitation for traumatic brain injury. *Archives of Physical Medicine and Rehabilitation* 98(8):1606-1613.

Hsia, R. Y., A. J. Markowitz, F. Lin, J. Guo, D. Y. Madhok, and G. T. Manley. 2018. Ten-year trends in traumatic brain injury: A retrospective cohort study of California emergency department and hospital revisits and readmissions. *BMJ Open* 8(12):e022297.

IOM (Institute of Medicine). 2001. *Crossing the quality chasm: A new health system for the 21st century.* Washington, DC: National Academy Press.

Iverson, K. M., A. M. Hendricks, R. Kimerling, M. Krengel, M. Meterko, K. L. Stolzmann, E. Baker, T. K. Pogoda, J. J. Vasterling, and H. L. Lew. 2011. Psychiatric diagnoses and neurobehavioral symptom severity among OEF/OIF VA patients with deployment-related traumatic brain injury: A gender comparison. *Women's Health Issues* 21(4 Suppl):S210-S217.

Johnstone, B., T. Price, T. Bounds, L. Schopp, M. Schootman, and D. Schumate. 2003. Rural/urban differences in vocational outcomes for state vocational rehabilitation clients with TBI. *NeuroRehabilitation* 18(3):197-203.

Kane, W. G., D. A. Wright, R. Fu, and K. F. Carlson. 2014. Racial/ethnic and insurance status disparities in discharge to posthospitalization care for patients with traumatic brain injury. *Journal of Head Trauma Rehabilitation* 29(6):E10-E17.

Karb, R. A., S. V. Subramanian, and E. W. Fleegler. 2016. County poverty concentration and disparities in unintentional injury deaths: A fourteen-year analysis of 1.6 million U.S. fatalities. *PloS One* 11(5):e0153516.

Karriker-Jaffe, K. J., J. Witbrodt, A. Mericle, D. Polcin, and L. A. Kaskutas. 2020. Testing a socioecological model of relapse and recovery from alcohol problems. *Substance Abuse: Research and Treatment* 14:1178221820933631.

Kim, L. H., J. Quon, F. Sun, K. Wortman, M. Adamson, and O. Harris. 2018. Traumatic brain injury among female veterans: A review of sex differences in military neurosurgery. *Neurosurgical Focus* 45(6):E16.

Kontos, A. P., K. Jorgensen-Wagers, A. M. Trbovich, N. Ernst, K. Emami, B. Gillie, J. French, C. Holland, R. Elbin, and M. Collins. 2020. Association of time since injury to the first clinic visit with recovery following concussion. *JAMA Neurology* 77(4):435-440.

Langlois, J. A., W. Rutland-Brown, and K. E. Thomas. 2005. The incidence of traumatic brain injury among children in the United States: Differences by race. *Journal of Head Trauma Rehabilitation* 20(3):229-238.

Li, W., S. L. Risacher, T. W. McAllister, and A. J. Saykin. 2016. Traumatic brain injury and age at onset of cognitive impairment in older adults. *Journal of Neurology* 263(7):1280-1285.

Livingston, D. H., R. F. Lavery, A. C. Mosenthal, M. M. Knudson, S. Lee, D. Morabito, G. T. Manley, A. Nathens, G. Jurkovich, D. B. Hoyt, and R. Coimbra. 2005. Recovery at one year following isolated traumatic brain injury: A western trauma association prospective multicenter trial. *Journal of Trauma and Acute Care Surgery* 59(6):1298-1304; discussion 1304.

Marquez de la Plata, C. D., T. Hart, F. M. Hammond, A. B. Frol, A. Hudak, C. R. Harper, T. M. O'Neil-Pirozzi, J. Whyte, M. Carlile, and R. Diaz-Arrastia. 2008. Impact of age on long-term recovery from traumatic brain injury. *Archives of Physical Medicine and Rehabilitation* 89(5):896-903.

Master, C. L., B. Katz, K. Arbogast, M. McCrea, T. McAllister, P. Pasquina, M. Lapradd, W. Zhou, S. Broglio, and CARE Consortium Investigators. 2020. Differences in sport-related concussion for female and male athletes in comparable collegiate sports: A study from the NCAA-DoD Concussion Assessment, Research and Education (CARE) Consortium. *British Journal of Sports Medicine* 55(24):1387-1394.

Master, C. L., B. P. Katz, K. B. Arbogast, M. A. McCrea, T. W. McAllister, P. F. Pasquina, M. Lapradd, W. Zhou, S. P. Broglio, and CARE Consortium Investigators. 2021. Differences in sport-related concussion for female and male athletes in comparable collegiate sports: a study from the NCAA-DoD Concussion Assessment, Research and Education (CARE) Consortium. *British Journal of Sports Medicine* 55:1387-1394.

McHale, P., A. Pennington, C. Mustard, Q. Mahood, I. Andersen, N. K. Jensen, B. Burström, K. Thielen, L. Harber-Aschan, A. McAllister, M. Whitehead, and B. Barr. 2020. What is the effect of changing eligibility criteria for disability benefits on employment? A systematic review and meta-analysis of evidence from OECD countries. *PloS One* 15(12):e0242976.

McQuistion, K., Zens, T., Jung, H. S., Beems, M., Leverson, G., Liepert, A., Scarborough, J., and S. Agarwal. 2016. Insurance status and race affect treatment and outcome of traumatic brain injury. *Journal of Surgical Research* 205(2):261-271.

Meagher, A., C. Beadles, J. Doorey, and A. Charles. 2015. Racial and ethnic disparities in discharge to rehabilitation following traumatic brain injury. *Journal of Neurosurgery* 122:599-601.

Moore, M., G. Robinson, R. Mink, K. Hudson, D. Dotolo, T. Gooding, A. Ramirez, D. Zatzick, J. Giordano, D. Crawley, and M. S. Vavilala. 2015. Developing a family-centered care model for critical care after pediatric traumatic brain injury. *Pediatric Critical Care Medicine* 16(8):758-765.

Moore, M., K. M. Conrick, M. Fuentes, A. Rowhani-Rahbar, J. Graves, D. Patil, M. Herrenkohl, B. Mills, F. Rivara, B. Ebel, and M. S. Vavilala. 2019. Research on injury disparities: A scoping review. *Health Equity* 3(1):504-511.

MRC CRASH Trial Collaborators, P. Perel, M. Arango, T. Clayton, P. Edwards, E. Komolafe, S. Poccock, I. Roberts, H. Shakur, E. Steyerberg, and S. Yutthakasemsunt. 2008. Predicting outcome after traumatic brain injury: Practical prognostic models based on large cohort of international patients. *British Medical Journal* 336(7641):425-429.

NASEM (National Academies of Sciences, Engineering, and Medicine). 2016a. *A national trauma care system: Integrating military and civilian trauma systems to achieve zero preventable deaths after injury.* Washington, DC: The National Academies Press.

NASEM. 2016b. *Framing the dialogue on race and ethnicity to advance health equity.* Washington, DC: The National Academies Press.

NASEM. 2017. *Communities in action, pathways to health equity.* Washington, DC: The National Academies Press.

NASEM 2019a. *Health-focused public-private partnerships in the urban context.* Washington, DC: The National Academies Press.

NASEM. 2019b. *Improving access to and equity of care for people with serious illness.* Washington, DC: The National Academies Press.

NASEM. 2019c. *Vibrant and healthy kids: Aligning science, practice, and policy to advance health equity.* Washington, DC: The National Academies Press.

NASEM. 2021a. *Implementing high-quality primary care: Rebuilding the foundation of health care.* Washington, DC: The National Academies Press.

NASEM. 2021b. *The future of nursing 2020–2030: Charting a path to achieve health equity.* Washington, DC: The National Academies Press.

NINDS (National Institute of Neurological Disorders and Stroke). 2017. *Workshop summary: Understanding traumatic brain injury in women.* https://www.ninds.nih.gov/sites/default/files/tbi_workshop_summary_-_december_18-19_2017_508c_0.pdf (accessed September 27, 2021).

NQF (National Quality Forum). 2017. *A roadmap for promoting health equity and eliminating disparities: The four I's for health equity.* https://www.qualityforum.org/Publications/2017/09/A_Roadmap_for_Promoting_Health_Equity_and_Eliminating_Disparities__The_Four_I_s_for_Health_Equity.aspx (accessed September 27, 2021).

NRC and IOM (National Research Council and Institute of Medicine). 2013. *U.S. health in international perspective: Shorter lives, poorer health.* Washington, DC: The National Academies Press.

Odonkor, C., R. Esparza, L. Flores, M. Verduzco-Gutierrez, M. Escalon, R. Solinski, and J. Silver. 2021. Disparities in health care for black patients in physical medicine and rehabilitation in the United States: A narrative review. *Physical Medicine and Rehabilitation* 13(2):180-203.

Piatt, J. 2021. Racial disparities in mortality after severe traumatic brain injury in childhood: Mediators identified by Oaxaca-Blinder decomposition of trauma registry data. *Injury Epidemiology* 8(1):1.

Powers, W. J., A. Rabinstein, T. Ackerson, O. Adeoye, N. Bambakidis, K. Becker, J. Biller, M. Brown, B. Demaerschalk, B. Hoh, E. Jauch, C. Kidwell, T. Leslie-Mazwi, B. Ovbiagele, P. Scott, K. Sheth, A. Southerland, D. Summers, and D. L. Tirschwell. 2019. Guidelines for the early management of patients with acute ischemic stroke: 2019 update to the 2018 Guidelines for the Early Management of Acute Ischemic Stroke: A Guideline for Healthcare Professionals From the American Heart Association/American Stroke Association. *Stroke* 50(12):e344-e418.

Pugh, M. J., A. A. Swan, M. E. Amuan, B. C. Eapen, C. A. Jaramillo, R. Delgado, D. F. Tate, K. Yaffe, and C. P. Wang. 2019. Deployment, suicide, and overdose among comorbidity phenotypes following mild traumatic brain injury: A retrospective cohort study from the chronic effects of neurotrauma consortium. *PLoS One* 14(9):e0222674

Register-Mihalik, J. K., and C. E. Callahan. 2020. Postconcussion exertion evolution: Clinical and behavioral considerations. *Current Sports Medicine Reports* 19(4):151-156.

Ruet, A., E. Bayen, C. Jourdan, I. Ghout, L. Meaude, A. Lalanne, P. Pradat-Diehl, G. Nelson, J. Charanton, P. Aegerter, C. Vallat-Azouvi, and P. Azouvi. 2019. A detailed overview of long-term outcomes in severe traumatic brain injury eight years post-injury. *Frontiers in Neurology* 10.120. https://doi.org/10.3389/fneur.2019.00120.

Schiraldi, M., C. Patil, D. Mukherjee, B. Ugiliweneza, M. Nuño, S. Lad, and M. Boakye. 2015. Effect of insurance and racial disparities on outcomes in traumatic brain injury. *Journal of Neurological Surgery* 76(3):224-232.

Stippler, M., E. Holguin, and E. Nemoto. 2012. Traumatic brain injury in elders. *Annals of Long-Term Care: Clinical Care and Aging* 20(5):1-7.

Stubbs, J., A. Thornton, J. Sevick, N. Silverberg, A. Barr, W. Honer, and W. Panenka. 2020. Traumatic brain injury in homeless and marginally housed individuals: A systematic review and meta-analysis. *Lancet Public Health* 5(1):e19-e32.

Susman, M., S. M. DiRusso, T. Sullivan, D. Risucci, P. Nealon, S. Cuff, A. Haider, and D. Benzil. 2002. Traumatic brain injury in the elderly: Increased mortality and worse functional outcome at discharge despite lower injury severity. *Journal of Trauma and Acute Care Surgery* 53(2):219-223; discussion 223-224.

Tanielian, T., L. Jaycox, and D. M. Adamson. 2008. *Invisible wounds of war.* Santa Monica, CA: RAND Corporation.

Thompson, H. J., W. C. McCormick, and S. H. Kagan. 2006. Traumatic brain injury in older adults: Epidemiology, outcomes, and future implications. *Journal of the American Geriatrics Society* 54(10):1590-1595.

Tiesman, H., T. Young, J. C. Torner, M. McMahon, C. Peek-Asa, and J. Fiedler. 2007. Effects of a rural trauma system on traumatic brain injuries. *Journal of Neurotrauma* 24(7):1189-1197.

van Erp, R., I. Huijnen, M. Jakobs, J. Kleijnen, and R. Smeets. 2019. Effectiveness of primary care interventions using a biopsychosocial approach in chronic low back pain: A systematic review. *Pain Practice* 19(2):224-241.

Yue, J. K., J. W. Rick, M. R. Morrissey, S. R. Taylor, H. Deng, C. G. Suen, M. J. Vassar, M. C. Cnossen, H. F. Lingsma, E. L. Yuh, P. Mukherjee, R. C. Gardner, A. B. Valadka, D. O. Okonkwo, T. A. Cage, G. T. Manley, and TRACK-TBI Investigators. 2018. Preinjury employment status as a risk factor for symptomatology and disability in mild traumatic brain injury: A TRACK-TBI analysis. *NeuroRehabilitation* 43(2):169-182.

Yue, J. K., P. Upadhyayula, L. Avalos, and T. A. Cage. 2020. Rural-urban disparities and considerations. *Brain Sciences* 10(3):135.

4

Traumatic Brain Injury Prevention and Awareness

Chapter Highlights

- Prevention strategies aim to reduce the number and severity of traumatic brain injuries (TBIs) that occur. Effectively reducing the risk of injury minimizes the number of people who will need treatment after an injury occurs, reducing the burden of TBI for individuals, their families, and society.
- Despite its frequency, misunderstanding about TBI and its potential consequences remains common, demonstrating the need to increase awareness and knowledge.

This chapter focuses on the importance of preventing traumatic brain injury (TBI) from occurring through analysis of risk factors and the development and implementation of prevention strategies. It also addresses misconceptions about TBI among those who experience it and their families, health professionals, members of the public, and other groups and the need for greater awareness and education to support effective prevention and treatment.

THE ROLE OF PREVENTION

The statement of task for this study (Box 1-3 in Chapter 1) did not explicitly include producing a review of or recommendations for the prevention of TBI. Nonetheless, prevention is an integral part of the landscape of TBI, and any systematic approach to improving TBI care and research needs to address the full continuum from prevention through longer-term care needs and recovery.

The importance and leverage of prevention are great enough that omitting it from consideration entirely would be inappropriate. Effective prevention of injury would dwarf the effectiveness of even an optimal system of acute and long-term TBI care for two simple and obvious reasons. First, an uninjured brain is at least as good as an injured and repaired one, often better. Second, despite decades of important progress in understanding the mechanics, biology, and neurology of TBI, dramatically effective treatments to "cure" TBI remain undiscovered. Instead, available treatments focus on addressing symptoms after injury and on implementing rehabilitation interventions to slow, stop, or help reverse impairments. Patients deserve the best science can offer, but even the best-known TBI treatments to date are not completely restorative; rather, they are supportive and rehabilitative, and buy time for natural healing processes to play out. In short, prevention "works" far better than treatment given the current level of knowledge.

Both theory (such as the Haddon Matrix, described below) and evidence exist regarding the effectiveness of many prevention strategies, such as use of protective equipment, prevention of falls, improved engineering and infrastructure designs, and incentive-oriented policies. Given effective prevention tactics, it is almost certainly less costly at a population level and from a societal perspective to reduce the risk of injury than to treat injury and pay for its downstream consequences.

The types of effort needed to improve treatment and to improve prevention overlap. For example, reducing public and professional misunderstanding of the burden and profile of TBI can increase both proper detection of these injuries and interest in their prevention. Thus, a key to prevention of TBI is to increase public and professional understanding of its nature and consequences and the fact that it can and does occur, and actions can be taken to help avoid it. Such understanding can in turn build will for making the necessary investments in risk mitigation. Moreover, that same understanding can aid in proper identification and management of TBI after it occurs and help avoid costly misclassification of and misperceptions about these injuries. On the high school sports field, for example, a community's commitment to protecting players from injury through use of proper equipment, management of field conditions, and adherence to rules probably draws on the same base of awareness as the commitment to identifying injuries early, removing injured players from further hazard, and recognizing subtle behavioral and physical symptoms for what they may be—consequences of TBI.

In important ways, then, the committee's statement of task calls attention to social, educational, and psychological factors that are as important for prevention of TBI as they are for its proper management. At a deep level, the bio-psycho-socio-ecological lens that this report urges for TBI care and research (see Chapter 3) applies equally to the prevention of TBI in the first place, warranting this chapter's brief review of some of the current science and evidence around TBI prevention.

The Haddon Matrix as a Framework for Injury Prevention

The Haddon Matrix is a widely used model for systematically identifying the factors that contribute to an injury to inform prevention (Haddon, 1980). The three rows of the matrix show different phases—preevent, event, and postevent—while the columns reflect influencing factors related to the person who experiences the injury, the agent that causes the injury, and the physical and social/economic environments in which the injury occurs. Table 4-1 shows one representative example of how the Haddon Matrix has been applied, in this case to brain injuries sustained during baseball and softball. As the table illustrates, the Haddon Matrix is a tool for identifying how and where one could intervene to prevent injuries and mitigate their effects. The matrix supports targeting of precursors that can prevent an injury from occurring in the first place and can thus decrease the number of people who need postinjury care.

TABLE 4-1 Example of Application of the Haddon Matrix: Brain Injuries Sustained during Baseball and Softball

Phase	Person	Agent	Physical Environment	Social/Economic Environment
Preinjury	• Velocity of pitch • Attitude of athlete (aggressive, competitive) • Athlete age and sex • Athlete strength	• Hardness/density of ball and bat • Inadequate protective gear • Design and type of helmet	• Maintenance of the field/grounds • Weather/time of year • Formal/informal setting	• Public perception of wearing protective gear • Costs of protective gear
Injury	• Unaware of the potential dangers of equipment (i.e., ball, bat) • Lack of supervision of younger athletes • Lack of education of children	• Hardness of the ball/bat • Association of bat and ball exit velocity	• Surface hardness • Obstacles on the field • Personal protective equipment	• Enforcement of rules and laws • Enforcement of protective gear use
Postinjury	• Knowledge to report symptoms • Compliance with return-to-play guidelines	• Engineering—improved helmet, bat, and ball design	• Access to a hospital or trauma center	• Expense/cost of medical system • Evaluation of surveillance systems • Insurance rates, fines • Social support • Community response to TBI

Source: Adapted from Cusimano and Zhu, 2017.

Selected Prevention Strategies Relevant to TBI

As detailed in Chapter 2, falls are the leading cause of hospitalization for TBI in the United States (almost 50 percent of cases of people with TBI). In 2017, falls caused roughly three-quarters of TBI-related hospitalizations and were the leading cause of TBI-related deaths among adults aged 65 and older (CDC, 2021). Intentional self-harm was the most common mechanism of TBI-related death among all adults over age 17 in 2016 and 2017, accounting for roughly a third of cases. Other leading causes of TBI hospitalization and TBI-related death in those years included motor vehicle crashes and assaults (CDC, 2021), the latter including such circumstances as fights, child maltreatment, intimate partner violence, and elder abuse. The Centers for Disease Control and Prevention's (CDC's) 2016 and 2017 surveillance data do not include TBI-related emergency department (ED) visits. However, approximately 2.5 million such visits were reported in 2014. Being struck by or against an object or person, including sports-related injuries, accounted for approximately 17 percent of these visits and were the second leading cause among children aged 0–17, after unintentional falls (CDC, 2019).

Extensive research has focused on the development of prevention strategies targeting common causes of TBI and how to reduce the likelihood of these injuries by changing factors in the three categories of the Haddon Matrix (person, agent, and physical and social/economic environments). Selected examples of prevention strategies relevant to TBI are highlighted in Table 4-2.

TABLE 4-2 Examples of Prevention Strategies for Common Causes of TBI in At-Risk Populations

At-Risk Population	Cause of TBI	Prevention Strategies
Children, aged 0–14 years	Falls	• Supervise children playing on or near fall hazards. • Place guards, gates, and screens around windows and stairs.
Older adults, aged 65 and up	Falls	• Improve home safety to reduce trip hazards, such as by using antislip rugs, in-home lighting, and grab bars along staircases. • Discuss fall risk and prevention with a health care provider. • Participate in exercises that improve balance, strength, coordination, and gait (e.g., Tai Chi).
Teens and young adults	Motor vehicle collisions	• Wear a seat belt, no matter how short the ride. • Wear a helmet when riding motorcycles, scooters, and bicycles. • Never drive while impaired. • Obey traffic laws, and exercise caution when driving in bad weather. • Enact and enforce laws related to impaired and distracted driving and other traffic safety issues. • Continue to develop advances in automobile engineering, such as antilock brakes and airbags.
	Sports and recreational activity injuries	• Adhere to safe play, and model a safe sports culture. • Wear well-maintained and properly fitting protective equipment, particularly helmets, for the activity. • Avoid hits to the head to the extent possible. • Implement rule changes (such as those limiting body checking or ball heading).

SOURCES: Adapted from CDC and NHTSA resources (all accessed October 13, 2021):
• Biomechanics and Trauma, https://www.nhtsa.gov/research-data/biomechanics-trauma.
• Traumatic Brain Injury & Concussion: Prevention, https://www.cdc.gov/traumaticbraininjury/prevention.html.
• Injury Prevention & Control: Let's Prevent Traumatic Brain Injury, https://www.cdc.gov/injury/features/traumatic-brain-injury/index.html.
• HEADS UP: Brain Injury Safety Tips and Prevention, https://www.cdc.gov/headsup/basics/concussion_prevention.html.
• Home and Recreational Safety: Important Facts About Falls, https://www.cdc.gov/homeandrecreationalsafety/falls/adultfalls.html.
• Protect the Ones You Love: Child Injuries Are Preventable: Fall Prevention, https://www.cdc.gov/safechild/falls/index.html.
• Transportation Safety, https://www.cdc.gov/transportationsafety.

Awareness-raising and information campaigns aimed at promoting these interventions include CDC's "Stopping Elderly Accidents, Injuries, and Deaths" (STEADI) and "HEADS UP" efforts focused on youth sports injuries.[1] The ThinkFirst National Injury Prevention Foundation has also been a leader in education and awareness to prevent traumatic injuries, operating programs for children, teens, young adults, and older adults on actions to reduce risk.[2] And professional societies and sports associations have issued statements in support of prevention efforts and produced materials and toolkits.[3]

Maas and colleagues (2017) discuss a number of population-based and targeted prevention strategies that may reduce the occurrence of TBI. Strategies for preventing TBIs caused

---

[1] For information on STEADI, see https://www.cdc.gov/steadi/index.html (accessed September 9, 2021). For information on HEADS UP, see https://www.cdc.gov/headsup/index.html (accessed September 9, 2021).

[2] See https://www.thinkfirst.org (accessed November 1, 2021).

[3] As just two examples, see the 2019 "Statement on Older Adult Falls and Falls Prevention" by the American College of Surgeons Committee on Trauma (https://www.facs.org/about-acs/statements/119-older-falls [accessed September 9, 2021]) and Sports Concussion Resources, produced by the American Academy of Neurology, including materials created in collaboration with the NFL Players Association (https://www.aan.com/concussion [accessed September 9, 2021]).

by falls include improved in-home lighting, use of stair handrails, and assessments of balance and gait in older persons. Strategies for preventing TBIs caused by traffic accidents and collisions include protected bicycle lanes, helmets for cyclists, seat belt wearing for car passengers, and hands-free phone use to reduce distracted driving. In sports and recreation, the risk of TBI can be reduced when participants use appropriate protective gear, especially helmets, and safe competitive play is enforced. In addition, participants who experience a blow to the head should be evaluated for signs of a concussion before returning to play.

A variety of interventions aimed at reducing falls and related injuries have been found effective (Stevens, 2010), and such interventions have the potential to be cost-effective in reducing health care expenditures (Carande-Kulis et al., 2015; Stevens and Lee, 2018).[4] Likewise, widespread use of and improvements in helmet design have been shown to reduce severe TBI and mortality. Bicycle helmets reduce the risk of severe TBI by nearly 70 percent (Olivier and Creighton, 2017), while use of helmets reduces the risk of TBI in motorcycle crashes by 69 percent (Liu et al., 2008). With respect to TBI-related deaths due to motor vehicle crashes, CDC (2013) reported an approximately 40 percent decrease, due in part to safety regulations and efforts around such issues as seat belt, helmet, and alcohol use and advances in auto engineering. For military service members, helmets can protect against penetrating head wounds from ballistic weapons. At the same time, it is important to recognize that helmet wearing may mitigate risk but not fully protect against the types of forces that can cause concussion, highlighting the continued importance of engineering advances to improve helmet efficacy in such situations as concussion and blast injuries (NASEM, 2014; Op't Eynde et al., 2020; Sone et al., 2017).

AWARENESS AND MISUNDERSTANDING OF TBI

Failure to understand the nature of TBI can undermine efforts to prevent and treat it effectively. Misunderstanding, inaccurate information, and lack of awareness about TBI can have a host of deleterious effects on people with TBI during their treatment, rehabilitation, and reintegration into the community. People who experience these injuries may not receive support and accommodations that can support their recovery process, and many TBI survivors face stigmatization and discrimination from the general public, educators, providers of social and community services, and health professionals that can further hamper their recovery. Misunderstanding among survivors themselves and their families and caretakers can lead to feelings of frustration and inadequacy that can worsen treatment outcomes (Gurusamy et al., 2019). Misunderstanding can also undermine efforts to prevent the occurrence of TBI. For instance, a common misbelief is that seat belts cause as many brain injuries as they prevent (Springer et al., 1997).

A substantial body of evidence reveals that misunderstanding, inaccurate information, and lack of awareness about brain injury are common among patients and families, the public, educators, student athletes, health professionals without expertise in brain injury, and other groups. Qualitative interview-based studies, as well as survey-based studies, have assessed knowledge and attitudes about TBI across different groups, nearly all of which reported inaccurate views about various facets of TBI. The "Common Misconceptions about Traumatic Brain Injury" (CM-TBI) 40-item questionnaire developed by Springer and colleagues (1997) has been used across the United States and in other countries to survey respondents' understanding of TBI. Some of the most commonly held false beliefs about TBI reported in the literature are listed in Box 4-1.

---

[4] CDC is supporting analysis of the implementation and cost-effectiveness of its STEADI initiative. See https://www.norc.org/Research/Projects/Pages/evaluating-the-cost-effectiveness-of-steadi-older-adult-fall-prevention-in-primary-care-settings.aspx (accessed September 24, 2021).

BOX 4-1   COMMON MISCONCEPTIONS ABOUT TBI

- A TBI cannot cause brain damage unless the person is knocked unconscious.
- Whiplash injuries to the neck cannot cause brain damage.
- Wearing seat belts causes as many brain injuries as it prevents.
- People with brain damage look obviously different from people without brain damage.
- It is uncommon for a person with brain injury to have a change in personality, to be irritable or easily angered, or to feel depressed or hopeless.
- It is not common for people with brain damage to have problems with speech or walking.
- When a person with brain injury can walk again, his/her brain is almost fully recovered.
- A second blow to the head can help people remember things they had forgotten.
- How quickly people recover from TBI depends on how hard they work at it.
- Most people who are knocked unconscious wake up quickly and have no lasting effects.
- After a TBI, people can forget who they are and not recognize others, but be perfect in every other way.
- A person with a brain injury will be "just like new" in a few months.
- People who have one brain injury are not more likely to have a second.

SOURCE: Adapted excerpts from Springer et al., 1997.

Swift and Wilson (2001) interviewed TBI patients, caregivers, and health professionals and identified several major themes. For example, inaccurate beliefs about the recovery time for brain injuries and the possible extent of recovery were prevalent. Respondents showed a lack of awareness of the range of cognitive and behavioral sequelae associated with brain injuries. Furthermore, people living with brain injury reported encountering misunderstandings about their capabilities often associated with the visibility or invisibility of their injury, including their being misidentified as mentally ill or learning disabled. In another qualitative study, TBI patients reported perceiving a lack of knowledge about TBI among the health professionals they encountered during their care (Dams-O'Connor et al., 2018). For example, certain cognitive and behavioral sequelae of TBI—such as disinhibition and risk-taking behaviors—can contribute to a higher likelihood of substance misuse (Brown and Harr, 2019). Accordingly, TBI patients with a substance misuse disorder benefit from individualized treatment that takes into account the convergence of neurobehavioral factors underlying such symptoms as aggression, low motivation, and cognitive deficits, including difficulty with comprehension and problem solving. However, many professionals providing addiction treatment have gaps in their training that can impede their ability to address these challenges effectively.

Although the public appears to be increasingly aware of the consequences of brain injuries, a qualitative study found that members of the general public still tended to characterize survivors of brain injury using such negative descriptors as aggressive, dependent, and unhappy (Linden and Boylan, 2010). The apparent etiology of a person's brain injury can also affect the public's attitudes. One study found that stigmatization and negative attitudes were more common if the person's behavior was perceived as contributing to the injury—for instance, when the injury was due to a fight rather than a car crash (Redpath and Linden, 2004). These public attitudes about TBI underlie some of the challenges faced by survivors as they seek to reintegrate into their community. A seminal systematic review evaluated 20 studies investigating the public's knowledge and attitudes about brain injury, finding that survivors tended to be vulnerable to discrimination and stigma (Ralph and Derbyshire, 2013). Misconceptions about survivors' postinjury symptoms, recovery, memory issues, and vulnerability to subsequent brain injury were common. This study also echoed the finding that public attitudes were more negative toward survivors who were perceived as being responsible for their brain injuries. The authors highlight the need for government and media campaigns to educate the public about brain injury and encourage greater inclusiveness for survivors in society.

Certain racial, ethnic, cultural, and socioeconomic factors have been associated with a greater likelihood of holding mistaken beliefs about TBI, and thus need to be considered when developing educational interventions. For instance, a survey conducted in the United States found that being born outside the United States, being Spanish speaking, having lower educational status, and actively practicing religion were associated with reporting a greater number of TBI misconceptions on the CM-TBI (Pappadis et al., 2011). A single-session educational intervention designed to increase knowledge about TBI among Black and Latinx patients has shown promise in decreasing misconceptions about the recovery process, common symptoms, and strategies for dealing with symptoms (Pappadis et al., 2017).

Despite the prevalence of TBI among children aged <18 years—estimated to include 812,000 TBI-related ED visits, 23,075 hospitalizations, and 2,529 deaths in the United States in 2014 (CDC 2019)—studies conducted in the United States and abroad have found that educators lack knowledge about TBI and may endorse mistaken beliefs about the condition (Ettel et al., 2016; Farmer and Johnson-Gerard, 1997; Hux et al., 1996; Linden et al., 2013). A survey of K–12 educators' knowledge about TBI found that they demonstrated a "reasonable" understanding of its symptoms and immediate effects (McKinlay and Buck, 2019). However, misunderstandings were common about the emotional, cognitive, and social sequelae, as well as the heightened risk of subsequent injuries. Another survey of educators found that those who had previously taught a child with brain injury had greater knowledge about the condition (Linden et al., 2013). The results of a survey of U.S. youth athletes and their parents indicated that they had a high level of awareness about concussion (Bloodgood et al., 2013), although another study among U.S. high school athletes found that fewer than half of their concussion events had been appropriately reported to a supervising adult (Register-Mihalik et al., 2013). Moreover, fewer than 18 percent of children who sustain a long-term injury due to TBI are referred for special education services, even though it has been considered a special education disability category since the 1990s in the United States (Ettel et al., 2016). Gaps in knowledge about TBI among educators—particularly general educators and speech-language pathologists—have likely contributed to the underidentification of students with TBI, leaving many of them with academic and behavioral needs that are unmet by the education system. These findings suggest that preservice training and professional development for educators about pediatric brain injuries could improve their ability to support the educational needs of students with TBI (McKinlay and Buck, 2019).

CONCLUSIONS

Prevention strategies to decrease the risks of TBI are integral to any system for advancing TBI care and research. Prevention efforts also can increase public and professional understanding of the nature and consequences of this condition. However, the studies cited in this chapter and elsewhere in this report provide evidence of a lack of awareness and understanding about brain injury among many of the people encountered by a person with TBI along the recovery pathway, from acute care, to rehabilitation, to reintegration into the community, highlighting the need for further evidence-informed efforts to

- increase public awareness about the symptoms and longer-term consequences of TBI through educational interventions and campaigns;
- inform the design of accommodations to support survivors of TBI as they reintegrate into their community environments—schools, workplaces, and interactions in the health care system with providers who are lacking expertise in TBI; and
- strengthen TBI prevention efforts by dispelling myths and misunderstandings about how TBI occurs and the consequences of a brain injury of any degree of severity.

REFERENCES

Bloodgood, B., D. Inokuchi, W. Shawver, K. Olson, R. Hoffman, E. Cohen, K. Sarmiento, and K. Muthuswamy. 2013. Exploration of awareness, knowledge, and perceptions of traumatic brain injury among American youth athletes and their parents. *Journal of Adolescent Health* 53(1):34-39.

Brown, J., and D. Harr. 2019. Perceptions of traumatic brain injury (TBI) among professionals providing drug and alcohol addiction treatment. *Journal of Neurology & Neuromedicine* 4(3).

Carande-Kulis V., J. A. Stevens, C. S. Florence, B. L. Beattie, and I. Arias. 2015. A cost-benefit analysis of three older adult fall prevention interventions. *Journal of Safety Research* 52:65-70.

CDC (Centers for Disease Control and Prevention). 2013. CDC grand rounds: Reducing severe traumatic brain injury in the United States. *Morbidity and Mortality Weekly Report* 62(27):549-552.

CDC. 2019. *Surveillance report of traumatic brain injury-related emergency department visits, hospitalizations, and deaths—United States, 2014*. Atlanta, GA: Department of Health and Human Services.

CDC. 2021. *Surveillance report of traumatic brain injury-related hospitalizations and deaths by age group, sex, and mechanism of injury—United States, 2016 and 2017*. Atlanta, GA: Department of Health and Human Services.

Cusimano, M. D., and A. Zhu. 2017. Systematic review of traumatic brain injuries in baseball and softball: A framework for prevention. *Frontiers in Neurology* 8:492.

Dams-O'Connor, K., A. Landau, J. Hoffman, and J. St De Lore. 2018. Patient perspectives on quality and access to healthcare after brain injury. *Brain Injury* 32(4):431-441.

Ettel, D., A. Glang, B. Todis, and S. Davies. 2016. Traumatic brain injury: Persistent misconceptions and knowledge gaps among educators. *Exceptionality Education International* 26:1-18.

Farmer, J., and M. Johnson-Gerard. 1997. Misconceptions about traumatic brain injury among educators and rehabilitation staff: A comparative study. *Rehabilitation Psychology* 42:273-286.

Gurusamy, J., S. Gandhi, S. Amudhan, K. B. Veerabhadraiah, P. Narayanasamy, S. T. Sreenivasan, and M. Palaniappan. 2019. Misconceptions about traumatic brain injury among nursing students in India: Implications for nursing care and curriculum. *BMC Nursing* 18:64.

Haddon W., Jr. 1980. Advances in the epidemiology of injuries as a basis for public policy. *Public Health Reports* 95(5):411-421.

Hux, K., M. Walker, and D. D. Sanger. 1996. Traumatic brain injury. *Language, Speech, and Hearing Services in Schools* 27(2):171-184.

Linden, M. A., and A. M. Boylan. 2010. "To be accepted as normal": Public understanding and misconceptions concerning survivors of brain injury. *Brain Injury* 24(4):642-650.

Linden, M. A., H. J. Braiden, and S. Miller. 2013. Educational professionals' understanding of childhood traumatic brain injury. *Brain Injury* 27(1):92-102.

Liu, B. C., Ivers, R., Norton, R., Boufous, S., Blows, S., and S. K. Lo. 2008. Helmets for preventing injury in motorcycle riders. *Cochrane Database of Systematic Reviews* (1):CD004333.

Maas, A., D. K. Menon, P. D. Adelson, N. Andelic, M. J. Bell, A. Belli, P. Bragge, et al. 2017. Traumatic brain injury: integrated approaches to improve prevention, clinical care, and research. *Lancet Neurology* 16(12):987-1048.

McKinlay, A., and K. Buck. 2019. Misconceptions about traumatic brain injury among educators: Has anything changed over the last 20 years? *Disability and Rehabilitation* 41(12):1419-1426.

NASEM (National Academies of Sciences, Engineering, and Medicine). 2014. *Sports-related concussions in youth: Improving the science, changing the culture*. Washington, DC: The National Academies Press.

Olivier, J., and P. Creighton. 2017. Bicycle injuries and helmet use: A systematic review and meta-analysis. *International Journal of Epidemiology* 46(1):278-292.

Op't Eynde, J., A. W. Yu, C. P. Eckersley, and C. R. Bass. 2020. Primary blast wave protection in combat helmet design: A historical comparison between present day and World War I. *PloS One* 15(2):e0228802.

Pappadis, M. R., A. M. Sander, M. A. Struchen, P. Leung, and D. W. Smith. 2011. Common misconceptions about traumatic brain injury among ethnic minorities with TBI. *Journal of Head Trauma Rehabilitation* 26(4):301-311.

Pappadis, M. R., A. M. Sander, B. Łukaszewska, M. A. Struchen, P. Leung, and D. W. Smith. 2017. Effectiveness of an educational intervention on reducing misconceptions among ethnic minorities with complicated mild to severe traumatic brain injury. *Archives of Physical Medicine and Rehabilitation* 98(4):751-758.

Ralph, A., and C. Derbyshire. 2013. Survivors of brain injury through the eyes of the public: A systematic review. *Brain Injury* 27(13-14):1475-1491.

Redpath, S. J., and M. A. Linden. 2004. Attitudes towards behavioural versus organic acquisition of brain injury. *Brain Injury* 18(9):861-869.

Register-Mihalik, J. K., K. M. Guskiewicz, T. C. McLeod, L. A. Linnan, F. O. Mueller, and S. W. Marshall. 2013. Knowledge, attitude, and concussion-reporting behaviors among high school athletes: A preliminary study. *Journal of Athletic Training* 48(5):645-653.

Sone, J. Y., D. Kondziolka, J. H. Huang, and U. Samadani. 2017. Helmet efficacy against concussion and traumatic brain injury: a review. *Journal of Neurosurgery* 126(3):768-781.

Springer, J. A., J. E. Farmer, and D. E. Bouman. 1997. Common misconceptions about traumatic brain injury among family members of rehabilitation patients. *Journal of Head Trauma Rehabilitation* 12(3):41-50.

Stevens, J. A. 2010. *A CDC compendium of effective fall interventions: What works for community-dwelling older adults*. 2nd ed. Atlanta, GA: National Center for Injury Prevention and Control, Centers for Disease Control and Prevention.

Stevens, J. A., and R. Lee. 2018. The potential to reduce falls and avert costs by clinically managing fall risk. *American Journal of Preventive Medicine* 55(3):290-297.

Swift, T. L., and S. L. Wilson. 2001. Misconceptions about brain injury among the general public and non-expert health professionals: An exploratory study. *Brain Injury* 15(2):149-165.

5

Acute Care After Traumatic Brain Injury

Chapter Highlights

- In the immediate stages after traumatic brain injury (TBI), care focuses on assessing the nature and initial severity of the injury, medically stabilizing the person if needed, and preventing the occurrence of further physical and neurological damage.
- Not everyone who experiences a TBI is screened and diagnosed at the time of injury, and not everyone receives the best evidence-based care.
- Elements including strength of evidence, provider attitudes, and institutional culture around the implementation and use of care guidelines affect variations in care.
- The current TBI clinical taxonomy, reduced to the categories of mild, moderate, and severe, is insufficient for purposes of both care and research.
- Drawing on multiple measures of brain injury severity to classify TBI—Glasgow Coma Scale, neuroimaging, and blood-based biomarkers—can improve precision diagnostic and prognostic models and inform a new generation of triage and treatment guidelines for TBI.

Acute injury management immediately following traumatic brain injury (TBI) focuses on minimizing complications, identifying sequelae, and optimizing long-term outcomes. This chapter provides an overview of care during the initial assessment of TBI, as well as acute-stage care after the injury. The chapter summarizes current practices and identifies clinical needs and knowledge gaps.

OVERVIEW OF CARE PROVIDED DURING THE ACUTE PHASE AFTER TBI

Because there are so many types of TBI, varying widely in severity and occurring in many different settings, patients with TBI may encounter the health care system in very different ways (see Figure 5-1). Many factors affect a person's pathway of care from entry to exit, as well as the health care providers engaged along the way. Immediately after a TBI, patients may be treated by first responders and prehospital care practitioners, such as emergency medical services (EMS) personnel and paramedics. During the acute care process, patients are often transferred in and out of settings that include the injury site, emergency medical transport vehicles, emergency departments (EDs), hospital intensive care units (ICUs), operating rooms (ORs), and hospital wards. In other cases, a person with a TBI may be evaluated outside of EMS and trauma care settings, may be seen in an urgent care clinic or a primary care office, or may receive no immediate medical care after the injury. This second pathway is more likely if the initial injury was less severe. In a population-based survey in Colorado, approximately 38 percent of people who reported experiencing a TBI were seen in an ED, 23 percent were hospitalized, 10 percent were seen in a physician's office, and 28 percent

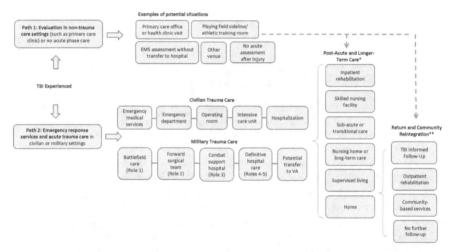

FIGURE 5-1 People who experience a TBI may follow different pathways for evaluation and potential care. Path 1: Many people who experience a TBI do not interact with the trauma care system, particularly if their initial injury is considered mild. For example, on-site evaluation may indicate that they do not require transport to a hospital, or they may report an incident or symptoms to a primary care provider. Some people will nevertheless require follow-up and further services in the post-acute and longer-term period. Path 2: Other people with a TBI require acute medical care through civilian or military trauma care systems. This pathway is most likely if the injuries sustained are more severe. After discharge from an acute care hospital stay, a further series of pathways are possible for care and community reintegration (see Chapter 6).

* After acute care hospitalization, a person may receive care from multiple types of facilities and in multiple care combinations (e.g., inpatient rehabilitation, to transitional care, to home; or discharge, to skilled nursing facility, to long-term care). The path taken by any given person depends on factors including injury severity and anticipated outcomes.

** Follow-up and support services available to people with TBI and their families once they are home or in a community setting also vary widely (e.g., from interdisciplinary and TBI-specialized outpatient rehabilitation, to supported employment services, to nothing).

did not seek care (Whiteneck et al., 2016). While some patients die as a result of their injury, many will move past the acute phase of care (see Chapter 6).

The pathway followed by an individual after TBI is determined by the injury mechanism and severity, as well as local resources. Injury severity and presenting symptoms guide decisions on whether to transport patients to EDs and trauma centers, as well as on the medical interventions provided. Acute care management emphasizes the prevention and mitigation of secondary injuries that increase morbidity and mortality, such as hypotension, hypoxia, and increased intracranial pressure that may occur because of the primary insult to the brain (Vella et al., 2017). If the injury requires surgery, acute management will typically involve attempts to reduce intracranial pressure prior to the operation. The medical condition of patients also may deteriorate during the acute care phase, requiring clinical reassessment and escalation of the care provided. Knowing how to provide the best care in this complex system of specialists and care settings requires accurate diagnostic assessment, triage, and information coordination among providers.

TBI CLASSIFICATION

Classification is fundamental to the study of the natural history of disease and can provide a taxonomy for diagnosis, prognosis, and treatment. For nearly 50 years, the Glasgow Coma Scale (GCS) has provided a practical method for assessing and classifying TBI patients for clinical care and research. Patients are assessed and assigned a numerical score for each of the three components of the scale—based on eye opening (E), verbal response (V), and motor response (M). Their GCS score then is communicated as three numbers (e.g., E4V4M6) (Teasdale and Jennett, 1974). See Figure 5-2 for an overview of the GCS scoring elements.

The summing of these separate subscale scores into a single sum, or total, score (e.g., GCS 14) was initially used for research, but was quickly adopted by clinicians as a convenient shorthand. This led to less precise individual patient information and created issues surrounding sum scores when a subscale component was untestable or missing (e.g., verbal response for an intubated patient). In time, these GCS sum scores were further reduced to the categories of mild TBI (GCS 13–15), moderate TBI (GCS 9–12), and severe TBI (GCS 3–8). While this was meant to simplify TBI classification, the widespread use of these broad categories has had unintended consequences for TBI clinical care and research. Similar to cancer and other complex diseases, TBI is a heterogeneous condition with many pathoanatomical subtypes that cannot be fully captured or characterized in a singular GCS composite score. Today, one could not imagine classifying cancer as "mild, moderate, and severe" for diagnosis, treatment, and prognosis. Changes to TBI classification approaches are already being implemented in some areas. In the setting of sport-related concussion, for example, guidelines have abandoned former "grading scales" in favor of multidimensional assessment to determine injury severity, track recovery, and inform a stepwise protocol for return to play.

When the full range of the GCS sum score (GCS 3–15) is used, in the absence of confounders, it is associated with a variety of other measures of TBI severity, recovery, and prognosis. Lower GCS values are associated with the occurrence of loss of consciousness (LOC) and longer duration of posttraumatic amnesia (PTA), a clinically important measure of injury severity (McMillan et al., 1996). Although the GCS was developed before computed tomography (CT) and magnetic resonance imaging (MRI), a lower GCS value is associated with a higher likelihood of TBI-related CT and MRI abnormalities (Amyot et al., 2015). Associations also are found between lower GCS values and higher levels of blood-based biomarkers of glial (such as glial fibrillary acidic protein [GFAP]) and neuronal (such as ubiquitin carboxy-terminal hydrolase L1 [UCH-L1]) injury (Okonkwo et al., 2013; Papa et al., 2012), even among

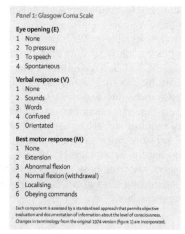

FIGURE 5-2 Glasgow Coma Scale
NOTE: The minimum Glasgow Coma Scale score is 3, while the maximum score is 15, indicating that a person is awake and responsive.
SOURCE: Reprinted from Teasdale et al., 2014, with permission from Elsevier.

those at the mildest end of the TBI continuum (GCS 15) (McCrea et al., 2020). However, a number of confounders, such as intoxication, sedation, intubation, dementia, and language issues that can affect the validity of the GCS score obtained, limit use of the GCS as a stand-alone measure for TBI classification (Zuercher et al., 2009). These confounders contribute to what is thought to be excessive use of CT imaging for the diagnosis of TBI, despite the fact that the CT result is often normal and is not as sensitive as MRI (Yue et al., 2019; Yuh et al., 2013).

Not only is the current classification of acute TBI as mild, moderate, or severe crude, but it also promotes bias that can limit care. Patients with "mild TBI" often receive no follow-up care based on the assumption that spontaneous full recovery will occur, despite the growing realization that a subset of these patients experience persistent symptoms and impairments after mild TBI (Nelson et al., 2019). Conversely, a nihilistic approach is taken to many individuals with "severe" injury, including early withdrawal of life-sustaining therapy, despite evidence that some of these patients can achieve significant improvement in global functional outcome (McCrea et al., 2021) (see the section on disorders of consciousness below). While mild, moderate, and severe as categories for TBI are diagnostically blunt, they also fail to characterize the pathoanatomical type and extent of injury. Such coarse categorization of TBI undercuts prognostic utility with respect to predicting the course of recovery and outcome for individual TBI patients. These categories may also have contributed to multiple failed clinical trials in TBI (Samadani, 2016). In a recent article, Haarbauer-Krupa and colleagues (2021, p. 3242) conclude that "work is needed to use the diverse existing data available to develop a taxonomy of TBI that incorporates injury mechanisms and early biomarkers to develop standard phenotypes and improve symptom trajectories."

Results from large-scale studies over the last decade support the use of imaging and blood-based biomarkers, along with the GCS, in the evolution of a more precise and informative classification system for TBI. This evolution is analogous to that of cancer classification. Cancer was initially characterized based on primary site or organ, tumor size, lymph node involvement, and presence of metastases. With increasing cohort sizes and extensive research, protein expression was included (e.g., epidermal growth factor receptor), and now genetic and epigenetic features are commonplace in the classification of cancer for targeted treatment.

CT imaging remains the workhorse of TBI assessment in the ED because it provides objective evidence of acute injury and identifies pathoanatomical features that require different types of clinical management. In fact, findings of CT imaging are the most important factor in hospital triage and surgical decision making in TBI (Bullock et al., 2006; Ratcliff et al., 2014). CT imaging features are also well-known prognostic biomarkers in patients with more significant injury (GCS 3–12), and more recently, the prognostic importance of CT imaging features has been extended to patients historically described as having sustained mild TBI (GCS 13–15) (Yuh et al., 2021). The diagnostic and prognostic utility of CT imaging helps explain why it is overused, even though the risks of radiation exposure are known (Kirsch et al., 2011). Although CT imaging is fast and readily available, the use of MRI is slowly increasing because it is more sensitive and safer. MRI can identify TBI-related pathology when the CT scan is normal, and emerging evidence supports its prognostic utility (Yue et al., 2019), although MRI is not as widely available as CT, may require intrahospital transport, and takes longer to perform. When available, however, both of these imaging modalities provide information that can contribute to a more precise TBI classification system.

There is also increasing evidence for the inclusion of blood-based biomarkers in an improved TBI classification system. Recent studies demonstrate that blood biomarkers can reliably predict the presence of intracranial bleeding on head CT, which could potentially reduce the volume of unnecessary CT studies in acute care settings. As discussed further below, these and other data helped support recent Food and Drug Administration (FDA) approval of GFAP and UCH-L1 as biomarkers for use in ruling out the need for head CT (Wang et al., 2021). Furthermore, blood biomarkers are associated with the type and extent of specific TBI pathologies (e.g., contusion, diffuse axonal injury) in neurotrauma patients, which is a critically important step toward achieving a precision medicine model for TBI (Okonkwo et al., 2020; Yue et al., 2019). Blood biomarkers also have prognostic utility, including an association between GFAP/UCH-L1 levels acutely (<24 hours postinjury) and functional outcome out to 12 months post-TBI (Okonkwo et al., 2013). Broader evidence suggests that blood biomarkers have diagnostic and prognostic utility across the full spectrum of TBI severity, from concussion to coma. Blood-based biomarkers provide prognostic information that is above and beyond information from a clinical exam (Frankel et al., 2019). In addition to data on patients with more severe TBI treated at Level 1 trauma centers, recent studies demonstrate significantly elevated levels of GFAP and UCH-L1 in athletes with sport-related concussion and in military service members with mild TBI (all GCS 15) that are also predictive of time to return to activity after injury (Giza et al., 2021; McCrea et al., 2020; Pattinson et al., 2020).

Although GCS values, neuroimaging, and blood-based biomarkers are strongly correlated, they each provide unique and complementary information, and an ideal classification system is therefore one that leverages all three measures of brain injury severity. Blood-based biomarkers of glial and neuronal injury quantify the extent of brain cell injury irrespective of the injury's location or functional consequences. Neuroimaging also provides information on the extent of brain cell and vascular injury, but it also provides information on the location and anatomic consequences of the injury (e.g., midline shift). The GCS score provides information on the functional consequences of the injury. Therefore, the incorporation of all three measures into a composite classification system would allow a multifaceted characterization of the injury, thereby reducing this heterogeneous condition to more homogeneous subsets that could become more focused targets for therapeutic intervention. Incorporating additional information from such sources as blood-based biomarkers could also aid decision making around when to use CT and/or MRI scans.

Collectively, extensive research over the past two decades supports the concept that the full range of GCS values, imaging findings, and blood biomarker results can be incorporated into a more accurate and sophisticated TBI classification model to aid in more precise pathoanatomical characterization, inform individualized treatment, and aid in predicting long-term outcome after TBI.

TOOLS FOR ACUTE EVALUATION OF TBI

Additional diagnostic tools are needed for acute-stage evaluation and risk stratification of TBI. Beyond the GCS and the brain CT scan, there are no standardized tools for assessing TBI in the ED. In the context of mild TBI or concussion, symptom assessments, such as the Rivermead Postconcussion Questionnaire (RPQ), are often used to evaluate patients in non-ED outpatient settings. For patients who are military service members or athletes, acute evaluation of TBI also includes the use of standardized assessment tools. These tools include short batteries of neurocognitive tests, neuropsychiatric tests, and symptom inventories, such as the Standardized Assessment of Concussion (SAC), the Sports Concussion Assessment Tool (SCAT5) (Echemendia et al., 2017; McCrea, 2001), and the Military Acute Concussion Evaluation 2 (MACE 2).[1] However, there are no standardized tools for assessing civilian TBI in the ED. The SAC, SCAT5, and MACE 2, among others, have not been validated for use in the ED because, relative to military and athlete patient populations, an ED typically sees more severely injured patients with a higher prevalence of comorbid conditions and patients who are injured by more varied injury mechanisms. As a consequence, TBI is often underdiagnosed in the ED (Blostein and Jones, 2003; Powell et al., 2008). Patients who have a negative head CT result are often told they are fine, and in more than 50 percent of cases, a diagnosis of TBI is not indicated on the patient's chart (Powell et al., 2008). While many of those who experience a mild TBI do indeed recover, some experience ongoing symptoms, and tools are needed to help emergency medicine providers identify which patients are unlikely to recover quickly on their own.

THE ROLE OF CLINICAL PRACTICE GUIDELINES IN INFORMING ACUTE TBI CARE

Clinicians draw on evidence-based clinical practice guidelines (CPGs), where available, to inform their choices about patient care and interventions across the range of TBI severity. According to the Institute of Medicine, "clinical practice guidelines are statements and recommendations intended to optimize patient care and are informed by systematic reviews of evidence and assessment of the benefits and harms of alternative care options" (IOM, 2011, p. 15). For example, the "Guidelines for Guidelines" from the Department of Veterans Affairs (VA) outlines how key questions are formulated, what types of evidence will be considered, how the strength of the evidence will be graded, how disclosures of conflict of interest will be handled, how literature reviews will be conducted, and how Veteran/patient input will be reviewed, among other parameters (VA, 2019). The results of guideline development processes by such entities as the VA, medical associations, professional societies, expert panels, the Brain Trauma Foundation, and other nonprofit organizations inform standards of care for patient populations with TBI (see Box 5-1).

---

[1] See https://health.mil/Reference-Center/Publications/2020/07/30/Military-Acute-Concussion-Evaluation-MACE-2 (accessed September 24, 2021).

BOX 5-1	SELECTED CLINICAL CARE GUIDELINES ADDRESSING PREHOSPITAL AND HOSPITAL-BASED ACUTE CARE OF TBI

- Brain Trauma Foundation's *Guidelines for Prehospital Management of TBI*, 2nd edition (Badjatia et al., 2008)
- Centers for Disease Control and Prevention's (CDC's) *Guidelines for Field Triage of Injured Patients* (Sasser et al., 2012)
- Department of Veterans Affairs'/Department of Defense's *Clinical Practice Guideline for the Management of Concussion-Mild Traumatic Brain Injury* (VA, 2016)
- *Guidelines for the Management of Severe Traumatic Brain Injury*, 4th Edition (Carney et al., 2017)
- Concussion in Sport Group's *Consensus Statement on Concussion in Sport* (McCrory et al., 2017)
- CDC's *Guideline on the Diagnosis and Management of Mild Traumatic Brain Injury among Children* (Lumba-Brown et al., 2018)
- *Guidelines for the Management of Pediatric Severe Traumatic Brain Injury*, 3rd Edition: Update of the Brain Trauma Foundation Guidelines (Kochanek et al., 2019)
- *Living Guideline for Diagnosing and Managing Pediatric Concussion* (Ontario Neurotrauma Foundation, 2019)
- *Guidelines for the Management of Severe Traumatic Brain Injury: 2020 Update of the Decompressive Craniectomy Recommendations* (Hawryluk et al., 2020)
- Excellence in Prehospital Injury Care (EPIC) guidelines (Spaite et al., 2019)

PREHOSPITAL EVALUATION AND TREATMENT OF TBI

The initial evaluation and treatment of TBI often begin at the scene of injury, which may be a war zone, roadside, sideline of a sporting event, or dark alley. Given that half of the deaths from TBI occur within 2 hours of injury, acute care in that crucial early window is a critical determinant of survival (Boto et al., 2006). Prehospital providers are often responsible for the rapid evaluation, initial resuscitation, and timely transport of suspected TBI patients. They must also contend with the resource constraints of a prehospital clinical examination, which may include lack of access to needed medical supplies; the need to attend to multiple trauma across organ systems; lack of time to perform a procedure; and the need to account for any special circumstances that may call for a different course of clinical care for individual patients, such as age, intoxication, allergic sensitivity, known medical history, and preexisting conditions. Note that in focusing on the care pathways of those TBI patients who receive acute emergency and hospital-based care, this chapter references other important types of TBI, but it does not delve in detail into out-of-hospital care provided by athletic trainers or other sports medicine practitioners, as is common in the management of sport-related concussion.

Assessing TBI

As noted earlier, EMS personnel are often the first health care providers to evaluate and stabilize TBI patients before they are transported to the hospital. Assessment of TBI in the prehospital setting involves monitoring vital signs, especially blood pressure and blood oxygen saturation; calculating the GCS score or pediatric GCS score; and examining the pupils for dilation and reactivity. These parameters may be assessed repeatedly to monitor clinical improvement or deterioration. Although other TBI classifications exist, management and transportation decisions are often based on the patient's GCS score in the prehospital setting.

The GCS score has limitations as a metric for assessing TBI in the prehospital setting, however. The score is based on the patient's subjective responses to questions (or those of a witness speaking on the patient's behalf), which may not be an accurate reflection of their status, and on a clinical examination for signs and symptoms that may be subtly present. TBI patients who initially present with a GCS score in the normal range may nonetheless harbor traumatic intracranial pathologies. However, prehospital providers lack tools with which to identify "hidden TBI" patients who would benefit from being transported to a trauma center for further evaluation and care. Novel point-of-care diagnostic tools beyond the GCS and clinical examination are needed to optimize prehospital care.

Prehospital Triage and Medical Transport

Prehospital evaluation and decisions about medical transport are informed by guidelines issued by the Centers for Disease Control and Prevention (CDC) and the Brain Trauma Foundation (Badjatia et al., 2008; Sasser et al., 2012). In general, the prehospital guidelines recommend transporting patients with GCS ≤12, those with penetrating head trauma, those experiencing high-risk falls or motor vehicle collisions, and those taking anticoagulant medications "to a facility that provides the highest level of care within the defined trauma system" (Sasser et al., 2012, p. 8). For example, because patients with low GCS scores have a high likelihood of harboring traumatic intracranial lesions and elevated intracranial pressure, guidelines generally recommend transporting these patients to facilities that offer immediate access to CT scans and neurosurgical care.

Individual jurisdictions determine how protocols for prehospital care are implemented within their jurisdiction. According to a recent report from the National Academies of Sciences, Engineering, and Medicine,

> Nationwide, there are an estimated 21,283 credentialed EMS agencies, comprising a mixture of private, public, and volunteer systems that often operate independently and sometimes at odds with each other. There is no one-size-fits-all configuration for EMS.... EMS providers generally follow medical protocols that may be local (applying only to a single agency), countywide, regional, or statewide. (NASEM, 2016, p. 82)

Significant differences in prehospital protocols across regions of the United States make both care coordination between the prehospital and hospital settings and triage of patients more challenging. This variability has particular effects on care management situations in which "optimal care of injured patients is delayed or limited by geography, weather, distance, or resources" (ACS, 2014, p. 94) or providers' lack of experience. Yet, standardizing emergency care is difficult because of the history of emergency care development and reliance on local physicians and local systems.[2]

In combat zones, as well as in remote or austere locations, medical evacuation from the injury scene may be delayed for hours or even days. Even when rapid evacuation is possible, transport time may be prolonged. For example, the transport of injured active duty service

---

[2] Robinson, J. 2021. TBI Care Gaps and Opportunities: Provider Perspectives on the Acute-Stage Continuum of Care. Panel discussion during virtual workshop for the Committee on Accelerating Progress in Traumatic Brain Injury Research and Care, March 18, 2021.

members by Critical Care Air Transport Teams[3] can take anywhere from 30 minutes to 16 hours or longer (Ingalls et al., 2014). Care en route is often challenged by loud ambient noise, heat, pressure, lack of appropriate equipment, and turbulence. Accordingly, emergency and frontline responders may need to manage patients who are sicker than they are accustomed to, for longer than they are equipped to handle, with fewer resources than what they have on hand, and in a challenging location. These conditions have given rise to the emerging concept of prolonged field care, which involves providing field medical care beyond the timelines conventionally called for in order to decrease patient mortality and morbidity (Shackelford et al., 2021).[4]

Prehospital Acute Care Management

While prehospital care is guided by the concept that care provided during the first 60 minutes following traumatic injury ("the Golden Hour") is critical in determining whether a patient survives the injury, it has become increasingly clear that secondary insults occurring beyond the Golden Hour increase the risk for mortality and disability (Stocchetti et al., 2017). Accordingly, constructs that guide care during the acute period are avoiding secondary injury, as well as aiding areas of the brain with reduced blood perfusion (the ischemic penumbra) to ensure maximum recovery.

The goals of acute TBI care management in the prehospital setting are to avoid the "3 Hs": hypoxia, hypotension, and hyper- or hypoventilation. Hypoxia (low blood oxygen level) can be corrected by providing supplemental oxygen, which may include intubating those patients with airway compromise (Vandromme et al., 2011). Hypotension (low blood pressure) is corrected by controlling hemorrhaging and administering fluids. Hypoventilation may be managed with mechanical ventilation. Hyperventilation can be avoided by controlling the number of breaths delivered during bag valve mask or mechanical ventilation. Prehospital care guidelines that highlight the importance of avoiding and treating the 3 Hs have been shown to improve the odds of a patient's surviving at least until admission to the hospital and decreasing overall mortality in persons with severe TBI (Spaite et al., 2019).

However, these interventions can come with risks, and there are also uncertainties in what is known about optimal prehospital care. For example, some studies indicate that when intubation is performed in a prehospital setting, unwanted side effects of hyperoxygenation and hypo- or hypercarbia increase the odds of poor patient outcomes (Davis et al., 2006). The literature on civilian urban trauma also has shown that patients have superior or similar outcomes if they are transported directly to a trauma center by means other than EMS (Demetriades et al., 1996; Winter et al., 2021). It is unclear why this is the case, but potential explanations include earlier arrival to definitive care or avoidance of interventions that have been associated with worse outcomes during transport (Schreiber et al., 2015). In another example, a recent study of 438 military patients evacuated out of theater during 2007 to 2014 found that patients with moderate to severe TBI were more likely to survive and return to duty if evacuated more than 3 days after injury, suggesting that a stabilization period may be beneficial prior to evacuation (Maddry et al., 2020). Further work would be needed to

---

[3] Critical Care Air Transport Teams (CCATTs) consist of an ICU-level physician, an ICU nurse, and a respiratory therapist. Transport is most frequently performed in two legs: from the origin country to Landstuhl, Germany, where the patient has an initial stay, and then from Germany to the continental United States. Transferring patients by CCATT is most similar to transporting ICU patients to the CT scanner and back in a hospital, except the transfer can take up to 16 hours.

[4] Further information about the concept of Prolonged Field Care is also available from the Special Operations Medical Association at http://www.specialoperationsmedicine.org/pages/pfcresources.aspx (accessed August 26, 2021).

understand this finding. Overall, there is a paucity of prehospital research on TBI, which makes it difficult to understand what works well for these patients in prehospital settings.[5] More research is needed to develop and implement guidelines and support best practices in prehospital settings so as to reduce adverse outcomes of TBI (Gravesteijn et al., 2020).

Telemedicine offers one opportunity to improve care prior to arrival at a definitive trauma center for advanced TBI care (Raso et al., 2021; Shah et al., 2020; Whiting et al., 2021). It enables expert clinicians to have both audio and visual access to the prehospital scene and provide real-time on-scene direction to EMS personnel. Such extension of the reach of expert clinicians may allow patients in low-resource areas, especially those in rural settings, to access care comparable to that provided at regional trauma centers. It may also prevent unnecessary transfers to trauma centers (Latifi et al., 2018). Further investigation of the feasibility of prehospital telemedicine consults in TBI and the effect of such consultation on clinical outcomes is warranted.

Handoff from Prehospital to Hospital-Based Care

If prehospital services indicate that a patient's injuries require further intervention, the patient may be transferred to a hospital or trauma center. Often, this handoff entails challenges of inadequate coordination, leading to discontinuities in patient care (Robertson et al., 2014). For example, there are currently no standardized processes for ensuring that key information is exchanged between dispatch and EMS personnel and between EMS and ED personnel (Reay et al., 2020; Stiell et al., 2003).

Another gap is the lack of integration of prehospital data with subsequent hospital and outpatient data. Data from care delivered in the prehospital setting are often not transmitted to the hospital in a structured, easy-to-use format (Martin et al., 2018; Wood et al., 2015). The lack of data integration and lack of a formal process for communication of key information from prehospital to ED providers limit the ability to deliver optimal care to TBI patients. The lack of data integration and the episodic nature of prehospital and hospital care also confound research on prehospital TBI care, and research in prehospital settings has been recognized as a critical challenge in both the United States and Europe (Maurin Söderholm et al., 2019). The Excellence in Prehospital Injury Care (EPIC) study—a large-scale public health effort to conduct prehospital research over multiple systems, patients, and years—may serve as a model for the conduct of prehospital research in TBI.[6] This study, in which more than 130 Arizona state and local EMS agencies participated, assessed the use and effectiveness of prehospital TBI guidelines for those with moderate to severe TBI (Spaite et al., 2019). Participants received training in the guidelines, and the study found that adherence to the guidelines increased survival to hospital admission.

HOSPITAL-BASED EVALUATION AND CARE

Emergency Department

Each year approximately 4.8 million ED visits occur in which people are evaluated for a potential TBI, and it is estimated that TBI is diagnosed in 2.5 million of these visits (Korley et al., 2016). In the ED, TBI severity is typically determined by clinical examination, including GCS, and by head CT imaging where available and indicated.

---

[5] Robinson, J. 2021. TBI Care Gaps and Opportunities: Provider Perspectives on the Acute-Stage Continuum of Care. Panel discussion during virtual workshop for the Committee on Accelerating Progress in Traumatic Brain Injury Research and Care, March 18, 2021.
[6] Ibid.

In the ED setting, evaluation for TBI focuses primarily on identifying life-threatening injuries. As a result, limited time and attention are devoted to identifying injuries that present with subtle signs and symptoms. People who are assessed as having a normal GCS score and do not appear significantly impaired may nonetheless have "hidden TBI" that may be revealed only with further imaging or testing, while patients with more substantial trauma may be resuscitated with limited attention to an underlying TBI. The American College of Surgeons' Advanced Trauma Life Support program offers limited guidance for resuscitation of TBI patients, focused in particular on controlling traumatic hemorrhage.[7] In patients with GCS <15 an evaluation is frequently multidisciplinary and may involve clinicians from the ED, trauma surgery, neurosurgery, and anesthesiology. Care includes managing the airway, blood oxygenation, intracranial pressure, and hemorrhaging. Standardized guidelines are especially needed on how to prevent hemodynamic deterioration in TBI patients during acute care.

In the ED, a brain CT scan is performed in 82 percent of TBI evaluations (Korley et al., 2016). Approximately 90 percent of suspected TBI patients who receive a head CT scan are classified as negative for TBI, with 9 percent showing traumatic intracranial lesions (Korley et al., 2016). Clinical decision rules exist for determining which patients to recommend for brain CT imaging (Haydel et al., 2000; Jagoda et al., 2008; Kuppermann et al., 2009; Shetty et al., 2016; Stiell et al., 2001); however, adherence to these decision rules is variable (DeAngelis et al., 2017).

As discussed above, FDA recently approved two blood-based biomarkers of TBI—GFAP and UCH-L1—that may be useful in guiding assessment in the ED, including the appropriate use of head CT scans. By January 2021, FDA had given the green light for clinicians to use a platform that measures these biomarkers at the point of care (see Phillips, 2021). Measurement of the blood-based biomarker troponin has revolutionized the emergent assessment of chest pain by providing a rapid test to facilitate diagnosis and triage (Gibbs and McCord, 2020). The expanding use of FDA-approved blood-based biomarkers for TBI similarly has the potential to transform TBI assessment.

The majority of research on TBI biomarkers to date has focused on diagnostic markers of acute TBI, including markers of blood–brain barrier integrity; neuroinflammation; and axonal, neuronal, astroglial, and vascular injury. (See Appendix B for additional information on biomarker research.) Clinical availability of blood-based biomarkers for TBI is expected to expand in 2022 and beyond, and studies are needed to determine the effectiveness of these tools in guiding TBI care and decreasing inappropriate use of head CT during TBI evaluation. Future studies will also be needed to explore biomarker profiles over time that may help in monitoring for longer-term sequelae of TBI.

As noted previously, emerging data suggest that MRI scans may also be useful in the acute risk stratification of TBI, being both safer and more sensitive than CT: approximately a third of TBI patients with negative head CT results have MRI findings of traumatic intracranial injuries that are associated with poorer outcomes (Yuh et al., 2013). Given that brain MRI often requires transport to a remote location in the hospital for a prolonged period, however—posing a potential safety risk, especially for the most severely injured patients—decision aids are needed to identify which TBI patients are likely to benefit from acute MRI brain imaging.

Care in the ICU and Hospital Ward

For moderate and severe TBI, hospital-based care may involve patient transfer from the ED to an ICU or medical ward. In the hospital, TBI management consists of the assessment and stabilization of vital signs, the assessment of severity based on the GCS; a neurologic

---

[7] See https://www.facs.org/quality-programs/trauma/atls (accessed September 24, 2021).

exam; and imaging of the brain, most commonly with a CT scan. In the ICU, additional monitoring of physiologic parameters may occur in hopes of preventing secondary brain injury. The monitoring may include intracranial pressure (ICP), cerebral perfusion pressure (CPP), partial brain tissue oxygenation ($PbtO_2$), brain metabolism, and brain activity.

Nearly all professional societies that publish guidelines on the treatment of TBI in the ICU use a similar stepwise algorithm. For example, current therapies sequentially involve elevating the head of the bed; using sedation and hyperosmolar fluids; avoiding fever; draining off cerebrospinal fluid to treat elevated ICP; and in cases of refractory elevated ICP and cerebral herniation, employing mild transient hyperventilation.

Traumatic intracranial lesions identified on CT scan include epidural, subdural, subarachnoid, and intraparenchymal hemorrhages; patients may have one type or a combination of these lesions, and different lesions have different prognoses (Yuh et al., 2021). For example, isolated epidural hemorrhages have an excellent prognosis if they are diagnosed early and treated with surgical evacuation, whereas subdural and subarachnoid hemorrhages are associated with disability and higher mortality. A person's prognosis is influenced by lesion size and location; time to diagnosis; and patient factors, including age, comorbid medical conditions, and use of anticoagulant/antiplatelet therapy. Approximately 25–60 percent of patients with traumatic intracranial lesions experience progression in lesion size, which may be detected by deterioration in clinical neurologic examination or on repeat brain CT scan (Allard et al., 2009; Narayan et al., 2008; Servadei et al., 2000). The incidence of lesion progression is influenced by the severity of the injuries in the patient population that is studied, and the risk for progression is greatest during the 24 hours following injury. A major barrier to delivering optimal management for these patients is the lack of objective tools for detecting lesion progression prior to the development of overt clinical signs or radiographic indication. Recently, a number of authors have questioned the utility of 6-hour repeat brain CT scans in GCS 13–15 TBI patients with traumatic intracranial lesions (Joseph et al., 2014; Rosen et al., 2018). Studies are needed to better define the subpopulation of TBI patients with traumatic intracranial lesions that are at risk for lesion progression and therefore warrant close monitoring.

Operating Room and Anesthesia Care

Patients with TBI requiring urgent surgical decompression spend varying amounts of time in the ED. Some patients receive rapid visual assessments followed by transport to the OR. Intraoperative CT scan prevents the need for transport to radiology suites for postoperative head CT scan and minimizes transport risks. Blood biomarkers are not currently used to evaluate treatment response during intraoperative TBI care.

The intraoperative goal for TBI care is to prevent secondary brain injury by optimizing such key physiologic parameters as CPP and brain tissue oxygenation. Doing so involves optimizing systemic blood pressure and ICP and peripheral oxygenation status by providing a balanced anesthetic, continued resuscitation, continuous monitoring, and life-sustaining hemodynamic management. To these ends, intraoperative TBI care requires timely readiness of an OR, availability of needed equipment, and nursing support. Patients with TBI who present for emergent craniotomy often have polytrauma, requiring that craniotomy be performed simultaneously with control of other injuries, which in turn necessitates coordination among surgical, nursing, and anesthesiology teams.

Patients with TBI and extracranial injuries requiring surgical intervention during the acute period may have ICP monitors in place, which allows for determination and maintenance of CPP. Brain oxygen monitoring systems (such as Licox monitors) provide additional information for brain tissue monitoring.

For patients with mild or moderate TBI, optimizing brain physiology is important to prevent postoperative worsening of ICP and TBI. For patients with traditionally defined mild or moderate TBI, attention to contusion size and intraoperative ICP may drive the decision to extubate patients at the end of surgery.

Intrahospital Handoffs and Transport

Patients hospitalized with TBI can undergo a number of intrahospital transports. Handoffs from ED to OR or inpatient hospital staff present the risk of adverse events (Horwitz et al., 2009), as do handoffs from OR to ICU. Handoffs are accompanied by information on demographics, intraoperative blood loss, surgical procedures performed, complications, and anticipated events upon transfer. Patients can suddenly deteriorate during transfer, and monitoring standards may vary, presenting challenges for patient transport within the hospital. Ideally, transporting staff should have the ability and equipment to stabilize patients who deteriorate during intrahospital travel. Transport is often facilitated by nursing staff, and most hospitals have nursing guidelines on intrahospital transport of critically ill patients (Fanara et al., 2010; Nathanson et al., 2020; Warren et al., 2004). Monitor alarms are set using age-specific parameters to account for pediatric or geriatric physiology, and patients are typically monitored with an electrocardiogram (ECG) monitor, blood pressure monitor, and pulse oximetry during transport. Similarly, during hospitalization in acute care and while transitioning to post-acute care, referral to specialists may not occur. Thresholds for consultation are not uniform and the process is often delayed, which results in suboptimal care and outcomes.

VARIATION IN CONTENT OF AND ADHERENCE TO CLINICAL CARE GUIDELINES

In addition to ensuring that the best available evidence is used to guide therapy, adherence to clinical care guidelines limits unwarranted variation in practice while not precluding personalized care. Absent more comprehensive clinical care guidelines, the provision of optimal care for acute TBI faces multiple challenges (Brolliar et al., 2016; Carney et al., 2017; Kochanek et al., 2019). Limited data on certain topics and variable adherence to existing guidelines both contribute to gaps in acute care for TBI.

Adherence to clinical care guidelines and protocols has been shown to improve outcomes following TBI. A 2007 study found that adherence to Brain Trauma Foundation guidelines resulted in better health outcomes for adult patients (Faul et al., 2007). In a study of children with severe brain injuries, adherence to pediatric guidelines was associated with survival at discharge and improved scores on the Glasgow Outcome Scale. Each percentage increase in guideline adherence was associated with a 6 percent lower risk of death (Vavilala et al., 2014). A study on adherence to return-to-play protocols for children experiencing sport-related TBI similarly found that "increased adherence to protocols predicted successful return to sport without symptom exacerbation" (DeMatteo et al., 2020, p. 7).

Guideline adherence is variable, however, with one review finding a range of 18–100 percent (Cnossen et al., 2021). This variability can be driven by a combination of guideline, provider, and institutional factors (Brolliar et al., 2016), including the strength of evidence supporting the guidelines, provider attitudes and experience, and the institution's culture around the implementation of care guidelines. The existence of multiple guidelines directed at different medical specialties caring for different types of TBI populations and covering different topics or using different standards of evidence for what is included or excluded from the guidelines also contributes to variability in the choices made by care providers and in the care patients receive. Payer influences and clinician bias contribute to variability in adherence to guidelines as well.

Limitations of Care Guidelines for TBI: Example of Intracranial Pressure (ICP) Monitoring

Clinical practice guidelines can also be of limited utility in some circumstances. ICP monitoring is the standard of care for severe TBI and is used frequently (Liu et al., 2015). However, monitoring of ICP has not been proven beneficial for improving patient outcomes (Marehbian et al., 2017; Shafi et al., 2008). Moreover, there is no standardization regarding indications and methods for ICP monitoring, and monitoring practices vary, including whether to use intraparenchymal or external ventricular drains to help regulate a patient's ICP (Cnossen et al., 2017; Van Cleve et al., 2013). Accordingly, parenchymal pressure monitors and external ventricular drains are routinely used interchangeably in trauma centers.

A number of other approaches are used to manage ICP, many of which carry risks and have side effects. These approaches include catecholamine drugs, barbiturates, surgical decompression, abdominal decompression, brain tissue oxygenation, resuscitation, provision of adequate cerebral perfusion, osmolar therapy, decompressive craniectomies, and nutrition support (Aarabi et al., 2006; Cook et al., 2008; Joseph et al., 2004). More work is needed to identify which patients are most likely to benefit from any or all of these approaches. Given that other TBI tests and treatments are predicated on ICP monitoring, the lack of standardization in this aspect of care results in unwarranted variability in acute TBI management.

More robust clinical care guidelines are also needed to address important aspects of TBI care that lack a clear consensus, such as the use of tranexamic acid (Maas et al., 2021), the use of a high fraction of inspired oxygen, the optimal target partial pressure of carbon dioxide, optimal anesthesia care, the order of prioritization of surgical interventions for different organ systems in polytrauma, and optimal blood transfusion thresholds.

Limitations of Care Guidelines for TBI: Example of Cerebral Perfusion Pressure (CPP) Management

Weak adherence to TBI guidelines may be affected by the lack of compelling clinical data on whether interventions are beneficial, leading to greater variability in case-by-case management. As an example, the choice of vasopressors to augment CPP is based largely on clinician or institutional preference. Even when vasopressors are used, standard resuscitation targets for both ICP and CPP are lacking.

PREPARATION FOR TRANSFER TO POST-ACUTE CARE

Patients with TBI often need early rehabilitation after hospital admission or discharge to inpatient and outpatient rehabilitation. Integrating rehabilitation consultation early in acute care has been shown to improve patient outcomes (see Chapter 6), but the timing and structure of rehabilitation consultations vary, and rehabilitation interventions are variably introduced during the acute care period. Referrals to rehabilitation services and the availability of follow-up care after TBI are also highly variable and frequently absent, particularly for vulnerable populations and patients without access to primary care. These issues are discussed further in Chapter 6.

Prior to discharge, patients with TBI need to be screened for discharge to a safe environment. By the time of discharge, acute care providers also need to have provided materials and resources on the person's brain injury to the person with TBI and their family. Providing education and support to persons with TBI and caregivers starting in the acute care phase is especially important for those patients being discharged to home. And while the military has systems of care to provide post-acute services and long-term rehabilitation, patients can experience loss of continuity when transitioning from Department of Defense (DoD) to Department of Veterans Affairs (VA) health systems (Randall, 2012). Care coordinators or patient navigators can facilitate smoother transitions for patients and families, but they are not routinely used in civilian medicine (Livergant et al., 2021; Natale-Pereira et al., 2011).

SPECIAL CHALLENGES IN ACUTE TBI MANAGEMENT

Penetrating versus Blunt TBI

While both penetrating and blunt brain injury are classed as TBI, important differences are associated with these two injury types. Blunt brain injury is a diffuse disease in which the entire brain is typically affected. While injury to the bony skull may occur, the wounding mechanism is the concussive force that is applied to the brain. In penetrating brain injury, the wounding missile traverses the brain, causing injury in its path. Penetrating injuries can be caused by fragments from explosions, bullets, and other sources. Skull fracture is common, and additional injury may occur as shards of bone are driven into the brain, causing secondary injury. Outcomes from penetrating brain injury are worse than those from blunt injury, and the mortality rate is higher (Larkin et al., 2018; Orman et al., 2012; Skarupa et al., 2019). This may be due to the severity of the brain injury but also to other associated life-threatening injuries.

Treatment for penetrating brain injury has largely been supportive, and operative therapy has not been a mainstay of care. This may be changing, however. Observational research from the wars in Iraq and Afghanistan suggests that an aggressive management approach for penetrating brain injury, including through decompressive craniectomy, results in good outcomes compared with historical controls (Bell et al., 2010). Penetrating brain injury is also becoming a more important civilian issue. Rates of civilian penetrating brain injury have increased, with a recent review of trauma admissions indicating an increase from 3,042 per 100,000 population in 2010 to 7,578 per 100,000 in 2014 (Skarupa et al., 2019). This issue may become increasingly important given that suicide by firearm injury has become a leading cause of TBI-related mortality (Daugherty et al., 2019), and the occurrence of violence in the United States has been increasing. Further research will be needed to address prevention and clinical management specifically for penetrating TBI.

Multiple Trauma

Patients who have multiple types of trauma (multitrauma or polytrauma) and severe TBI are often critically ill and present a special challenge. For example, bleeding lowers blood pressure, which can worsen outcomes of TBI. Sites of blood loss must be quickly identified and bleeding controlled, with surgery if necessary. The anesthesia needed for surgical procedures may also decrease blood pressure, potentially worsening secondary brain injury.

The inflammatory response to operative therapy, the so-called "second hit," may affect TBI outcome as well (Hinson et al., 2015). Specific injuries are often treated with medications to lower blood pressure, at least temporarily; such is the case, for example, with thoracic aortic injury, to prevent aortic rupture. The result is competing interests as clinicians attempt to treat both conditions.

As another example, patients who have suffered multiple injuries often have long-bone fractures. Ideal therapy involves early operative fracture fixation, but the ideal timing of fracture fixation in patients with TBI remains uncertain (Scalea et al., 1999, 2000). For patients with TBI who also have polytrauma, then, clarity is needed regarding the optimal timing of surgery for noncranial surgical procedures. Patients who have blunt trauma with combined hemorrhage and TBI present a dilemma in that they may require operations for hemorrhage control but at the same time may have life-threatening intracranial processes that are not diagnosed because they need to bypass the CT scanner on the way to the OR. Rapid methods of diagnosing intracranial hemorrhage and determining the optimal time to repair long-bone fractures are needed.

Confounding Factors and Comorbidities

During hospitalization and during the transition from acute to post-acute care for TBI, many patients have comorbidities and preexisting conditions that require ancillary services in addition to TBI care. In addition to other types of traumatic injuries, such comorbidities and preexisting conditions commonly include cardiovascular risk factors, such as hypertension, and mental health disorders, among others. A review of TBI hospitalizations in Canada found a trend toward increasing age, along with a trend toward "increasing severity, comorbidity, and length of stay among TBI hospitalizations" (Fu et al., 2015, p. 452).

Clinicians may give inadequate attention to comorbidities and preexisting conditions or fail to consider strategies for minimizing side effects, such as pain, during TBI care. Although pain is one of the leading complaints among patients with TBI (Nampiaparampil, 2008), a systematic and holistic approach to pain management for these patients is seldom the norm. Clinicians do not have many options for adjunctive treatments to offer patients. Patients with TBI are also at increased risk of substance use disorders, and the American College of Surgeons' (ACS's) guidance requires ACS-verified trauma centers to undertake injury prevention efforts and to screen patients for alcohol abuse (ACS, 2014). However, substance abuse screening is not performed consistently.

Disorders of Consciousness and Withdrawal of Life-Sustaining Therapies

Making prognostic judgments in cases of severe TBI can be challenging, and it is therefore important to avoid making definitive predictions too early on while aiming to minimize unnecessary interventions.

> Severe impairment in the short term did not portend poor outcomes in a substantial minority of patients with [moderate to severe] TBI. When discussing prognosis during the first 2 weeks after injury, clinicians should be particularly cautious about making early, definitive prognostic statements suggesting poor outcomes and withdrawal of life-sustaining treatment. (McCrea et al., 2021, p. E1)

It has been reported that 40 percent of patients thought to be unconscious actually are found to retain conscious awareness when they are reevaluated, and that five examinations can bring the rate of misdiagnosis down to 5 percent, highlighting the importance of serial examination.[8] An ethical framework has also been proposed for identifying covert consciousness, or consciousness that is not readily observed in hospitalized TBI patients (Edlow and Fins, 2018). However, many acute care providers are unaware of the available data on long-term functional progress after prolonged disorders of consciousness (DOC). It has been reported that life-sustaining treatment is withdrawn in 26 percent of severe TBI patients within 72 hours of injury, whereas many patients with severe TBI display signs of consciousness only 1–2 months after injury.[9] Similarly, Edlow and Fins (2018, p. 2) note that in patients with DOC, "withdrawal of life-sustaining therapy accounts for up to 70% of TBI deaths in the intensive care unit (ICU), with decisions often made within 3 days of admission." Diagnostic accuracy is improved through the use of evidence-based practice guidelines, which provide specific guidance on diagnostic assessment (Giacino et al., 2018); however, these guidelines still need to be widely translated into clinical practice.

Making prognostic and treatment judgments in cases of severe TBI also poses ethical challenges when a patient cannot engage in the decision-making process and exercise his or her agency, as is the case in patients with DOC. The sudden nature of traumatic injuries means that preplanning or advance care directives are often not in place, and family members may be uncomfortable with making health decisions for their loved ones.[10] Decisions can be made that potentially result in withdrawing life-sustaining therapies too soon, especially when care teams are less familiar with the emerging evidence in patients with DOC.[11]

ADDITIONAL CONSIDERATIONS

Importance of Multidisciplinary Consultations

Optimal care for trauma patients involves consultation from many specialized services. Patients with severe TBI require transport to multiple sites, such as the OR or radiology suite. In acute care, trauma surgeons often must evaluate input from consultants in orthopedics, anesthesiology, maxillofacial surgery, interventional or trauma radiology, and neurocritical care to ensure that care is safe and coordinated, decide whether operative care is needed, and determine whether and how to place monitoring devices. In addition to physicians, care commonly also involves nurses, social workers, pharmacists, psychologists, physical therapists, occupational therapists, and speech therapists.

However, coordination of care among these specialists during acute care and between acute and post-acute care falls short of optimal. Given the many health science disciplines involved in acute care for patients with TBI, an interdisciplinary approach is required for optimal care and outcomes, with care being coordinated on a timeline of anticipated trajectories across disciplines. Such an approach entails, for example, obtaining a nutrition consult early after admission to optimize brain metabolism and recovery, and, again soon after admission, consulting the appropriate specialists to optimize resources, care, and outcomes. Yet, while recognized as a best practice, teamwork in the care of TBI patients is not always rewarded by health systems, which can contribute to less than optimal collaboration across disciplines.

---

[8] Giacino, J., R. Nakase-Richardson, and J. Whyte. 2021. Disorders of Consciousness After Traumatic Brain Injury: A Virtual Workshop for the Committee on Accelerating Progress in Traumatic Brain Injury Research and Care, May 24, 2021.

[9] Ibid.

[10] Allen Davis, J. 2021. System Challenges for TBI Care. Panel discussion during virtual workshop for the Committee on Accelerating Progress in Traumatic Brain Injury Research and Care, March 30, 2021.

[11] Ibid.

Communication in handoffs between practitioners is critical to ensure that information is exchanged clearly and accurately, as dropped information can be disastrous.

Pediatric and Geriatric TBI

Special considerations apply for evaluation and/or treatment of TBI in both pediatric and geriatric populations. A number of special considerations are important for acute TBI management in pediatric patients (Kochanek et al., 2019). Because the center of gravity in young people lies in their head, their falls produce a TBI more commonly relative to other age groups. In addition to falls, pediatric TBI can result from abusive head trauma (shaking) and from nonaccidental and accidental trauma. As a result, "clinicians must always consider abuse in differential diagnosis when evaluating and treating children, when the mechanism of injury is unclear or reported history does not match injuries or [the child's] age" (Smith et al., 2019, p. 119). Special factors pertinent to children also include the need for age-dependent hemodynamic management and reference to the pediatric TBI guidelines for care.

Care for TBI in older adults entails additional considerations. It must be stressed, moreover, that while there are guidelines for acute care of adults with severe TBI, data on geriatric TBI care and outcomes remain insufficient (Gardner et al., 2018). For example, few or no guidelines address the management of dangerous blood clotting in older adult patients. Geriatric patients often have some degree of cerebral atrophy due to advanced age. Therefore, significant bleeding or clots can initially accumulate with minimal symptoms. These patients often develop severe symptoms quickly when the accumulated blood causes cerebral herniation. The use of anticoagulation, common in older patients, can exacerbate intracranial hemorrhage. A major care gap for geriatric TBI patients is a lack of consensus on the need for reversing the effects of modern anticoagulation drugs and antiplatelet agents to avoid progression of intracranial bleeding (Gardner et al., 2018). Other geriatric TBI considerations during surgery include attention to elderly physiology and frailty.

In both pediatric and geriatric populations, assessing brain injury and its progression can be extremely challenging when the patient is nonverbal, cognitively impaired, or cognitively delayed. TBI commonly clouds the sensorium, and patients may be unable to cooperate with standard neurological testing.

Other Considerations for Patient-Centered Care

Patients who are nonbinary or noncisgender are vulnerable to clinicians' lack of experience in addressing their concerns.[12] Transgender people may be at greater risk for violence compared with cisgender people, and individuals who are nonbinary or non-gender-conforming need to receive unbiased care. In addition, much remains unknown about the role of biological sex hormones in TBI outcomes, including potential effects of hormone therapies (Duncan and Garijo-Garde, 2021).

Since TBI may render patients with or without limited English proficiency unable to provide consent, preoperative discussions with family members may be needed. In a study of family-centered care after pediatric TBI, for example, families with limited English proficiency recalled a variety of acute care communication and coordination challenges (Moore et al., 2015). It is important for care providers to be sensitive to the varied circumstances and needs of their patients.

---

[12] Moore, M. 2021. Disparities in TBI Outcomes. Presentation and panel discussion during virtual workshop for the Committee on Accelerating Progress in Traumatic Brain Injury Research and Care, March 16, 2021.

CONCLUSIONS

It is critically important for clinicians to avoid missing a diagnosis of TBI during acute care evaluation for trauma-related injuries. A missed diagnosis is a missed opportunity to inform patients about recovery from TBI and to provide a referral to inpatient or outpatient rehabilitation or further follow-up. Missed diagnoses also contribute to underestimating the true burden of TBI at the population level. However, an improved classification system for TBI is needed. A TBI taxonomy reduced to "mild, moderate, and severe" is insufficient diagnostically, is of limited value prognostically, and fails to stratify patients adequately into TBI clinical trials.

Patient-centered care during the acute period after a TBI has been sustained needs to achieve an appropriate balance between reducing unwanted variation and enabling the provision of medicine personalized by age, sex, patient preferences, and other factors. However, many patients do not benefit from the best evidence-based care after experiencing a TBI. All patients with TBI should receive guideline-based care, where available. However, guideline, provider, and institutional factors all affect variations in TBI care. Care recommendations and decision tools exist for mild and severe TBI in pediatric and adult populations, but implementation of these guidelines is variable, and the existing guidelines vary significantly with respect to the topics covered, the level of detail, and the criteria for inclusion of studies in evidence syntheses.

A number of additional knowledge gaps and clinical care challenges continue to constrain prompt and accurate diagnosis and management of acute-stage TBI in prehospital and hospital settings. Needs include further incorporating biomarkers and multimodal information in diagnostic and outcome prediction tools to provide greater personalization and improvement in care after TBI; filling evidence gaps in such areas as prehospital stabilization, surgical timing, and optimal management in the context of comorbidities, potential medical interactions, and multiple trauma; and fostering effective information exchange and coordination across the multiple locations and phases of care and among the different specialties involved.

REFERENCES

Aarabi, B., D. Hesdorffer, E. Ahn, C. Aresco, T. Scalea, and H. Eisenberg. 2006. Outcome following decompressive craniectomy for malignant swelling due to severe head injury. *Journal of Neurosurgery* 104(4):469-479.

ACS (American College of Surgeons) Committee on Trauma. 2014. *Resources for optimal care of the injured patient,* 6th ed. https://www.facs.org/-/media/files/quality-programs/trauma/vrc-resources/resources-for-optimal-care.ashx (accessed August 3, 2021).

Allard, C. B., S. Scarpelini, S. Rhind, A. Baker, P. Shek, H. Tien, M. Fernando, L. Tremblay, L. Morrison, R. Pinto, and S. Rizoli. 2009. Abnormal coagulation tests are associated with progression of traumatic intracranial hemorrhage. *Journal of Trauma* 67(5):959-967.

Amyot, F., D. B. Arciniegas, M. P. Brazaitis, K. C. Curley, R. Diaz-Arrastia, A. Gandjbakhche, P. Herscovitch, S. R. Hinds 2nd, G. T. Manley, A. Pacifico, A. Razumovsky, J. Riley, W. Salzer, R. Shih, J. G. Smirniotopoulos, and D. Stocker. 2015. A review of the effectiveness of neuroimaging modalities for the detection of traumatic brain injury. *Journal of Neurotrauma* 32(22):1693-1721.

Badjatia, N., N. Carney, T. Crocco, M. E. Fallat, H. Hennes, A. Jagoda, S. Jernigan, P. Letarte, E. B. Lerner, T. Mortiarty, P. Pons, S. Sasser, T. Scalea, C. Schleien, D. Wright, Brain Trauma Foundation, and BTF Center for Guidelines Management. 2008. *Prehospital Emergency Care* 12(Suppl 1):S1-S52.

Bell, R. S., C. Mossop, M. Dirks, F. Stephens, L. Mulligan, R. Ecker, C. Neal, A. Kumar, T. Tigno, and R. Armonda. 2010. Early decompressive craniectomy for severe penetrating and closed head injury during wartime. *Neurosurgical Focus* 28(5):E1.

Blostein, P., and S. J. Jones. 2003. Identification and evaluation of patients with mild traumatic brain injury: Results of a national survey of level I trauma centers. *Journal of Trauma* 55(3):450-453.

Boto, G., P. Gómez, J. De La Cruz, and R. Lobato. 2006. Severe head injury and the risk of early death. *Journal of Neurology, Neurosurgery, and Psychiatry* 77(9):1054-1059.

Brolliar, S., M. Moore, H. Thompson, L. Whiteside, R. Mink, M. Wainwright, J. Groner, M. Bell, C. Giza, D. Zatzick, R. Ellenbogen, L. Boyle, P. Mitchell, F. Riara, and M. Vavilala. 2016. A qualitative study exploring factor associated with provider adherence to severe pediatric traumatic brain injury guidelines. *Journal of Neurotrauma* 33(16):1554-1560.

Bullock, M. R., R. Chesnut, J. Ghajar, D. Gordon, R. Hartl, D. W. Newell, F. Servadei, B. C. Walters, and J. E. Wilberger. 2006. Guidelines for the Surgical Management of Traumatic Brain Injury. *Neurosurgery* 58(3):S2-vi–S2-3

Carney, N., A. Totten, C. O'Reilly, J. Ullman, G. Hawryluk, M. Bell, S. Bratton, R. Chesnut, O. Harris, N. Kissoon, A. Rubiano, L. Shutter, R. Tasker, M. Vavilala, J. Wilberger, D. Wright, and J. Ghajar. 2017. Guidelines for the management of severe traumatic brain injury, 4th ed. *Neurosurgery* 80(1):6-15.

Cnossen, M. C., J. Huijben, M. van der Jagt, V. Volovici, T. van Essen, S. Polinder, D. Nelson, A. Ercole, N. Stocchetti, G. Citerio, W. Peul, A. Maas, D. Menon, E. Steyerberg, H. Lingsma, and CENTER-TBI investigators. 2017. Variation in monitoring and treatment policies for intracranial hypertension in traumatic brain injury: A survey in 66 neurotrauma centers participating in the CENTER-TBI study. *Critical Care* 21(1):233.

Cnossen, M. C., A. C. Scholten, H. F. Lingsma, A. Synnot, E. Tavender, D. Gantner, F. Lecky, E. W. Steyerberg and S. Polinder. 2021. Adherence to guidelines in adult patients with traumatic brain injury: A living systematic review. *Journal of Neurotrauma* 3(8):1072-1085.

Cook, A. M., A. Peppard, and B. Magnuson. 2008. Nutrition considerations in traumatic brain injury. *Nutrition in Clinical Practice* 23(6):608-620.

Daugherty, J., D. Waltzman, K. Sarmiento, and L. Xu. 2019. Traumatic brain injury–related deaths by race/ethnicity, sex, intent, and mechanism of Injury—United States, 2000-2017. *Morbidity and Mortality Weekly Report* 68:1050-1056.

Davis, D. P., A. Idris, M. Sise, F. Kennedy, A. Eastman, T. Velky, G. Vilke, and D. B. Hoyt. 2006. Early ventilation and outcome in patients with moderate to severe traumatic brain injury. *Critical Care Medicine* 34(4):1202-1208.

DeAngelis, J., V. Lou, T. Li, H. Tran, P. Bremjit, M. McCann, P. Crane, and C. Jones. 2017. Head CT for minor head injury presenting to the emergency department in the era of choosing wisely. *Western Journal of Emergency Medicine* 18(5):821-829.

DeMatteo, C., E. Bednar, S. Randall, and K. Falla. 2020. Effectiveness of return to activity and return to school protocols for children postconcussion: A systematic review. *BMJ Open Sport & Exercise Medicine* 6(1):e000667. https://doi.org/10.1136/bmjsem-2019-000667.

Demetriades, D., L. Chan, E. Cornwell, H. Belzberg, T. Berne, J. Asensio, D. Chan, M. Eckstein, and K. Alo. 1996. Paramedic vs private transportation of trauma patients: Effect on outcome. *Archives of Surgery* 131(2):133-138.

Duncan, K. A., and S. Garijo-Garde. 2021. Sex, genes, and traumatic brain injury (TBI): A call for a gender inclusive approach to the study of TBI in the lab. *Frontiers in Neuroscience* 15:681599.

Echemendia, R. J., W. Meeuwisse, P. McCrory, G. Davis, M. Putukian, J. Leddy, M. Makdissi, et al. 2017. The Sport Concussion Assessment Tool 5th Edition (SCAT5): Background and rationale. *British Journal of Sports Medicine* 51(11):848-850.

Edlow, B. L., and J. J. Fins. 2018. Assessment of covert consciousness in the intensive care unit: Clinical and ethical considerations. *Journal of Head Trauma Rehabilitation* 33(6):424-434.

Fanara, B., C. Manzon, O. Barbot, T. Desmettre, and G. Capellier. 2010. Recommendations for the intra-hospital transport of critically ill patients. *Critical Care* 14(3):R87. https://doi.org/10.1186/cc9018.

Faul, M., M. Wald, W. Rutland-Brown, E. Sullivent, and R. W. Sattin. 2007. Using a cost-benefit analysis to estimate outcomes of a clinical treatment guideline: Testing the Brain Trauma Foundation guidelines for the treatment of severe traumatic brain injury. *Journal of Trauma* 63(6):1271-1278.

Frankel, M., L. Fan, S. D. Yeatts, A. Jeromin, P. E. Vos, A. K. Wagner, B. J. Wolf, et al. 2019. Association of very early serum levels of S100B, glial fibrillary acidic protein, ubiquitin C-terminal hydrolase-L1, and spectrin breakdown product with outcome in ProTECT III. *Journal of Neurotrauma* 36(20):2863-2871.

Fu, T. S., R. Jing, S. McFaull, and M. D. Cusimano. 2015. Recent trends in hospitalization and in-hospital mortality associated with traumatic brain injury in Canada: A nationwide, population-based study. *Journal of Trauma and Acute Care Surgery* 79(3):449-454.

Gardner, R. C., K. Dams-O'Connor, M. Morrissey, and G. T. Manley. 2018. Geriatric traumatic brain injury: Epidemiology, outcomes, knowledge gaps, and future directions. *Journal of Neurotrauma* 35(7):889-906.

Giacino, J. T., D. Katz, N. Schiff, J. Whyte, E. Ashman, S. Ashwal, R. Barbano, F. Hammond, S. Laureys, G. Ling, R. Nakase-Richardson, R. T. Seel, S. Yablon, T. Getchius, G. Gronseth, and M. J. Armstrong. 2018. Practice guideline update recommendations summary: Disorders of consciousness: Report of the Guideline Development, Dissemination, and Implementation Subcommittee of the American Academy of Neurology; the American Congress of Rehabilitation Medicine; and the National Institute on Disability, Independent Living, and Rehabilitation Research. *Neurology* 91(10):450-460.

Gibbs, J., and J. McCord. 2020. Chest pain evaluation in the emergency department: Risk scores and high-sensitivity cardiac troponin. *Current Cardiology Reports* 22:49.

Giza, C. C., M. McCrea, D. Huber, K. L. Cameron, M. N. Houston, J. C. Jackson, G. McGinty, G., et al. 2021. Assessment of blood biomarker profile after acute concussion during combative training among US military cadets: A Prospective study from the NCAA and US Department of Defense CARE Consortium. *JAMA Network Open* 4(2):e2037731.

Gravesteijn, B., C. Aletta Sewalt, D. Nieboer, D. Menon, A. Maas, F. Lecky, M. Klimek, and H. Floor Lingsma. 2020. Tracheal intubation in traumatic brain injury: A multicenter prospective observational study. *British Journal of Anaesthesia* 125(4):505-517.

Haarbauer-Krupa, J., M. Pugh, E. Prager, N. Harmon, J. Wolfe, and K. C. Yaffe. 2021. Epidemiology of chronic effects of traumatic brain injury. *Journal of Neurotrauma* 38(23):3235-3247.

Hawryluk, G., A. Rubiano, A. Totten, C. O'Reilly, J. Ullman, S. Bratton, R. Chesnut, O. Harris, N. Kissoon, L. Shutter, R. Tasker, M. Vavilala, J. Wilberger, D. Wright, A. Lumba-Brown, and J. Ghajar. 2020. Guidelines for the management of severe traumatic brain injury: 2020 update of the decompressive craniectomy recommendations. *Neurosurgery* 87(3):427-434.

Haydel, M., C. Preston, T. Mills, S. Luber, E. Blaudeau, and P. DeBlieux. 2000. Indications for computed tomography in patients with minor head injury. *New England Journal of Medicine* 343(2):100-105.

Hinson, H. E., S. Rowell, and M. Schreiber. 2015. Clinical evidence of inflammation driving secondary brain injury: A systematic review. *Journal of Trauma and Acute Care Surgery* 78(1):184-191.

Horwitz, L. I., T. Meredith, J. Schuur, N. Shah, R. Kulkarni, and G. Y. Jenq. 2009. Dropping the baton: A qualitative analysis of failures during the transition from emergency department to inpatient care. *Annals of Emergency Medicine* 53(6):701-710. https://doi.org/10.1016/j.annemergmed.2008.05.007.

Ingalls, N., D. Zonies, J. Bailey, K. Martin, B. Iddins, P. Carlton, D. Hanseman, R. Branson, W. Dorlac, and J. Johannigman. 2014. A review of the first 10 years of critical care aeromedical transport during Operation Iraqi Freedom and Operation Enduring Freedom: The importance of evacuation timing. *JAMA Surgery* 149(8):807-813.

IOM (Institute of Medicine). 2011. *Clinical practice guidelines we can trust.* Washington, DC: The National Academies Press.

Jagoda, A., J. Bazarian, J. Bruns Jr, S. Cantrill, A. Gean, P. Kunz Howard, J. Ghajar, S. Riggio, D. Wright, R. Wears, A. Bakshy, P. Burgess, M. Wald, R. Whitson, American College of Emergency Physicians, and Centers for Disease Control and Prevention. 2008. Clinical policy: Neuroimaging and decision making in adult mild traumatic brain injury in the acute setting. *Annals of Emergency Medicine* 52(6):714-748.

Joseph, D., R. Dutton, B. Aarabi, and T. Scalea. 2004. Decompressive laparotomy to treat intractable intracranial hypertension after traumatic brain injury. *Journal of Trauma* 57(4):687-693.

Joseph, B., H. Aziz, V. Pandit, N. Kulvatunyou, A. Hashmi, A. Tang, M. Sadoun, T. O'Keeffe, G. Vercruysse, D. J. Green, R. S. Friese, and P. Rhee. 2014. A three-year prospective study of repeat head computed tomography in patients with traumatic brain injury. *Journal of the American College of Surgeons* 219(1):45-51.

Kirsch, T. D., Y. H. Hsieh, L. Horana, S. G. Holtzclaw, M. Silverman, and A. Chanmugam. 2011. Computed tomography scan utilization in emergency departments: A multi-state analysis. *Journal of Emergency Medicine* 41(3):302-309.

Kochanek, P., R. Tasker, N. Crney, A. Totten, P. D. Adelson, N. Selden, C. Davis-O'Reilly, E. Hart, M. Bell, S. Bratton, G. Grant, N. Kissoon, K. Reuter-Rice, M. Vavilala, and M. Wainwright. 2019. Guidelines for the management of pediatric severe traumatic brain injury, third edition: Update of the Brain Trauma Foundation Guidelines. *Pediatric Critical Care Medicine* 20(3S):S1-S82.

Korley, F., G. Kelen, C. Jones, and R. Diaz-Arrastia. 2016. Emergency department evaluation of traumatic brain injury in the. United States, 2009-2010. *Journal of Head Trauma Rehabilitation* 31(6):379-387.

Kuppermann, N., J. Holmes, P. Dayan, J. Hoyle Jr., S. Atabaki, R. Holubkov, F. Nadel, D. Monroe, R. Stanley, D. Borgialli, M. Badawy, J. Schunk, K. Quayle, P. Mahajan, R. Lichenstein, K. Lillis, M. Tunik, E. Jacobs, J. Callahan, M. Gorelick, T. Glass, L. Lee, M. Bachman, A. Cooper, E. Powell, M. Gerardi, K. Melville, J. P. Muizelaar, D. Wisner, S. J. Zuspan, J. M. Dean, S. Wootton-Gorges, and Pediatric Emergency Care Applied Research Network (PECARN). 2009. Identification of children at very low risk of clinically-important brain injuries after head trauma: A prospective cohort study. *Lancet* 374(9696):1160-1170.

Larkin, M. B., E. Graves, J. Boulter, N. Szuflita, R. Meyer, M. Porambo, J. Delaney, and R. Bell. 2018. Two-year mortality and functional outcomes in combat-related penetrating brain injury: Battlefield through rehabilitation. *Neurosurgical Focus* 45(6):E4.

Latifi, R., F. Olldashi, A. Dogjani, E. Dasho, A. Boci, and A. El-Menyar. 2018. Telemedicine for neurotrauma in Albania: Initial results from case series of 146 patients. *World Neurosurgery* 112:e747-e753.

Liu, H., W. Wang, F. Cheng, Q. Yuan, J. Yang, J. Hu, and G. Ren. 2015. External ventricular drains versus intraparenchymal intracranial pressure monitors in traumatic brain injury: A prospective observational study. *World Neurosurgery* 83(5):794-800.

Livergant, R. J., N. Ludlow, and K. A. McBrien. 2021. Needs assessment for the creation of a community of practice in a community health navigator cohort. *BMC Health Services Research* 21(1):657.

Lumba-Brown, A., K. Yeates, K. Sarmiento, M. Breiding, T. Haegerich, G. Gioia, M. Turner, E. Benzel, S. Suskauer, C. Giza, M. Joseph, C. Broomand, B. Weissman, W. Gordon, D. Wright, R. Scolaro Moser, K. McAvoy, L. Ewing-Cobbs, A-C. Duhaime, M. Putukian, B. Holshouser, D. Paulk, S. Wade, S. Herring, M. Halstead, H. Keenan, M. Choe, C. Christian, K. Guskiewicz, P. Raksin, A. Gregory, A. Muha, H. G. Taylor, J. Callahan, J. DeWitt, M. Collins, M. Kirkwood, J. Ragheb, R. Elenbogen, T. Spinks, T. Ganiats, L. Sabelhaus, K. Altenhofen, R Hoffman, T. Getchius, G. Gronseth, Z. Donnell, R. O'Connor, and S. Timmons. 2018. Centers for Disease Control and Prevention guidelines on the diagnosis and management of mild traumatic brain injury among children. *JAMA Pediatrics* 172(11):e182853. https://doi.org/10.1001/jamapediatrics.2018.2853.

Maas, A. I. R., E. Steyerberg, and G. Citerio. 2021. Tranexamic acid in traumatic brain injury: Systematic review and meta-analysis trumps a large clinical trial? *Intensive Care Medicine* 47:74-76.

Maddry, J. K., A. Arana, C. Perez, K. Medellin, J. Paciocco, A. Mora, W. Holder, W. Davis, P. Herson, and V. S. Bebarta. 2020. Influence of time to transport to a higher-level facility on the clinical outcomes of US combat casualties with TBI: A multicenter 7-year study. *Military Medicine* 185(1-2):e138-e145. https://doi.org/10.1093/milmed/usz178.

Marehbian, J., S. Muehlschlegel, B. Edlow, H. Hinson, and D. Y. Hwang. 2017. Medical management of the severe traumatic brain injury patient. *Neurocritical Care* 27(3):430-446.

Martin, T. J., M. Ranney, J. Dorroh, N. Asselin, and I. N. Sarkar. 2018. Health information exchange in emergency medical services. *Applied Clinical Informatics* 9(4):884-891.

Maurin Söderholm, H., H. Andersson, M. Andersson Hagiwara, P. Backlund, J. Bergman, L. Lundberg, and B. A. Sjöqvist. 2019. Research challenges in prehospital care: the need for a simulation-based prehospital research laboratory. *Advances in Simulation* 4:3. https://doi.org/10.1186/s41077-019-0090-0.

McCrea, M. 2001. Standardized mental status testing on the sideline after sport-related concussion. *Journal of Athletic Training* 36(3):274-279.

McCrea, M., S. P. Broglio, T. W. McAllister, J. Gill, C. C. Giza, D. L. Huber, J. Harezlak, et al. 2020. Association of blood biomarkers with acute sport-related concussion in collegiate athletes: Findings from the NCAA and Department of Defense CARE Consortium. *JAMA Network Open* 3(1):e1919771.

McCrea, M. A., J. Giacino, J. Barber, N. Temkin, L. Nelson, H. Levin, S. Dikmen, et al. 2021. Functional outcomes over the first year after moderate to severe traumatic brain injury in the prospective, longitudinal TRACK-TBI study. *JAMA Neurology* 78(8):982-992.

McCrory, P., W. Meeuwisse, J. Dvořák, M. Aubry, J. Bailes, S. Broglio, R. Cantu, et al. 2017. Consensus statement on concussion in sport-the 5th international conference on concussion in sport held in Berlin, October 2016. *British Journal of Sports Medicine* 51(11):838-847.

McMillan, T. M., E. L. Jongen, and R. J. Greenwood. 1996. Assessment of post-traumatic amnesia after severe closed head injury: retrospective or prospective? *Journal of Neurology, Neurosurgery, and Psychiatry* 60(4):422-427.

Moore, M., G. Robinson, R. Mink, K. Hudson, D. Dotolo, T. Gooding, A. Ramirez, D. Zatzick, J. Giordano, D. Crawley, and M. S. Vavilala. 2015. Developing a family-centered care model for critical care after pediatric traumatic brain injury. *Pediatric Critical Care Medicine* 16(8):758-765.

Nampiaparampil, D. E. 2008. Prevalence of chronic pain after traumatic brain injury: A systematic review. *Journal of the American Medical Association* 300(6):711-719.

Narayan, R. K., A. Maas, F. Servadei, B. Skolnick, M. Tillinger, L. Marshall, and Traumatic Intracerebral Hemorrhage Study Group. 2008. Progression of traumatic intracerebral hemorrhage: A prospective observational study. *Journal of Neurotrauma* 25(6):629-639.

NASEM (National Academies of Sciences, Engineering, and Medicine). 2016. *A national trauma care system: Integrating military and civilian trauma systems to achieve zero preventable deaths after injury.* Washington, DC: The National Academies Press.

Natale-Pereira, A., K. Enard, L. Nevarez, and L. A. Jones. 2011. The role of patient navigators in eliminating health disparities. *Cancer* 117(15 Suppl):3543-3552.

Nathanson, M. H., J. Andrzejowski, J. Dinsmore, C. Eynon, K. Ferguson, T. Hooper, A. Kashyap, J. Kendall, V. McCormack, S. Shinde, A. Smith, and E. Thomas. 2020. Guidelines for safe transfer of the brain-injured patient: Trauma and stroke, 2019: Guidelines from the Association of Anaesthetists and the Neuro Anaesthesia and Critical Care Society. *Anaesthesia* 75(2):234-246.

Nelson, L. D., N. R. Temkin, S. Dikmen, J. Barber, J. T. Giacino, E. Yuh, H. S. Levin, et al., 2019. Recovery after mild traumatic brain injury in patients presenting to US level I trauma centers: A Transforming Research and Clinical Knowledge in Traumatic Brain Injury (TRACK-TBI) study. *JAMA Neurology* 76(9):1049-1059.

Okonkwo, D. O., J. K. Yue, A. M. Puccio, D. M. Panczykowski, T. Inoue, P. J. McMahon, M. D. Sorani, E. L. Yuh, H. F. Lingsma, A. I. Maas, A. B. Valadka, G. T. Manley, and Transforming Research and Clinical Knowledge in Traumatic Brain Injury (TRACK-TBI) Investigators. 2013. GFAP-BDP as an acute diagnostic marker in traumatic brain injury: results from the prospective transforming research and clinical knowledge in traumatic brain injury study. *Journal of Neurotrauma* 30(17):1490-1497.

Okonkwo, D. O., R. C. Puffer, A. M. Puccio, E. L. Yuh, J. K. Yue, R. Diaz-Arrastia, F. K. Korley, et al. 2020. Point-of-care platform blood biomarker testing of glial fibrillary acidic protein versus S100 calcium-binding protein B for prediction of traumatic brain injuries: A Transforming Research and Clinical Knowledge in Traumatic Brain Injury Study. *Journal of Neurotrauma* 37(23):2460-2467.

Ontario Neurotrauma Foundation. 2019. *Living guideline for diagnosing and managing pediatric concussion.* https://braininjuryguidelines.org/pediatricconcussion (accessed August 3, 2021).

Orman, J. A., D. Geyer, J. Joes, E. Schneider, J. Grafman, M. Pugh, and J. DuBose. 2012. Epidemiology of moderate to severe penetrating versus closed traumatic brain injury in the Iraq and Afghanistan wars. *Journal of Trauma and Acute Care Surgery* 73(6S):S496-S502.

Papa, L., L. M. Lewis, J. L. Falk, Z. Zhang, S. Silvestri, P. Giordano, G. M. Brophy, J. A. Demery, N. K. Dixit, I. Ferguson, M. C. Liu, J. Mo, L. Akinyi, K. Schmid, S. Mondello, C. S. Robertson, F. C. Tortella, R. L. Hayes, and K. K. Wang. 2012. Elevated levels of serum glial fibrillary acidic protein breakdown products in mild and moderate traumatic brain injury are associated with intracranial lesions and neurosurgical intervention. *Annals of Emergency Medicine* 59(6):471-483.

Pattinson, C. L., T. B. Meier, V. A. Guedes, C. Lai, C. Devoto, T. Haight, S. P. Broglio, et al. 2020. Plasma biomarker concentrations associated with return to sport following sport-related concussion in collegiate athletes: A Concussion Assessment, Research, and Education (CARE) Consortium study. *JAMA Network Open* 3(8):e2013191.

Phillips, C. 2021. *Army announces FDA clearance of field deployable TBI blood test.* https://health.mil/News/Articles/2021/03/12/Army-Announces-FDA-Clearance-of-Field-Deployable-TBI-Blood-Test (accessed September 14, 2021)

Powell, J. M., J. Ferraro, S. Dikmen, N. Temkin, and K. R. Bell. 2008. Accuracy of mild traumatic brain injury diagnosis. *Archives of Physical Medicine and Rehabilitation* 89(8):1550-1555.

Randall, M. J. 2012. Gap analysis: Transition of health care from Department of Defense to Department of Veterans Affairs. *Military Medicine* 177(1):11-16.

Ratcliff, J. J., O. Adeoye, C. J. Lindsell, K. W. Hart, A. Pancioli, J. T. McMullan, J. K. Yue, et al. 2014. ED disposition of the Glasgow Coma Scale 13 to 15 traumatic brain injury patient: Analysis of the Transforming Research and Clinical Knowledge in TBI study. *American Journal of Emergency Medicine* 32(8):844-850.

Raso, M., F. Arcuri, S. Liperoti, L. Mercurio, A. Mauro, F. Cusato, L. Romania, S. Serra, L. Pignolo, P. Tonin, and A. Cerasa. 2021. Telemonitoring of patients with chronic traumatic brain injury: A pilot study. *Frontiers in Neurology* 12:598777.

Reay, G., J. Norris, L. Nowell, K. Hayden, K. Yokom, E. Lang, G. Lazarenko, and J. Abraham. 2020. Transition in care from EMS providers to emergency department nurses: A systematic review. *Prehospital Emergency Care* 24(3):421-433.

Robertson, E. R., L. Morgan, S. Bird, K. Catchpole, and P. McCulloch. 2014. Interventions employed to improve intrahospital handover: A systematic review. *BMJ Quality & Safety* 23(7):600-607.

Rosen, C. B., D. Luy, M. Deane, T. Scalea, and D. Stein. 2018. Routine repeat head CT may not be necessary for patients with mild TBI. *Trauma Surgery & Acute Care Open* 3(1):e000129.

Samadani, U. 2016. When will a clinical trial for traumatic brain injury succeed? *AANS Neurosurgeon* 25(3). https://aansneurosurgeon.org/will-clinical-trial-traumatic-brain-injury-succeed (accessed September 24, 2021).

Sasser, S., R. Hunt, M. Faul, D. Sugerman, W. Pearson, T. Dulski, M. Wad, G. Jurkovich, C. Newgard, E.B. Lerner, and Centers for Disease Control and Prevention. 2012. Guidelines for field triage of injured patients: Recommendations of the National Expert Panel on Field Triage. 2011. *Morbidity and Mortality Weekly Report* 61(RR-1):1-20.

Scalea, T., J. Scott, R. Brumback, A. Burgess, K. Mitchell, J. Kufera, C. Turen, and H. Champion. 1999. Early fracture fixation may be "just fine" after head injury: No difference in central nervous system outcomes. *Journal of Trauma* 46(5):839-846.

Scalea, T., S. Boswell, J. Scott, K. Mitchell, M. Kramer, and A. Pollak. 2000. External fixation as a bridge to intramedullary nailing for patients with multiple injuries and with femur fractures: Damage control orthopedics. *Journal of Trauma* 48(4):613-621.

Schreiber, M. A., E. Meier, S. Tisherman, J. Kerby, C. Newgard, K. Brasel, D. Egan, W. Witham, C. Williams, M. Daya, J. Beeson, B. McCully, S. Wheeler, D. Kannas, S. May, B. McKnight, D. Hoyt, and ROC Investigators. 2015. A controlled resuscitation strategy is feasible and safe in hypotensive trauma patients: results of a prospective randomized pilot trial. *Journal of Trauma and Acute Care Surgery* 78(4):687-697.

Servadei, F., G. Murray, K. Penny, G. Teasdale, M. Dearden, F. Iannotti, F. Lapierre, A. Maas, A. Karimi, J. Ohman, L. Persson, N. Stocchetti, T. Trojanowski, and A. Unterberg, A. 2000. The value of the "worst" computed tomographic scan in clinical studies of moderate and severe head injury. European Brain Injury Consortium. *Neurosurgery* 46(1):70-77.

Shackelford, S. A., D. Del Junco, J. Riesberg, D. Powell, E. Mazuchowski, R. Kotwal, P. Loos, H. Montgomery, M. Remley, J. Gurney, and S. Keenan. 2021. Case-control analysis of prehospital death and prolonged field care survival during recent US military combat operations. *Journal of Trauma and Acute Care Surgery* 91(2S Suppl 2):S186-S193.

Shafi, S., R. Diaz-Arrastia, C. Madden, and L. Gentilello. 2008. Intracranial pressure monitoring in brain-injured patients is associated with worsening of survival. *Journal of Trauma* 64(2):335-340.

Shah, S., G. Yang, D. Le, C. Gerges, J. Wright, A. Parr, J. Cheng, and L. Ngwenya. 2020. Examining the Emergency Medical Treatment an Active Labor Act: Impact on telemedicine for neurotrauma. *Neurosurgical Focus* 49(5):E8. https://doi.org/10.3171/2020.8.FOCUS20587.

Shetty, V. S., M. Reis, J. Aulino, K. Berger, J. Broder, A. Choudhri, A. Kendi, M. Kessler, C. Kirsch, M. Luttrull, L. Mechtler, J. Prall, P. Raksin, C. Roth, A. Sharma, O. West, M. Wintermark, R. Cornelius, and J. Bykowski. 2016. ACR appropriateness criteria head trauma. *Journal of the American College of Radiology* 13(6):668-679.

Skarupa, D. J., M. Khan, A. Hsu, M. Madbak, D. Ebler, B. Yorkitis, G. Rahmatulla, D. Alcindor, and B. Joseph. 2019. Trends in civilian penetrating brain injury: A review of 26,871 patients. *American Journal of Surgery* 218:255-269.

Smith, E. B., J. Lee, M. Vavilala, and S. A. Lee. 2019. Pediatric traumatic brain injury and associated topics: An overview of abusive head trauma, nonaccidental trauma, and sports concussions. *Anesthesiology Clinics* 37(1):119-134.

Spaite, D., B. Bobrow, S. Keim, B. Barnhart, V. Chikani, J. Gaither, D. Sherrill, K. Denninghoff, T. Mullins, P. D. Adelson, A. Rice, C. Viscusi, and C. Hu. 2019. Association of statewide implementation of prehospital traumatic brain injury treatment guidelines with patient survival following traumatic brain injury: The Excellence in Prehospital Injury Care (EPIC) Study. *JAMA Surgery* 154(7):e191152. https://doi.org/10.1001/jamasurg.2019.1152.

Stiell, I. G., G. Wells, K. Vandeemheen C. Clement, H. Lesiuk, A. Laupacis, R. D. McKnight, R. Verbeek, R. Brison, D. Cass, M. Eisenhauer, G. Greenberg, and J. Worthington. 2001. The Canadian CT head rule for patients with minor head injury. *Lancet* 357(9266):1391-1396.

Stiell, A., A. Forster, I. Stiell, and C. van Walraven. 2003. Prevalence of information gaps in the emergency department and the effect on patient outcomes. *Canadian Medical Association Journal* 169(10):1023-1028.

Stocchetti, N., M. Carbonara, G. Citerio, A. Ercole, M. Skrifvars, P. Smielewski, T. Zoerle, and D. Menon. 2017. Severe traumatic brain injury: Targeted management in the intensive care unit. *Lancet Neurology* 16(6):452-464.

Teasdale, G., and B. Jennett. 1974. Assessment of coma and impaired consciousness. A practical scale. *Lancet* 2(7872):81-84.

Teasdale, G., A. Maas, F. Lecky, G. Manley, N. Stocchetti, and G. Murray. 2014. The Glasgow Coma Scale at 40 years: Standing the test of time. *Lancet Neurology* 13(8):844-854.

VA (Department of Veterans Affairs). 2016. *VA/DoD clinical practice guideline for the management of concussion-mild traumatic brain injury*. Department of Defense. https://www.healthquality.va.gov/guidelines/rehab/mtbi/mtbicpgfullcpg50821816.pdf (accessed August 3, 2021).

VA. 2019. *Guideline for Guidelines*. 2019. Department of Defense. Revised January 29, 2019. https://www.healthquality.va.gov/documents/GuidelinesForGuidelinesRevised013019.pdf (accessed August 3, 2021).

Van Cleve, W., M. Kernic, R. Ellenbogen, J. Wang, D. Zatzick, M. Bell, M. Wainwright, J. Groner, R. Mink, C. Giza, L. Boyle, P. Mitchell, F. Rivara, M. Vavilala, and PEGASUS (Pediatric Guideline Adherence and Outcomes) Project. 2013. National variability in intracranial pressure monitoring and craniotomy for children with moderate to severe traumatic brain injury. *Neurosurgery* 73(5):746-752.

Vandromme, M., S. Melton, R. Griffin, G. McGwin, J. Weinberg, M. Minor, L. Rue III, and J. Kerby. 2011. Intubation patterns and outcomes in patients with computer tomography-verified traumatic brain injury. *Journal of Trauma* 71(6):1615-1619.

Vavilala, M. S., M. A. Kernic, J. Wang, N. Kannan, R. Mink, M. Wainwright, J. Groner, M. Bell, C. Giza, D. Zatzick, R. Ellenbogen, L. Boyle, P. Mitchell, F. Rivara, and Pediatric Guideline Adherence and Outcomes Study. 2014. Acute care clinical indicators associated with discharge outcomes in children with severe traumatic brain injury. *Critical Care Medicine* 42(10):2258-2266.

Vella, M. A., M. Crandall, and M. B. Patel. 2017. Acute management of traumatic brain injury. *Surgical Clinics of North America* 97(5):1015-1030.

Wang, K., F. Kobeissy, Z. Shakkour, and J. A. Tyndall. 2021. Thorough overview of ubiquitin C-terminal hydrolase-L1 and glial fibrillary acidic protein as tandem biomarkers recently cleared by US Food and Drug Administration for the evaluation of intracranial injuries among patients with traumatic brain injury. *Acute Medicine & Surgery* 8(1):e622. https://doi.org/10.1002/ams2.622.

Warren, J., R. Fromm Jr., R. Orr, L. Rotello, H. Horst, and American College of Critical Care Medicine. 2004. Guidelines for the inter- and intrahospital transport of critically ill patients. *Critical Care Medicine* 32(1):256-262.

Whiteneck, G. G., J. Cuthbert, J. Corrigan, and J. A. Bogner. 2016. Prevalence of self-reported lifetime history of traumatic brain injury and associated disability: A statewide population-based Survey. *Journal of Head Trauma Rehabilitation* 31(1):E55-E62.

Whiting, D., G. Simpson, F. Deane, S. Chuah, M. Maitz, and J. Weaver. 2021. Protocol for a phase two, parallel three-armed non-inferiority randomized controlled trial of acceptance and commitment therapy (ACT-Adjust) comparing face-to-face and video conferencing delivery to individuals with traumatic brain injury experiencing psychological distress. *Frontiers in Psychology* 12:652323. https://doi.org/10.3389/fpsyg.2021.652323.

Winter, E., A. Hynes, K. Shultz, D. Holena, N. Malhotra, and J. W. Cannon. 2021. Association of police transport with survival among patients with penetrating trauma in Philadelphia, Pennsylvania. *JAMA Network Open* 4(1):e2034868. https://doi.org/10.1001/jamanetworkopen.2020.34868.

Wood, K., R. Crouch, E. Rowland, and C. Pope. 2015. Clinical handovers between prehospital and hospital staff: Literature review. *Emergency Medicine Journal* 32(7):577-581.

Yue, J. K., E. L. Yuh, F. K. Korley, E. A. Winkler, X. Sun, R. C. Puffer, H. Deng, et al. 2019. Association between plasma GFAP concentrations and MRI abnormalities in patients with CT-negative traumatic brain injury in the TRACK-TBI cohort: A prospective multicentre study. *Lancet Neurology* 18(10):953-961.

Yuh, E. L., P. Mukherjee, H. Lingsma, J. Yue, A. Ferguson, W. Gordon, A. Valadka, D. Schnyer, D. Okonkwo, A. Maas, G. Manley, and TRACK-TBI Investigators. 2013. Magnetic resonance imaging improves 3-month outcome prediction in mild traumatic brain injury. *Annals of Neurology* 73(2):224-235.

Yuh, E. L., S. Jain, X. Sun, D. Pisica, M. Harris, S. R. Taylor, A. J. Markowitz, et al. 2021. Pathological computed tomography features associated with incomplete recovery and unfavorable outcome after mild traumatic brain injury: A TRACK-TBI study. *JAMA Neurology* 78(9):1137-1148.

Zuercher M., W. Ummenhofer A. Baltussen, and B. Walder. 2009. The use of Glasgow Coma Scale in injury assessment: A critical review. *Brain Injury* 23:371-384.

6

Rehabilitation and Long-Term Care Needs After Traumatic Brain Injury

Chapter Highlights

- People who experience traumatic brain injury (TBI) may follow multiple care pathways and receive multiple types of interventions to assist them in recovering from the physical, cognitive, emotional, and behavioral consequences of their injuries. Care options include inpatient and/or outpatient rehabilitation, nursing home care, and community-based services. Some people need lifelong care, while others may benefit from periodic follow-up to anticipate factors that could lead to decline.
- Evidence supports the efficacy and cost-effectiveness of TBI rehabilitation. Although many patients with moderate to severe TBI would benefit from comprehensive interdisciplinary inpatient rehabilitation, most are discharged to home or to skilled nursing facilities that may not provide intensive, comprehensive, or specialized therapy and that offer limited opportunities for reevaluation.
- Barriers to accessing comprehensive inpatient rehabilitation include the need for insurance preauthorization, lack of available beds in rehabilitation facilities, location of a facility far from a person's home and family, inconsistent quality of rehabilitation services, and hesitancy on the part of facilities to take patients who may not be able to be discharged home after rehabilitation.
- Lack of access to TBI-informed outpatient physical and mental health services and lack of awareness or resources to address needs among those returning to work and school after TBI can hinder the recovery process for those with less severe TBI.
- TBI affects the families and caregivers of those who experience the injury. Families need culturally competent information on their loved one's injury and likely course of recovery, as well as strategies for reducing burdens commonly reported by families and caregivers. TBI rehabilitation interventions need to prioritize patient-centered outcomes and consider not only the person with injury but also the person's family or caregiver(s).

Once acute interventions have stabilized the condition of a person experiencing traumatic brain injury (TBI) (see Chapter 5), the need for rehabilitation and follow-up services becomes paramount. This chapter begins by identifying target outcomes for people with TBI as they move to post-acute care, rehabilitation, and recovery or long-term care. The chapter describes care pathways and types of care a person may receive during this period. The past decade has seen growing awareness of the longer-term consequences of TBI, including concussion and so-called "mild TBI," along with increasing recognition that persons with TBI can require long-term services and supports. The chapter highlights the needs of persons with TBI, as well as their families and caregivers, in the rehabilitation and recovery process.

Based on current evidence, guidelines, and best practices, the chapter summarizes the features that form part of an optimal system for post-acute and longer-term TBI care. However, the current TBI post-acute care and rehabilitation system is fragmented, is not accessible to many patients, and is not optimally designed to meet the evolving needs of many people with TBI and their families. The chapter concludes by identifying the key gaps that contribute to these challenges and will need to be addressed to improve care and outcomes for TBI patients.

TARGET GOALS AND OUTCOMES OF CARE

When a TBI patient transitions to the post-acute phase of care, clinical outcomes different from those of the acute care phase become important. While the initial focus of TBI care is on sustaining life and minimizing secondary damage to the brain, post-acute care focuses on the optimization of a person's day-to-day function and the ability to return to community living. In addition, treatment during these later phases of care aims to minimize post-TBI complications, the development of adverse sequelae, and negative interactions between the effects of TBI and any comorbidities the person may have.

While evidence indicates that earlier initiation of rehabilitation for TBI results in the greatest improvements in function, even patients who start rehabilitation therapy later after injury can still make tremendous strides in recovery. Box 6-1 conceptualizes target outcomes in the immediate, medium, and long terms after acute care.

BOX 6-1 **TARGET OUTCOMES FOR PERSONS WITH TBI IN THE IMMEDIATE, MEDIUM, AND LONG TERMS**

Immediate (upon discharge from acute rehabilitation)

- Medical stability
- Optimized functional outcome at discharge
- Discharge to community (versus institutional setting)
- Prepared and educated family

Medium (upon discharge from post-acute rehabilitation or during first years postinjury)

- Vocational/avocational activities
- Community participation/integration
- Stable mood

BOX 6-1   CONTINUED

- Family engagement in rehabilitation and recovery
- Supportive relationships with family and friends
- Cognitive function (optimization of cognitive function with awareness of abilities and deficits)
- Continued improvement in function and supports for sustainability of gains (needs for and success of support given, assistive technology, ongoing therapy, and follow-up)
- Sufficient and affordable resources to access needed medical care, interventions, and services
- Self-efficacy and subjective well-being
- Maximized brain health and recovery through healthy behaviors and avoidance of unhealthy behaviors (e.g., risky substance use)
- Economic stability for individual and family

Long-term and chronic (living with TBI)

- Maintained upward or at least stable trajectory (avoiding decline) across all domains (family, partner relationships, medical, functional, etc.)
- Access to needed services and follow-up
- Maintained brain health
- Maintained stable mental health
- Attained self-identified life goals (self-actualization)

CURRENT CARE PATHWAYS AFTER ACUTE TBI CARE

Multiple care pathways are possible after a person experiences a TBI. Ideally, the course of treatment would be based on the initial severity of the TBI and any other sustained injuries, how those injuries developed or changed over time, and how the injuries affected the person's capacity for self-care. The sections below describe the types of facilities that provide rehabilitation and longer-term care after the acute phase of care (see Chapter 5).

Overview of Civilian and Military Care Pathways

For civilians, the care pathway experienced by TBI patients is strongly influenced by whether they underwent an initial hospital-based evaluation. For those who start their care pathway with hospital-based treatment, acute rehabilitative services may begin within 24–72 hours of injury. Subsequent stages of the journey can involve referrals to different types of care facilities, including additional inpatient rehabilitation, outpatient rehabilitation, nursing homes, and residential care facilities (see Box 6-2). Patients with severe injuries may be referred to a long-term acute care hospital or to inpatient rehabilitation followed by support services that allow them to return to the home environment, and/or may be transferred to a nursing home or residential care facility. Meanwhile, patients returning to home may receive further in-home or outpatient rehabilitation with physician follow-up. For those who start their care pathway without hospital-based treatment, the type and extent of follow-up are highly variable. Some individuals with TBI may never see a health care provider for evalu-

---

BOX 6-2   SELECTED TYPES OF CARE FACILITIES FOR PATIENTS WITH TBI

A variety of facilities provide inpatient support should a person with TBI require ongoing levels of care after discharge from an acute hospital stay. A long-term acute care hospital (LTACH) may be required if the patient is stable enough not to require an intensive care unit (ICU) but requires hospital-level clinical care for longer than can generally be provided by a regular hospital—often on a timeline of several weeks rather than several days of hospital-based care. A comprehensive inpatient rehabilitation facility (IRF) (and some LTACHs) provides the patient with intensive and tailored rehabilitation, including 3 hours per day of occupational and/or physical therapy, plus speech therapy or prosthetics/orthotics. A rehabilitation physician oversees the stay and meets with the patient at least three times per week. The interdisciplinary team meets at least weekly and includes a case manager and/or social worker and a rehabilitation nurse. Patients may also receive care in alternative types of subacute, transitional, or skilled nursing settings. For example, a skilled nursing facility (SNF) provides continuing medical support at a less intensive level than that offered by a hospital and may also provide therapy, though not at the level available through specialized IRFs. Notably, the Centers for Medicare & Medicaid Services' (CMS's) Patient-Driven Payment Model, implemented in 2019, was associated with a 30 percent decrease in therapy provided each day in SNFs, from approximately 1.5 hours to 1 hour per day.*

Care facilities providing rehabilitation and longer-term care and services for TBI patients are frequently accredited by the Commission on Accreditation of Rehabilitation Facilities (CARF), an independent, nonprofit organization that publishes quality standards for business and service practices and that operates an accreditation process through which providers and programs can demonstrate conformance with such practices. The Brain Injury Specialty Program accreditation is reserved for systems of care that provide interdisciplinary services to address the unique needs of patients with acquired brain injury. These facilities must demonstrate the use of rehabilitation methods based on current evidence and provide patient- and family-centered care within an integrated system designed to maximize recovery and community reintegration. The integrated system may include components—comprehensive integrated inpatient rehabilitation, outpatient medical rehabilitation, home and community services, residential rehabilitation services, and vocational services—that in nonspecialized settings could be individually accredited. Persons with substantial deficits that preclude return to home may benefit from a residential rehabilitation program, which typically provides rehabilitation over a longer period of time to achieve goals related to community integration, regulation of behavior and social relations, and productive activity.

---

* See https://medicareadvocacy.org/cms-confirms-steep-decline-in-therapy-at-nursing-facilities (accessed August 17, 2021).
SOURCES: CARF International and 2020 Medical Rehabilitation Program Descriptions, http://www.carf.org and http://www.carf.org/Programs/Medical (accessed August 17, 2021). Centers for Medicare & Medicaid Services, *Place of Service Code Set*, https://www.cms.gov/Medicare/Coding/place-of-service-codes/Place_of_Service_Code_Set (accessed August 17, 2021).

---

ation of their injury, while others may be evaluated and referred for additional post-TBI rehabilitation or follow-up.

In the military, the Joint Trauma System (JTS) organizes and delivers trauma care. For service members who experience a TBI in combat theater, there are five levels or "roles" of care, each with progressively greater resources and capabilities: on-site treatment by initial field responders (role 1), surgical resuscitation by forward emergency medical care teams (role 2), treatment at combat support hospitals (role 3), and off-theater evacuation to definitive care facilities (roles 4 and 5).[1] Unique challenges faced by military trauma services include

---

[1] Lee, K. 2021. System Challenges for TBI Care. Panel discussion during virtual workshop for the Committee on Accelerating Progress in Traumatic Brain Injury Research and Care, March 30, 2021.

the frequency of blast-related injuries, the likelihood of patients having severe multisystem injuries (multitrauma), the complexity of providing care in a combat environment, and the provision of care that can be discontinuous across locations and time as service members are transferred across JTS roles rather than being housed within a single trauma center (NASEM, 2016). Post-acute and rehabilitative services for service members and Veterans with TBI are provided through Department of Veterans Affairs (VA) centers.

Even with these differences, the civilian and military care pathways for the post-acute and recovery stages after TBI encompass a generally similar range of inpatient and outpatient care settings and potential types of rehabilitation interventions. However, access to care may vary between the two systems. Veterans with TBI are able to access care through the VA Polytrauma System of Care, whereas in the private sector, civilians may experience substantial care gaps and difficulty accessing rehabilitation services (discussed later in this chapter).

Care Pathways for Persons with TBI Who Are Able to Care for Themselves at Discharge from Acute Care

The return home after brain injury can be complex. Many individuals look forward to continuing their recovery in a familiar, comforting, and secure environment near their loved ones (BIAUSA, 2021). Individuals who are discharged home after acute care for TBI may receive a recommendation to follow up with a brain trauma clinic or their primary care provider. Targeted rehabilitation may include cognitive rehabilitation, speech-language pathology services, physical or occupational therapy, vestibular and oculomotor rehabilitation, cervical strain treatment, treatments for specific symptoms (e.g., persistent dizziness), and psychotherapy for mental health concerns.

Although many people with concussion and "mild TBI" may recover fully without rehabilitation, others would benefit from receiving post-acute care. In 2019, the Ontario Neurotrauma Foundation issued Standards for High Quality Post-Concussion Services and Concussion Clinics to inform patients, families, and care providers (ONF, 2017a). The Post-Concussion Care Pathway described by the Foundation suggests that about 55 percent of patients who experience a concussion will improve toward recovery within 1–2 weeks; about 30 percent will experience symptoms that resolve over a longer period; and about 15–20 percent will experience persisting symptoms that require longer-term, interdisciplinary management (ONF, 2017b).

In pockets of the country, these patients may have access to evidence-based, comprehensive concussion management programs that provide specialized rehabilitation and recovery services, such as comprehensive assessment by a coordinating health care provider, symptom monitoring and neuropsychological assessment, referral for multidisciplinary rehabilitation tailored to individual needs, and treatment of comorbidities that affect progress (Bailey et al., 2019; Ellis et al., 2018). The timing of the services is important. Several studies have found that earlier evaluation and access to specialized care after sports-related concussion improves recovery (Desai et al., 2019; Kontos et al., 2020; Master et al., 2020). And while biological sex differences in concussion injury and recovery have been reported, research also indicates that "sex-based differences in recovery disappeared when controlling for time to presentation to specialty care" (Desai et al., 2019, p. 361). This finding suggests that the timing of rehabilitation treatment is a strong factor in recovery—the earlier, the better.

Although specialized concussion centers improve functional outcomes for those patients who need them, these facilities are not available in all areas of the country, and the field of concussion care is not highly regulated. The emergence of private concussion clinics over the past decade has been described by some as a "Wild West" (see, e.g., Crowe, 2016). The interventions these clinics offer are not standardized, and not all interventions provided to patients have demonstrated efficacy. For example, a 2017 study of the websites of concussion care providers found that "there are few concussion healthcare providers or clinics with access to the complete complement of multidisciplinary professionals required to meet the diverse needs of concussion patients … [and] providers are offering a diverse number of services to concussion patients, some of which are provided by experts with suboptimal training and some that have a limited base of supportive evidence" (Ellis et al., 2017, p. 4).

Care Pathways for Persons with TBI Who Do Not Achieve Independent Functioning Prior to Discharge from Acute Care

For patients who cannot return home safely after post-acute care, transfer to a care setting that provides interdisciplinary comprehensive inpatient rehabilitation is most beneficial (DaVanzo et al., 2014; Nehra et al. 2016). For some patients with complex medical needs, an intermediate stepdown setting may be required before admission to comprehensive rehabilitation. For example, the setting may provide care through a Commission on Accreditation of Rehabilitation Facilities (CARF)-accredited brain injury specialty program designed to meet the complex needs of the patient with TBI. Medicare patients with medical necessity who can tolerate 3 hours of therapy per day or 15 hours per week are eligible for admission to an inpatient rehabilitation facility (IRF), where most CARF-accredited programs are located.[2] Long-term acute care hospitals (LTACHs) and residential rehabilitation facilities with brain injury specialty designations are also available in some areas for those patients who require longer lengths of stay, as well as interdisciplinary rehabilitation (see Box 6-2).

However, only about 13–25 percent of patients who survive moderate, severe, or penetrating TBI receive comprehensive, interdisciplinary inpatient rehabilitation, and even fewer receive TBI-specialized rehabilitation care (Corrigan et al., 2012). Instead, patients are often discharged to home, where they may or may not receive home health services, or to skilled nursing facilities (SNFs) that do not provide intensive, comprehensive, or specialized therapy and that often limit physician visits to as infrequently as once per month. Acute care hospitals need to open up patient beds as quickly as possible, and may discharge a patient to an alternative care facility with relatively less substantial requirements for preauthorization or prescreening,[3] such as an SNF, or to home, expecting the patient's family to provide care.

Factors affecting the discharge of people with moderate to severe TBI to inpatient rehabilitation, to home, or to care settings such as nursing homes include the severity of injury; such characteristics as age, sex, and race/ethnicity; and payment source (Cuthbert et al., 2011). Injury severity factors play primary roles in decisions to discharge to home, while such sociobiologic and socioeconomic factors as age and race affect decisions to discharge to rehabilitation rather than to sub-acute care. The impact on outcomes for those who do not receive inpatient rehabilitation for TBI has not been sufficiently studied; however, a well-controlled comparison of persons with stroke who received rehabilitation at an IRF versus a

---

[2] Medicare coverage requirements for care in an IRF are described at https://www.cms.gov/Medicare/Medicare-Fee-for-Service-Payment/InpatientRehabFacPPS/Coverage (accessed August 25, 2021). The Complete List of IRF Clarifications for the Coverage Requirements linked from the website states, "the generally accepted standard by which the intensity of these services is typically demonstrated in inpatient rehabilitation facilities (IRFs) is by the provision of intensive therapies at least 3 hours per day at least 5 days per week" (p. 26), while recognizing the possibility of meeting the requirement in other ways. See https://www.cms.gov/Medicare/Medicare-Fee-for-Service-Payment/InpatientRehabFacPPS/Downloads/Complete-List-of-IRF-Clarifications-Final-Document.pdf (accessed August 25, 2021).

[3] Hammond, F. 2021. TBI Care Gaps and Opportunities: Provider Perspectives on the Post-Acute Continuum of Care. Panel discussion during virtual workshop for the Committee on Accelerating Progress in Traumatic Brain Injury Research and Care, March 18, 2021.

SNF found better outcomes for the IRF (Hong et al. 2019). Taken together, this evidence suggests an important role for high-quality inpatient rehabilitation after moderate to severe TBI.

Whichever care pathway patients follow, the expectation is that they will ultimately return home. Many will continue to require comprehensive interdisciplinary rehabilitation on an outpatient basis to maintain and expand the gains observed in inpatient rehabilitation. In addition, persons living with more severe TBI often have continuing lifetime needs, such as assistance with return to work, assistance with self-care, accessible housing, and treatment of mental health disorders. Unfortunately, for most patients, TBI-informed care and assistance drop off over time. Families rarely report any source of ongoing support, especially after the first year following TBI.[4]

Access to Post-Acute Care and Services

Health insurance coverage is a major determinant of whether a person with TBI receives rehabilitative services. Unlike acute clinical care, rehabilitation services generally require prior authorization by the health insurance payer. During its information-gathering sessions, the committee heard from patients and families, patient advocacy organizations, and care providers that patients and families often must advocate with insurance companies for coverage of TBI rehabilitation and post-acute care.

Acute care teams encounter multiple barriers when attempting to discharge a person with TBI to a comprehensive, interdisciplinary inpatient rehabilitation facility. Physicians and case managers may lack awareness of the differences in quality of care and outcomes across different types of post-acute care facilities, and therefore can be limited in their ability to address these barriers and secure an optimal discharge disposition for the person. Barriers include the following:

- Securing preauthorization for comprehensive inpatient rehabilitation can sometimes take several days (days that could be used to serve other acute care patients). Even when preauthorization is not required, a preadmission screening may need to be conducted with review by a rehabilitation physician to ensure that the person meets requirements for admission. These requirements are more stringent than those for discharge to SNFs.
- Rehabilitation facilities often require assurance that the individual can be discharged home after rehabilitation. The ability to discharge to home helps ensure that the facility will receive the full federal prospective payment for Medicare patients (lump sum payment per discharge); however, making that prognostication prior to the start of rehabilitation may not be possible. When it is not possible to discharge home, provisions for a per diem payment are in place.
- Patients' families may be reluctant to have them sent to rehabilitation facilities that may be far from their home. Comprehensive inpatient rehabilitation facilities are usually located in urban centers, which could be several hours away from an individual's home (and may not even be in the same state). Some families lack access to transportation from such a distance.
- Other factors that affect access to evidence-based TBI rehabilitation include such social determinants of health as age, sex, and race/ethnicity. A lack of diversity in

---

[4] Sander, A. 2021. Family Impacts from TBI and Engagement in TBI Care. Panel discussion during virtual workshop for the Committee on Accelerating Progress in Traumatic Brain Injury Research and Care, March 16, 2021.

the field of physical medicine and rehabilitation and a general lack of cultural competence may also undermine the trust of patients from diverse backgrounds.

- Finally, the length of stay in inpatient rehabilitation facilities is typically short, with pressure to move patients out of the program or to sub-acute care facilities.[5]

Individuals who are active duty service members or Veterans may have easier access to a more comprehensive system of post-acute care relative to civilians. A number of key features of the VA's Polytrauma System of Care that support high-quality, evidence-based rehabilitation and functional recovery after TBI are highlighted in Chapter 7. However, another major barrier to accessing rehabilitation is the so-called "3-hour rule." The "3-hour rule"—a Centers for Medicare & Medicaid Services (CMS) practice that requires that patients have sufficient energy and endurance to engage actively in occupational, speech, or physical therapy for 3 hours per day, 5 days per week (or 15 hours per week). Most insurers will cover comprehensive inpatient rehabilitative services for a patient only if this "3-hour rule" is met (Forrest et al., 2019). While exceptions may be possible, most private insurers and the VA consider this metric when authorizing rehabilitation services. Meanwhile, admission to sub-acute rehabilitation at an SNF does not come with this requirement. In response to the lengthier preapproval process for inpatient rehabilitation and because they may need to vacate space for new incoming patients, acute care facilities may opt to discharge their TBI patients to an SNF rather than to a comprehensive inpatient rehabilitation program, even when the patient might have benefited from the latter. This practice constrains access to and coverage for specialized, comprehensive interdisciplinary rehabilitation care that is generally available only at IRFs (and some LTACHs).

Limited evidence supports use of a fixed "3-hour rule" in determining eligibility for rehabilitation. Beaulieu and colleagues (2019) found that the "level of effort" made by TBI patients undergoing inpatient rehabilitation had a positive effect on outcomes, but that compliance with the 3-hour policy did not. Another study found that "patients whose care was consistent with the rule did not have more improvement in function or shorter length of stay than patients whose care was not consistent with the 3-hour rule" (Forrest et al., 2019, p. 1). In sum, widespread use of the "3-hour rule" as a requirement for payer coverage of comprehensive interdisciplinary rehabilitation programs is a significant barrier to care for patients who have difficulty meeting this requirement at the time of evaluation, but may nonetheless experience improved functional outcomes as a result of this intervention.

Types of Rehabilitation Interventions

Persons with TBI experience a variety of new or persisting symptoms, and multiple interventions may be provided to address their cognitive, sensory, behavioral, and physical difficulties and support their recovery. The process of preparing a person with TBI to return to independent functioning often begins in the acute care setting, and the use of practice guidelines and standardization along all phases of the care continuum is receiving increased emphasis (see Box 6-3). Such guidelines aid therapists in homing in on specific treatment components to better support the individual patient's recovery. It is increasingly recognized that rehabilitation should start with asking patients what matters to them. In addition to addressing the patient's symptoms and health conditions, care is enhanced by asking ques-

[5] Esquenazi, A. 2021. TBI Care Gaps and Opportunities: Provider Perspectives on the Post-Acute Continuum of Care. Panel discussion during virtual workshop for the Committee on Accelerating Progress in Traumatic Brain Injury Research and Care, March 18, 2021.

BOX 6-3   GUIDELINES INFORMING REHABILITATION CARE FOR TBI

A number of clinical guidelines summarize the state of evidence and provide recommenda-tions regarding the use of rehabilitation interventions during recovery from TBI. The importance and impact of rehabilitation for patients with TBI in the acute care setting is well established and is incorporated in the American College of Surgeons' (ACS's) Committee on Trauma guide *Resources for Optimal Care of the Injured Patient,* which states "the rehabilitation of injured patients should begin the first hospital day" (ACS, 2014, p. 88). The ACS recommendations encompass trauma centers located in various settings and providing various levels of trauma care (Level I, II, and III facilities). The recommendations cover care initiation; recommended services and their frequency; policies regarding transfers, including requirements related to rehabilitation transfer agreements; and goals of rehabilitation in this setting, stating, for example:

> In Level I and II trauma centers, rehabilitation services must be available within the hospital's physical facilities or as a freestanding rehabilitation hospital, in which case the hospital must have transfer agree-ments (CD 12-1). In any case, a clear understanding of rehabilitation capabilities should be incorporated into the trauma program. Rehabilitation needs in the critical care unit are sometimes overlooked. Rehabilitation consultation services, occupational therapy, speech therapy, physical therapy, and social services are often needed in the critical care phase and must be available in Level I and II trauma cen-ters.... Policies for proper transfer into a rehabilitation facility and proper follow-up after discharge from the rehabilitation facility should be a component of all trauma programs. (ACS, 2014, p. 92)

A number of additional guidelines address post-acute care and recovery from TBI. Examples include the following:

- American Academy of Neurology's *Practice Guideline Update: Disorders of Consciousness* (Giacino et al., 2018)
- American Congress of Rehabilitation Medicine's *Cognitive Rehabilitation Manual: Translating Evidence-Based Recommendations into Practice* (Haskins et al., 2012)
- *INCOG Guidelines for Cognitive Rehabilitation Following Traumatic Brain Injury* (Bayley et al., 2014)
- Ontario Neurotrauma Foundation and Institut National d'Excellence en Santé et en Services Sociaux's *Clinical Practice Guideline for the Rehabilitation of Adults with Moderate to Severe TBI* (INESSS-ONF, 2015)
- Ontario Neurotrauma Foundation's *Guideline for Concussion/Mild Traumatic Brain Injury & Prolonged Symptoms, 3rd Edition, for Adults Over 18 Years of Age* (ONF, 2018)
- Ontario Neurotrauma Foundation's *Living Guideline for Diagnosing and Managing Pediatric Concussion* (ONF, n.d.)
- Department of Veterans Affairs (VA)/Department of Defense (DoD) *VA/DoD Clinical Practice Guideline for the Management and Rehabilitation of Post-Acute Mild Traumatic Brain Injury* (VA, 2021)

---

tions regarding personal goals and other non-health-related objectives. Functional training that is patient-centered and context-relevant is thought to be most likely to engage the patient and facilitate generalization to the home setting (Bogner et al., 2019b).

Examples of the variety of therapies and interventions provided after TBI are briefly described below. As noted, functional rehabilitation after TBI needs to be patient-centered and relevant to the person's context, and rehabilitation clinicians combine components of treatment into strategies designed to address the person's specific functional needs. Guides such as the *Manual for Rehabilitation Treatment Specification* (Hart et al., 2018) provide advice on the targets, mechanisms of action, and design of rehabilitation treatment programs for patients.[6]

Overall, many questions remain regarding which patients will benefit from which rehabilitation interventions and when and how to use them to optimize outcomes. Research in this area has been hampered by inconsistencies in definitions of injury severity, limited durations of follow-up, and the heterogeneity of TBI. Patients may also receive multiple types of therapies, making it challenging to assess the effects of any one type of intervention. Assessments of progress need to consider not only how a person is improving at a certain task in the therapy setting, but also whether the person is acquiring strategies that can be applied to contexts that are most relevant to that individual's daily settings. For example, people with more subtle effects from mild TBI may realize a need for services when they reencounter complex tasks requiring high levels of executive functioning or multitasking as part of daily living.[7] As advances in tools and knowledge are achieved, translating this knowledge rapidly and broadly beyond the research arena remains a challenge.

Rehabilitation Therapies

Examples of therapies for persons recovering from TBI are listed below. As with so many aspects of TBI care, whether patients receive a particular type of treatment and for how long on average they receive it per week are variable.

- *Cognitive rehabilitation therapy* focuses on restoring cognitive function through interventions or tools designed to improve memory, focus, and other cognitive skills. Neuropsychological assessments can be used to identify treatment targets and strengths that can be leveraged to optimize function.
- *Speech-language therapy* aims to treat difficulties with communication and language, including reading, speaking, and pragmatic communication, as well as other challenges involving movement of the tongue, mouth, and throat, such as difficulty swallowing.
- *Physical therapy* is focused on improving movement, reducing pain, and otherwise managing issues associated with mobility, balance, gait, and strength, including use of assistive devices such as canes and wheelchairs.
- *Occupational therapy* is directed at increasing a person's ability to participate in everyday activities, including such activities of daily living as grooming and dressing; to engage in meaningful activities; and to reintegrate within the community.
- *Vocational rehabilitation* provides services to facilitate a person's ability to work or return to work, and can include such services as training and job coaching. *Supported employment* can also be used to assist a person with significant disabilities in holding or maintaining employment to the maximum extent of their abilities.
- *Psychotherapy* and *behavior therapy* assist with cognitive, emotional, behavioral, and social-environmental challenges or barriers to community participation and adjustment to disability.

[6] Frey, K., Y. Goverover, K. McCulloch, T. Pogoda, and D. Porcello. 2021. Accelerating Progress in Traumatic Brain Injury Research and Care: Webinar on Rehabilitation Care and Research, June 15, 2021.
[7] Ibid.

Symptom Management

No Food and Drug Administration (FDA)-approved pharmaceutical treatments are available for TBI recovery; however, care can be aimed at mitigating or managing symptoms and addressing modifiable factors associated with TBI sequelae, including sleep, pain, nutrition, and mental health. A significant proportion of people with TBI—including 30–70 percent of people who experience a "mild TBI"—experience sleep disturbances (Viola-Saltzman and Watson, 2012). For these patients, "good sleep hygiene," use of medications for insomnia, treatments to reduce sleep apnea, and other interventions may be used during recovery. Significant numbers of people with TBI also report headaches, pain, dizziness, and other concerns that may be mitigated with medication, as well as nonpharmaceutical approaches. Modifying or structuring the person's environment and implementing new cognitive strategies are examples of strategies that can be used to help accommodate some types of post-TBI symptoms.

Interactions with Physiological Systems

A noted previously, TBI patients frequently experience multisystem trauma, complicating their treatment requirements. Because the brain and central nervous system play important roles in other body systems, TBI can lead to metabolic and endocrine dysfunction (Li and Sirko, 2018). Apart from the effects of other injuries, brain injury causes inflammation, and the duration of post-TBI inflammation and its effects on brain and body functions continue to be investigated (Irvine and Clark, 2018; Schimmel et al., 2017). Drugs that have anti-inflammatory properties or modulate inflammatory responses may prove useful and are being investigated as well (Begemann et al., 2020). The brain and central nervous system also communicate with cells in the gut (the "gut–brain axis"). The gut microbiome is an important source of neurotransmitters, but little is known about how this relates to brain function in TBI (Opeyemi et al., 2021).

Complementary and Integrative Health Approaches

VA-approved whole-health complementary and integrative approaches for treatment of health and well-being issues for Veterans include acupuncture, biofeedback, clinical hypnosis, and massage therapy, while approved approaches for well-being include meditation, guided imagery, Tai Chi, Qigong, and yoga.[8] A current area of focused analysis of the outcomes of these approaches has been chronic pain, including its impact on opioid use and mental health challenges, such as depression. Evaluation of the potential benefits of such whole-health interventions for patients with TBI may be a focus area for future research.

Self-Help and Empowerment

Patients can benefit from guidance on what to expect in the future and advice on such pragmatic questions as when they will be able to drive again and when to seek further assistance should sequelae develop or change. Enhancing self-efficacy while the person is in the hospital and supporting the person's ability to self-advocate may improve near- and long-term outcomes (Hawley et al., 2021).

---

[8] A complete list of VA Health Services Research and Development studies on these approaches can be found at https://www.hsrd.research.va.gov/cyberseminars/catalog-archive.cfm?#Archived.

Family and Caregiver Involvement in Rehabilitation

Research, albeit limited, suggests that family engagement in rehabilitation is associated with better patient outcomes. For example, one study found that "family involvement during inpatient rehabilitation may improve community participation and cognitive functioning up to 9 months after discharge" (Bogner et al., 2019a, p. 1801). In this sample of 1,835 patients during a first-time inpatient TBI rehabilitation stay, patients whose family members attended at least 10 percent of therapy sessions were significantly more engaged in their communities at 3 and 9 months after discharge compared with those whose families attended less than 10 percent of sessions. Although not meeting statistical significance in all analyses, improved cognitive functioning at 9 months was associated with increased family attendance. The benefits of family involvement were echoed in a qualitative study of 20 TBI survivors in Denmark, who described the importance of family involvement in their TBI care and reported that family support was crucial to their recovery in terms of navigating the health care system and coordinating rehabilitation (Graff et al., 2018). According to these studies, patient and family/caregiver engagement is at the heart of care that transitions patients successfully back into society.

New Types of Therapies and Interventions

New treatment approaches supporting rehabilitation and recovery after TBI continue to be explored. Increasing evidence supports the use of such therapies as vestibular and vision therapy and earlier initiation of heart-rate-targeted exercise in managing concussion (Leddy et al., 2018; Mucha et al., 2018). Repetitive transcranial magnetic stimulation (rTMS) is being investigated for its potential to reduce posttraumatic depression and cognitive deficits. Current evidence in support of rTMS is based primarily on studies with rats, however, and the limited human studies have shown mixed results (Nardone et al., 2020). Research has also investigated the use of rTMS to reduce such symptoms as headache, overall pain, depressive symptoms, and problems with executive function following mild to severe TBI, with mixed results (Anderson et al., 2020). Few studies have examined outcomes beyond 6 weeks, and they did not find significant differences from controls. Other neuromodulation therapies under study for treatment after TBI include transcranial direct current stimulation, epidural electrical cortical stimulation, and deep brain stimulation (Hofer and Schwab, 2019).

Discharge Planning and Communication with Patients and Their Families and Caregivers

The sequelae of TBI can have a profound impact not only on the injured person but also on the person's family and caregivers. It is estimated that 5.3 million people in the United States live with brain injury–related disabilities,[9] and that 2.5 million military and civilian families and caregivers are caring for a person with TBI (Malec et al., 2017). Family members and caregivers of persons with TBI have been described both as "hidden victims" because they report significant stress and burden, and as the "hidden heroes" of TBI because the support and care they provide is critical for their loved ones (Ramchand et al., 2014).

Planning for discharge and for longer-term TBI management needs to begin in advance of the person's return home, with close involvement of the family and caregivers. Patients requiring inpatient care often remain hospitalized for only a few weeks, and this may not be

---

[9] See https://www.cdc.gov/traumaticbraininjury/pubs/tbi_report_to_congress.html (accessed August 30, 2021).

sufficient time to educate patients and their families/caregivers about the experiences they will face after returning home. Care organizations and providers thus need to pay attention to the importance of communication with all individuals involved to prepare them for postdischarge care needs. Some health systems offer support groups for families/caregivers while patients are in the hospital, but in many cases, there is no streamlined continuation of support postdischarge. A variety of educational materials and resources have been published to help persons with TBI and their families and caregivers understand the injury, the potential course of recovery, and longer-term management of the condition (see Box 6-4).

Not all patients and families may be aware of the available high-quality resources; some may have difficulty accessing them online, or materials may not be available in multiple languages. More than half of participants in one survey of people with TBI and their families reported not receiving sufficient information on the nature and consequences of the injuries (Biester et al., 2016). Culturally resonant messaging about care trajectories, potential complications, and resources are also lacking. Data are currently limited on which dissemination strategies can best achieve the goal of educating and empowering patients and families with respect to the care needed upon discharge, and their preferences for consumption of information remain largely unknown.

LONG-TERM AND COMMUNITY-BASED SERVICES

After discharge from health care settings, persons with TBI and their families commonly need access to a variety of services, depending on the nature of the injury and anticipated longer-term functional outcomes.

BOX 6-4   **EXAMPLES OF EDUCATIONAL MATERIALS AND RESOURCES ON TBI**

Selected examples of available resources include the following:

- *Traumatic Brain Injury: A Guide for Caregivers of Service Members and Veterans, Back to School: Guide to Academic Success After Traumatic Brain Injury,* and other resources published by the military's Traumatic Brain Injury Center of Excellence (https://www.health.mil/Military-Health-Topics/Centers-of-Excellence/Traumatic-Brain-Injury-Center-of-Excellence/Patient-and-Family-Resources)
- National Brain Injury Information Center from the Brain Injury Association of America (BIAA), a staffed helpline, extensive website materials and FAQs (https://www.biausa.org), and such resources as *Moderate to Severe Brain Injury: A Practical Guide for Families* (https://shop.biausa.org/product/LWBIPG18/moderate-to-severe-brain-injury-a-practical-guide-for-families)
- *Caregiver Journey Map* from the Elizabeth Dole Foundation, the Department of Veterans Affairs, Philips, and the Wounded Warrior Project (https://caregiverjourney.elizabethdolefoundation.org/about)
- HEADS UP initiative and website from the Centers for Disease Control and Prevention, with information on symptoms of and recovery from concussion, including returning to school and to sports (https://www.cdc.gov/headsup)
- WETA-TV website, Brainline.org, a multimedia site that promotes education and awareness about brain injury (https://www.brainline.org)

NOTE: Accessed January 24, 2022.

Follow-Up and Services via Telehealth

Telehealth encompasses the use of technology, telecommunications, and information systems to support long-distance assessment and clinical care of patients (Mashima and Doarn, 2008; ONC, 2021). This evolving mode of care includes use of the telephone, email, videoconferencing, web-based platforms, mobile health apps, wearable sensors, virtual reality, and other technologies.

Telerehabilitation for any individual needs to be practical, motivational, feasible, and structured (De Luca et al., 2020). It provides a mechanism for addressing problems with communication and social interaction outside the rehabilitation environment; evaluating the everyday-life context; recognizing long-term negative outcomes and functional limitations of depression, social isolation, and unemployment; and providing efficient service delivery in particular for individuals from underserved populations (De Luca et al., 2020; Turkstra et al., 2012).

Several studies with small samples have evaluated the feasibility of using telehealth for *assessment* of persons with TBI. For example, telephone-administered cognitive testing was found to be feasible, efficient, and useful for persons with moderate to severe TBI at 1 and 2 years postinjury (Dams-O'Connor et al., 2018), while videoconferences were found to be equivalent to in-person recordings (in all but one dimension) for assessing conversational participation among people with TBI (Rietdijk et al., 2020). Similarly, Turkstra and colleagues (2012) found no significant differences in a comparison of in-person and teleconference assessments of discourse ability, supporting the use of telehealth for such assessment. Another study found that ecological momentary assessment (EMA) using smartphones was able to capture mood-related symptoms following TBI (Juengst et al., 2015).

Other studies have supported the feasibility of telehealth for *rehabilitation* of persons with TBI. Tsaousides and colleagues (2014) demonstrated the feasibility of delivering group therapy by videoconferencing to improve emotion regulation in persons with TBI. Ng and colleagues (2013) found it feasible to deliver the cognitive orientation to daily occupational performance (CO-OP) approach, a metacognitive intervention, via videoconferencing to adults with TBI, and observed trends toward increased community integration and fewer symptoms of cognitive dysfunction with its use. And a study by De Luca and colleagues (2020) supports the feasibility and usability of a virtual reality rehabilitation system for cognitive rehabilitation for patients with severe TBI and their caregivers during the patient's hospitalization, suggesting its potential therapeutic use at home.

Larger studies using more rigorous designs are beginning to build evidence for the efficacy of telehealth for persons with TBI. A review of studies published between January 1980 and April 2017 testing the efficacy of telerehabilitation yielded 13 eligible studies—10 randomized controlled trials (RCTs) and 3 pre-post group studies (Ownsworth et al., 2018). Although efficacy results were mixed, 4 of 5 RCTs comparing telephone-based interventions with usual care showed positive effects. Further rigorous research will be essential to better understand the effect of various telehealth interventions on rehabilitation care and outcomes.

Providing services via telehealth offers a number of advantages. Telehealth can increase access to care and reduce disparities in access to rehabilitation (WHO, 2015) for persons with TBI who live in rural areas, are geographically distant from rehabilitation services, or experience barriers to care related to social determinants of health. Furthermore, telerehabilitation services show evolving promise in facilitating access to specialized TBI follow-up and neurorestorative services in the home and community-based settings. Care for military service members ranging from acute management of TBI through recovery and rehabilitation currently incorporates telehealth modalities to extend subspecialty consultation to more remote sites and ensure high-quality standardized care.[10] Telemedicine systems within the VA provide monitoring and care for military Veterans isolated not only by geography but also by poverty and disability (Girard, 2007). In-home VA telehealth services result in decreased hospitalizations, emergency department visits, and lengths of hospital stays (Darkins, 2006). Varied VA and military telehealth services for patients with TBI are being used to assist in assessments, improve care coordination between remote sites, provide teleconsultation for medical management, deliver telerehabilitation, and offer training to patients and providers (Girard, 2007).

During the COVID-19 pandemic, expanded use of telehealth for civilians and Veterans offered an alternative to traditional in-person clinical visits for persons with TBI and other neuropsychological conditions (Wells et al., 2021). The accelerated adoption of telehealth during the pandemic demonstrates the platform's ability to expand access, reach more locations, improve interdisciplinary collaboration, and customize patient-centered care (Matsumoto et al., 2021). Continued CMS and private insurance coverage of telehealth services for civilians with TBI may be critical to supporting such expanded access longer-term.

Telehealth also has the potential to support family caregivers of persons with TBI; however, telehealth research involving caregivers is limited. In one RCT, an individualized education and problem-solving intervention delivered by telephone to caregivers of persons with moderate to severe TBI was compared with usual care (Powell et al., 2016). Caregivers in the telehealth group showed improved outcomes, particularly in emotional well-being, compared with the usual-care group at 6 months after discharge of the patient to the community. A review of published studies between 1999 and 2019 on telehealth interventions for caregivers of persons with TBI (nine RCTs and three quasi-experimental studies) found that more than half showed positive caregiver outcomes. However, study samples included little racial diversity, limiting the generalizability of results. Further development and evaluation of telehealth interventions to support the well-being of family caregivers with the inclusion of more diverse samples is an important direction for future research.

Accommodations and Further Community Services After TBI

As part of their reintegration into the community, many TBI survivors return to workplaces and schools that hire and teach persons who have experienced TBI and that may need to provide accommodations for them. Despite the large burden of TBI in the population, however, employers have no direct communication with health systems to learn about TBI, and there is no uniform requirement for workplaces, schools, social and community services organizations, or primary health care providers to undergo continued education around this injury. For children, many states do not require return-to-learn planning analogous to the return-to-play laws that have been enacted by all 50 U.S. states, and youth concussion laws in some states that include this requirement apply only to student athletes.[11] Several

---

[10] Personal communication from Francis L. McVeigh, Office of the Surgeon General, U.S. Army Medical Command, Gary L. Legault, Brook Army Medical Center, and Amy O. Bowles, Brooke Army Medical Center to Eric Schoomaker, November 23, 2021.

[11] See The Network for Public Health Law. Summary Matrix of State Laws Addressing Concussions in Youth Sports (https://www.networkforphl.org/wp-content/uploads/2019/11/Summary-of-State-Laws-Addressing-Concussions-in-Youth-Sports-5-28-19.pdf [accessed November 14, 2021]); National Conference of State Legislatures. "Return-to-Learn" State Laws for Students with Traumatic Brain Injuries (https://www.ncsl.org/research/health/-return-to-learn-state-laws-for-students-with-traumatic-brain-injuries.aspx [accessed November 14, 2021]); and Centers for Disease Control and Prevention. HEADS UP: Sports concussion policies and laws (https://www.cdc.gov/headsup/policy/index.html [accessed August 17, 2021]).

states have return-to-learn programs that are not mandated by law, and individual schools or school systems may incorporate procedures for students returning to academics after TBI, but these efforts are variable (Howland et al., 2021; Thompson et al., 2016). This variability in TBI awareness among school and work systems means that TBI recovery needs are not uniformly met within and by these systems.

For people with TBI and their families, other important community-based services might include vocational support, financial assistance, housing assistance, mental health or substance abuse treatment, or other services that support recovery and return to functioning. Supported employment and other vocational rehabilitation services, where available, can help a person with disability from TBI obtain or maintain employment, and such supported employment has demonstrated a return on investment in a limited number of studies (Fure et al., 2021). Other services include day programs and respite care to assist primary caregivers of persons with TBI.

People with TBI and their families who have the most serious needs may require long-term services and supports (LTSS) for months, years, or even their lifetime (see below). These supports are intended to assist recipients and their caregivers in performing tasks they are unable to accomplish on their own, including self-care (e.g., dressing, medication management), home care (e.g., housekeeping), and transportation.

Funding and infrastructure for post-TBI rehabilitation and community services vary widely by state, and the need for services to help patients and families meet long-term needs after TBI is not well addressed in many areas of the country. Even when some services are available in communities, persons with brain injury and their families may be unaware of them, be unable to access them, or find them not suitable without accommodations for cognitive and physical deficits.

The Long-Term Services and Supports Program

The range of state-provided services for persons with physical disabilities (including persons with TBI), older adults, and family caregivers is evaluated by the LTSS State Scorecard (Reinard et al., 2020). Eligibility criteria, coverage, and the services provided vary by state. The scorecard series started in 2011 as a means of measuring states' performance and providing data for informed policy making. State LTSS systems are evaluated based on (1) affordability and access, (2) choice of setting and provider, (3) quality of life and quality of care, (4) support for family caregivers, and (5) effective transitions. The 2020 scorecard indicated that "state performance remained largely flat across most of the indicators" (p. 16) at a time when demographic trends suggest that the demand for LTSS is increasing. Importantly, persons with TBI living in states with higher LTSS rankings have reported greater community participation and life satisfaction after individual-level differences and outcome fluctuation over time have been taken into account (Corrigan et al., 2021).

LTSS can be provided through Medicaid home- and community-based services (HCBS) waivers enabling people to receive services covered by Medicaid in their home or community rather than in an institutional setting. States request HCBS waivers from CMS. The waivers are generally designed for adult patients with limited financial resources who need the equivalent of inpatient or institutional-level services. While some states already use HCBS waivers to provide services to persons living with TBI and/or spinal cord injury, this use of these waivers is not universal. According to a recent report, fewer than 25,000 people with TBI were receiving LTSS through brain injury waivers in 2018, a figure representing less than 1 percent of persons living with disability due to TBI (Vaughn, 2018). States could explore further adapting existing HCBS waivers to the needs of persons living with TBI to address their chronic symptoms though education from TBI specialists and use of cognitive and physical accommodations.

Some states have access to additional funding for LTSS for persons with TBI through federal and state sources. Under the Traumatic Brain Injury Act, states can apply for grants to improve access to rehabilitation and community services. About 16 states have consistently secured these grants. Some states include line items in their state budgets, and some have developed trust funds generated from motor vehicle– or alcohol-related offenses (Vaughn, 2018). The funds available through these avenues and their uses vary greatly by state.

LONG-TERM CARE FOR TBI AS A CHRONIC CONDITION

The past decade has seen a shift from the assumption that persons with TBI achieve a life-long plateau following an initial period of recovery to recognition of the reality, first identified by Masel and Dewitt (2010), that a substantial portion of individuals experience late effects and evolving status. In some cases, patients experience recovery that is greater than initially expected, while in other cases, patients experience decline. As reported by Whiteneck and colleagues (2018, p. 5), "almost half of individuals experienced a change in their cognitive function between 1 and 5 years post-injury, with 24% improving and 24% declining." Long-term outcome studies of persons with moderate to severe TBI have similarly shown that about one-third decline after previously reaching a plateau (Corrigan and Hammond, 2013).

Functional decline and increased risk of later mortality have been observed after moderate to severe TBI, while findings after mild TBI appear to be sample dependent and possibly associated with preexisting lifestyle factors (Wilson et al., 2017). However, evidence suggests that even a single TBI can increase the risk for subsequent neurodegenerative disorders and stroke (Postupna et al., 2021; Smith et al., 2021). In addition, "injury to the brain can evolve into a lifelong health condition termed chronic brain injury (CBI). CBI impairs the brain and other organ systems and may persist or progress over an individual's lifespan. CBI must be identified and proactively managed as a lifelong condition to improve health, independent function and participation in society" (Corrigan and Hammond, 2013, p. 1199[12]). Recommendations from a consensus conference on this issue included the need for a disease management approach; further studies to identify those at greatest risk for decline; self-management training, including encouraging healthy behaviors; and periodic resumption of rehabilitation (Corrigan and Hammond, 2013).

Applying Models for Long-Term Care Coordination and Management of Chronic Conditions to TBI

The Chronic Care Model (CCM), a widely accepted model for the lifelong management of medical conditions, has been applied extensively to patients and their families experiencing such illnesses as diabetes and heart failure (Malec et al., 2013). Originally described by Wagner and colleagues (1999), the CCM frames the management of chronic medical conditions as a dynamic, interactive process whereby health system and community resources interact at the system and provider levels to support patient self-management and improve outcomes. When applied to TBI care, a model that incorporates long-term care for TBI as a chronic condition can inform the organization of health care system components, such as delivery system design, decision support, and clinical information systems. A key facet of

---

[12] Quoting from the 2012 Galveston Brain Injury Conference; see https://www.utmb.edu/cerpan/moody-prize/consensus (accessed September 27, 2021).

chronic care management is its focus on fostering productive, sustained working relationships between informed, activated patients and prepared, proactive providers.

Models for chronic care management aim to transform the approach to care for people living with chronic conditions from one that is case-specific and reactive to one that is population-based, planned, and proactive (Coleman et al., 2009). This ethos is well suited for application to patients with TBI, who often require active self-management or management by a caregiver while navigating a multitude of ongoing interactions with providers and payers within the health care system (Giacino et al., 2016). Application of chronic care management could also spur the needed transition in TBI practice toward consistent treatment of brain injury as a chronic condition. Broad application of chronic care management to TBI could help catalyze the development and implementation of a structured and comprehensive system for brain injury management to guide more effective assessment and treatment of patients across the continuum of care (Malec et al., 2013). Based on evidence of its benefit when applied to other chronic conditions, chronic care management has the potential to improve patients' quality of life, as well as providers' satisfaction, while reducing costs (Coleman et al., 2009). In addition to forging strong patient–provider relationships, applying chronic care management promotes integration and communication between providers and the community at large. This benefit could be of particular importance for persons with TBI, as many cognitive, behavioral, and emotional issues associated with brain injury affect communities through social and vocational vectors.

Despite the potential of chronic care management models to improve the health and well-being of people with TBI, however, their implementation would require establishing the necessary infrastructure and further developing the TBI knowledge base. Key knowledge gaps include the need to better understand long-term impairments and comorbidities associated with TBI, identify risk and protective factors, develop protocols for early detection and patient self-management, and prioritize evidence-based treatments (Corrigan and Hammond, 2013; Giacino et al., 2016). The authors of a study comparing application of chronic care management to cancer survivorship, diabetes management, and chronic TBI care concluded that a separate chronic care management model is needed to address the needs of and resources required by TBI survivors and their family caregivers (Heiden and Caldwell, 2018).

Some efforts are already under way to develop and implement chronic care management for TBI. In Canada, researchers are developing a Chronic Care Model for Neurological Conditions to improve the quality of care and enhance well-being for people with neurological conditions, including severe brain injury (Jaglal et al., 2014). A TBI Model Systems collaborative project led by Indiana University—BeHEALTHY Chronic Disease Management for TBI—is developing a chronic care management approach to support patients with TBI, their caregivers, and their health care providers.[13] The program aims to produce new knowledge to address evidence gaps in the management of brain injury as a chronic condition.

Although additional research is needed to test the components of a chronic care management model that are most effective for persons with TBI, the committee identified certain features that could be applied. These features include agencies and organizations utilizing collaborative care and integrated care models to optimize mental health outcomes and facilitate behavior change, along with providing person-centered case management and ongoing health care monitoring to persons with TBI experiencing significant sequelae. Such care is necessary to ensure that health needs and the social determinants of health are addressed, thereby optimizing recovery and minimizing the development of new or worsening sequelae. Other elements to support a chronic care management model for TBI include state policies

---

[13] See https://medicine.iu.edu/physiatry/research/behealthy (accessed December 10, 2021).

and resources to ensure that LTSS are available to all persons living with the effects of TBI, and the inclusion in medical and nursing school curricula—and respective board examinations—of modules on screening for lifetime exposure to TBI, recognition of TBI-related sequelae, and TBI management. Finally, a chronic care management model for TBI needs to engage social service agencies, which can screen for lifetime exposure to TBI in their intake processes, and social services providers, who need to receive training on providing accommodations for the sequelae of TBI.

The Role of Care Management

Navigating the complex and fragmented landscape of longer-term health and community services is daunting for people with TBI and their families and caregivers. Patient-centered case managers or care navigators can reduce this barrier by providing patients and families with valuable assistance in accessing care, and by educating providers in how to adapt their services to the unique needs of the person with TBI. A health care provider with expertise in the needs of persons with TBI can also continue to provide long-term follow-up for emerging needs. Unfortunately, many persons living with TBI and their families lack access to either a person-centered case manager or a provider who can offer ongoing follow-up care. Box 6-5 describes an example developed in the context of dementia to illustrate how this type of role might function for TBI. A study is currently examining the effectiveness for TBI patients and their families of a standard discharge plan compared with a plan providing follow-up and care management (by phone or video) from a TBI care manager for 6 months and 1 year after discharge (Fann et al., 2021). The investigators' hypothesis is that improving the transition from inpatient to outpatient care will support better results for patients and families.

Resource facilitation models have also been developed for persons with TBI, and a variety of terms have been used to describe programs aimed at addressing this need. Resource facilitation connects persons with TBI with services and supports to assist in their recovery and reintegration. Such programs draw on a resource facilitator to assist the person and family in identifying and navigating resources and in problem solving, as well as a team of

---

BOX 6-5   THE CARE ECOSYSTEM MODEL

The Care Ecosystem Model was developed in the context of dementia care. A multidisciplinary team of care providers is available to the patient–caregiver dyad, while a care team navigator plays the lead role in communicating with and supporting the patient and caregiver on such topics as reviewing medications, managing behaviors, offering advice regarding caregiving, and providing assistance around decision making. Demonstrated benefits of the approach include improved caregiver well-being, better patient quality of life, and reduced emergency visits. Isolated populations and groups of lower socioeconomic status reportedly have experienced the most profound improvements from the care team navigator approach, and use of a similar model may provide an opportunity for improving TBI patient and caregiver outcomes.

SOURCES: Possin et al., 2019; Miller, B., Comparative Systems of Care: Lessons from Other Disease Systems. Presentation and panel discussion during the virtual workshop on Accelerating Progress in Traumatic Brain Injury Research and Care, March 30, 2021.

rehabilitation specialists. Trexler and colleagues (2010) conducted one of the first RCTs of the effectiveness of a resource facilitation program for TBI, which demonstrated improved return to work for participants receiving this support.

ADDRESSING NEEDS OF SPECIFIC TBI POPULATIONS

TBI in Children and Adolescents

In pediatric TBI patients, coordinated long-term follow-up care is essential to maximize functional outcomes. Evidence has shown that children with moderate to severe TBI have improved long-term outcomes if they receive treatment from pediatric trauma centers, management by specialists, and active early rehabilitation (Fuentes et al., 2016; Potoka et al., 2000). As a result, access to these specialized services becomes paramount (CDC, 2018). However disparities in access to these services exist with regard to insurance and community settings. Uninsured children and children in rural locales have poorer access and worse subsequent outcomes (Greene et al., 2014; Haarbauer-Krupa et al., 2017; Lishner et al., 1996). Rural patients are also at greater risk for more dangerous, higher-energy mechanisms of injury with associated greater trauma and TBI severity compared with their urban counterparts (Yue et al., 2020). These factors, coupled with less access to pediatric trauma centers and postinjury specialist and mental health resources, result in higher health care costs and poorer outcomes in this context.

Attention to academic and school needs is an important focus for pediatric TBI, as most children with moderate to severe TBI and many with mild TBI require academic support and accommodation after injury (Hartman et al., 2015). While services including early intervention, special education, and academic support are technically legally available to children with TBI through a Section 504 plan, many patients and families experience challenges in obtaining this support (Glang et al., 2008; Haarbauer-Krupa, 2012). And even with this support, many patients and families find that educators lack training in how best to support children in the academic setting after injury (Ettel et al., 2016). Legislation mandating identification and removal from play in cases of concussion[14] and a standardized plan for return to play involving medical supervision has led to systematic improvement in the diagnosis and management of sport-related concussion and standardized return-to-play protocols (Bell et al., 2019; McCrory et al., 2017). Attention to the return to academics after concussion has lagged somewhat behind return to play, but awareness of the impact of concussion on academics is increasing, with progress made in terms of expert recommendations on how best to support students returning to school (Gioia, 2016; Halstead et al., 2013; Rose et al., 2015). During testimony at its public sessions, the committee heard that coordination between medical providers and schools is key to ensuring that children and adolescents with TBI can meet educational requirements during the recovery process.[15]

TBI in Older Adults

The increase in the aging population in the United States and the prevalence of TBI in this demographic group have led to growing recognition of TBI as an important issue for older adults (Flanagan et al., 2005; Peters, 2020). Yet the effects of age on recovery from TBI

---

[14] See National Conference of State Legislatures. Traumatic Brain Injury Legislation https://www.ncsl.org/research/health/traumatic-brain-injury-legislation.aspx (accessed March 3, 2022).

[15] Brandt, L., S. Hamilton, K. Primeau, A. Purser, and K. Swift. 2021. Patient Experiences with TBI Systems of Care. Panel discussion during virtual workshop for the Committee on Accelerating Progress in Traumatic Brain Injury Research and Care, March 16, 2021.

remain understudied, and clinical guidelines for care of elderly people with TBI are underdeveloped (Stein et al., 2018). For example, Gardner and colleagues (2018, p. 890) found that "despite the large and growing epidemic of older adults with incident TBI, there are few to no evidence-based geriatric TBI guidelines to inform complex medical decisions for ether acute or long-term management."

Of particular concern is the number of TBIs occurring in older adults as a result of falls. According to the Centers for Disease Control and Prevention (CDC), falls are the leading cause of TBI (51 percent) for older adults. Age-related changes, such as frailty, balance problems, joint problems, medical comorbidities, and medications, can increase fall risk (Cefalu, 2011). In addition, changes in the brain occur with aging (Gardner et al., 2018). Distinguishing between mild cognitive impairment due to aging and cognitive effects arising from a mild TBI can be challenging,[16] while underserved seniors can reportedly also be "misdiagnosed as having dementia and are deemed not candidates for intensive rehabilitation."[17] Pain is common in older adults with TBI as well (Kornblith et al., 2020).

Rehabilitation for TBI in older adults warrants approaches that distinguish it from standard rehabilitation (Narapareddy et al., 2019; Peters, 2016; Stein et al., 2018). A longer time period is often needed to accommodate a slower trajectory of improvement. Maintenance rehabilitation may also be required to sustain functioning over time (Stein et al., 2018). However, long-term longitudinal studies of rehabilitation in later life are generally lacking (Griesbach et al., 2018). Most research has been cross-sectional, with individuals of different ages being compared (Narapareddy et al., 2019), an approach that limits the ability to identify causative factors that could be modified.

A number of other knowledge gaps exist with regard to care and outcomes after TBI in older adults. Examining the unique features related to geriatric TBI could enable the development of new intervention methods or more effective implementation of existing methods. Questions to be addressed include the following:

- The relationship of changes that take place in the aging brain to TBI outcomes (Griesbach et al., 2018). Experiencing a TBI is a risk factor for the development of neurodegenerative diseases, such as dementia. However, further investigation of this risk is needed.[18] Studies of the connection between TBI and dementia are difficult, as such studies generally rely on self-recall of remote events or require longitudinal designs for a prolonged period.
- Identification and validation of biomarkers in older patients (Gardner et al., 2018). Studies may exclude elderly populations because of potentially different pathology or comorbidities that increasingly are observed in older samples. Few biomarker studies have examined differential biomarker profiles based on age and other factors, including comorbidities and common medications. Another key issue is the greater overlap with stroke pathology in older samples, as well as difficulty in diagnosing a TBI using computed tomography (CT) in older individuals.
- Understanding the role of preexisting conditions in TBI outcomes. Many earlier TBI studies failed to include patients with preexisting conditions, a gap that leads to the

---

[16] Frey, K., Y. Goverover, K. McCulloch, T. Pogoda, and D. Porcello. 2021. Accelerating Progress in Traumatic Brain Injury Research and Care: Webinar on Rehabilitation Care and Research, June 15, 2021.

[17] Connors, S. 2021. Family Impacts from TBI and Engagement in TBI Care. Panel discussion during virtual workshop for the Committee on Accelerating Progress in Traumatic Brain Injury Research and Care, March 16, 2021.

[18] Miller, B. 2021. Comparative Systems of Care: Lessons from Other Disease Systems. Presentation and panel discussion during virtual workshop for the Committee on Accelerating Progress in Traumatic Brain Injury Research and Care, March 30, 2021.

exclusion of older adults, decreases the generalizability of findings to this population (Peters and Gardner, 2018), and makes it impossible to identify factors that contribute to differential outcomes based on older age. In a recent review, Gardner and colleagues (2018) conclude that few studies have examined the role of preexisting comorbidities in TBI outcomes in older adults, and few have evaluated the role of pre-TBI functional status in predicting TBI outcomes.

• Understanding "mild TBI" in older adults. Compared with the number of studies of functional outcomes in all-severity or moderate to severe TBI, functional outcomes in in older adults with mild TBI have received little attention (Gardner et al., 2018). Diagnosis of mild TBI in older individuals may also be impeded by a lack of clear reporting by the patient or attribution to other factors, such as blood pressure and cognitive issues. Therefore, the actual prevalence of this condition in older adults may be higher than known, and may result in more morbidity than previously estimated.

Persons with Disorders of Consciousness

A severe TBI can result in disorders of consciousness (DOC), including coma, vegetative state, and minimally conscious state. Patients with severe TBI may not display signs of consciousness until 4–8 weeks postinjury (Giacino et al., 2020). For a sample of patients unable to follow commands at admission to rehabilitation, two-thirds were following commands by discharge from rehabilitation, and by 5 years, independent functioning ranged from 56 percent to 85 percent, depending on the functional domain (Whyte et al., 2013). Among patients who were unable to follow commands by rehabilitation discharge, independence at 5 years ranged from 19 percent to 36 percent, depending on functional domain (Whyte et al., 2013). An additional 31–69 percent were able to participate in a functional task by 5 years even if they were not fully independent. For patients who are minimally conscious, "rehabilitation during the first 6 months after traumatic brain injury may increase the chances of improving outcomes" (AAPM&R, 2021, para. 8). These results highlight the possibility of meaningful functional progress over time even in patients who experience very severe TBI.[19] Unfortunately, once discharged, a patient is unlikely to be evaluated again, despite research showing that recovery is a long-term process. Prognostication for persons who experience severe TBI and DOC needs to be improved. Patient heterogeneity and spontaneous recovery need to be better addressed, and more long-term outcome studies are needed as well. Once patients are medically stable, however, they are discharged from acute care to institutions, including sub-acute rehabilitation facilities and SNFs, that have little or no research infrastructure, as well as to home, which makes meeting these research needs challenging.

Models for care that is age- and ability-appropriate and long-term need to be developed for patients who experience DOC. Greater provider awareness of the possibility of better long-term prognosis than traditionally considered is an important need as well. One type of alternative care model could entail temporarily referring all TBI patients with DOC to intensive multidisciplinary rehabilitation programs for expert evaluation and prognostic assessment, followed by treatment plan recommendations that might include continued rehabilitation at an IRF or LTACH or an alternative pathway of care.

---

[19] Giacino, J., R. Nakase-Richardson, and J. Whyte. 2021. Disorders of Consciousness After Traumatic Brain Injury: A Virtual Workshop for the Committee on Accelerating Progress in Traumatic Brain Injury Research and Care, May 24, 2021.

In 2018, the American Academy of Neurology; the American Congress of Rehabilitation Medicine; and the National Institute on Disability, Independent Living, and Rehabilitation Research released a new guideline on caring for patients with DOC (Giacino et al., 2018). And in 2019, the Neurocritcal Care Society launched the Curing Coma Campaign to raise awareness of needs among this patient population and develop new treatment strategies (Provencio et al., 2020).

A variety of therapies—pharmacologic, neuromodulation, mechanical, and sensory—exist for persons with prolonged DOC (Edlow et al., 2021). The potential utility of regenerative (e.g., cell-based) therapies is also being explored (Cox, 2018). Studies of central nervous system and deep brain stimulation in patients with prolonged DOC have been promising, but many have had small sample sizes or limited rigor, and it is challenging to compare studies that used different time points, stimulation regimens, treatment durations, and other variables. RCTs have found that participants in minimally conscious states, but not participants in vegetative or unresponsive wakefulness states, show increased consciousness with use of the noninvasive neuromodulation method of transcranial direct current stimulation (tDCS) (Zaninotto et al., 2019). Other forms of neuromodulation have also been tested, including transcranial magnetic stimulation (TMS) and stimulation of the peripheral vagus nerve. Some moderate, transient adverse effects, as well as a potential increase in the risk of seizure, have been noted for noninvasive stimulation (Matsumoto and Ugawa, 2016; Oberman et al., 2020; Stultz et al., 2020).

Knowledge gaps remain for all forms of therapy for patients with DOC. Elements needed to fill these gaps include a conceptual framework for better understanding mechanisms of action and the identification of biomarkers for detecting subclinical effects in early-phase trials. Research needs identified as part of the Curing Coma Campaign include (Hammond et al., 2021)

- identifying meaningful and patient-centered outcomes and milestones for different patient groups based on biological features, treatment response, outcome probability, premorbid characteristics of the individual's health, biology, and other factors;
- improving prognostic accuracy through use of big data and identifying the best ways to communicate prognosis and its uncertainty in a culturally sensitive manner; and
- determining which health care delivery models will maximize recovery.

UNMET FAMILY AND CAREGIVER BURDENS

When people with TBI live with their families, as most do, family members often experience psychological distress, especially depression, and high levels of caregiver burden (Dillahunt-Aspillaga et al., 2013; Moriarty et al., 2016; Stevens et al., 2012). In one study, for example, 45 percent of family members of Veterans with TBI reported clinically significant levels of depressive symptoms (Moriarty et al., 2018). In addition to depression, family members may experience anxiety (Kreutzer et al., 1994, 2009; Nabors et al., 2002; Ponsford et al., 2003; Riley, 2007), social isolation (Marsh et al. 1998a,b, 2002; Romano, 1974), caregiver burden (Knight et al., 1998; Kreutzer et al., 1994; Marsh et al., 1998a), diminished quality of life (Verhaeghe et al., 2005), worse perceived health (McPherson et al., 2000), and financial distress (Riley, 2007). TBI also contributes to dysfunction and conflict in families (Bay et al. 2012; Ergh et al., 2002; Groom et al. 1998; Kreutzer et al. 1994), as well as communication (Tyerman and Booth, 2001) and marital problems (Peters et al., 1990). Family members often report that behavioral and emotional changes are the most difficult TBI-related symptoms for them (Ergh et al., 2002). These changes may cause family members to experience ambiguous loss—their loved one with TBI is alive, but the person they knew has been lost (Boss, 2005; Landau and Hissett, 2008). As one family member expressed it, "[he] was not the man that I had sent off to war, it was not the man who loved his children and loved being with them."[20]

Research has often focused on family caregivers of civilians with TBI, but research centered on family caregivers of Veterans with TBI is increasing (e.g., Griffin et al., 2017; Moriarty et al., 2016; Shepherd-Banigan et al., 2018; Winter and Moriarty, 2017). Family members of Veterans with TBI may be more vulnerable to caregiver stress relative to civilian families because stress from multiple and lengthy deployments had preceded the Veteran's return home (Dausch and Saliman, 2009; Stevens et al., 2017). In addition, Veterans with TBI often have other conditions, such as posttraumatic stress disorder (PTSD), depression, pain, and polytrauma, that may increase the family's vulnerability to stress (Hoge et al., 2008; Nampiaparampil, 2008; Tanielian et al., 2008).

A number of studies have shed light on the needs of families of TBI survivors. Family members have identified many unmet needs, particularly for emotional and instrumental support (Kreitzer et al., 2018; Norup et al., 2015). Family caregivers have frequently reported becoming socially isolated and being left on their own to support their loved ones with TBI and themselves.[21] The heavy toll imposed by the caregiving role may lead to family disintegration, with loss of this major source of support for the person with TBI (Kolakowsky-Hayner et al., 2001). The "emotion work" described by family care partners of Veterans with TBI encompasses "creating a new 'normal,'" "keeping things calm," and suppressing their emotions "to put on a brave face" (Abraham et al., 2021, p. 27). This intangible and often invisible work is typically not appreciated by others. Acknowledging and supporting family members around emotion work is an important and new direction for future practice and research. Family members also often struggle with high levels of burden from caregiving demands (Baker et al., 2017). In a scoping review of 21 intervention studies for TBI caregivers, Baker and colleagues (2017) concluded that interventions targeting family coping skills and functioning reduced the burden of care.

Recognizing TBI as a family affair, literature has underscored the need for interventions for both patient and family (Boschen et al., 2007; Foster et al., 2012; Kolakowsky-Hayner et al., 2001; Moriarty et al., 2016; Stejskal, 2012). However, a limited number of studies have evaluated family-inclusive interventions using rigorous methodology, and few evidence-based practice models that consider the needs of both patient and family have been identified as best treatments (Boschen et al., 2007; Verhaeghe et al., 2005). Although some interventions for TBI caregivers show promise, more research is needed to demonstrate their effectiveness in improving caregivers' mental health and quality of life, as well as outcomes for the person living with TBI.[22]

In their review, Boschen and colleagues (2007) identify only four intervention studies designed to reduce caregiver distress and conclude that no evidence exists to support the usefulness of any one psychosocial intervention for family caregivers of persons with TBI. A later review article (Kreitzer et al., 2018) concludes that few rigorous intervention studies have included the person with TBI and a family member or solely a family member. In one RCT with family caregivers of persons with TBI, Rivera and colleagues (2008) evaluated the impact of problem-solving training (PST) delivered through four in-home sessions and eight telephone sessions over 1 year and informed by cognitive-behavioral therapy. Compared with

---

[20] Rotenberry, E. 2021. Family Impacts from TBI and Engagement in TBI Care. Panel discussion during virtual workshop for the Committee on Accelerating Progress in Traumatic Brain Injury Research and Care, March 16, 2021.

[21] Sander, A. 2021. Family Impacts from TBI and Engagement in TBI Care. Panel discussion during virtual workshop for the Committee on Accelerating Progress in Traumatic Brain Injury Research and Care, March 16, 2021.

[22] Ibid.

caregivers in the education-only control group, family caregivers in the PST group reported significant decreases in depression, health complaints, and dysfunctional problem-solving style but no significant change in burden.

In another RCT, Backhaus and colleagues (2010) examined the effect of a 12-session cognitive-behavioral intervention that delivered psychoeducation, supportive psychotherapy, stress management, and problem-solving strategies for 20 persons with acquired or traumatic brain injury and their 20 respective family caregivers. Intervention participants showed a significant increase in perceived self-efficacy immediately posttreatment and at the 3-month follow-up compared with controls, but no significant difference in psychological distress. Findings were not described separately for the TBI survivors and family members.

Another RCT involving patients with TBI and family members found significant benefits of peer mentorship for both, including increased behavioral control and positive coping and better quality of life for patients, and increased community reintegration for family members (Hanks et al., 2012).

Finally, a more recent RCT (Moriarty et al., 2016) evaluated the effect of the Veterans' In-home Program (VIP), an in-home intervention for Veterans with TBI and their families. Veterans in VIP showed significantly increased community reintegration and ability to manage patient-identified TBI-related problems compared with controls who received usual clinic care (Winter et al., 2016a,b). Family caregivers in VIP experienced significantly fewer depressive symptoms and less burden compared with controls (Moriarty et al., 2016; Shepherd-Banigan et al., 2018).

Overall, gaps in knowledge needed to address unmet family and caregiver needs include the following:

- What are the most effective interventions to support family caregivers during the acute, post-acute, and chronic stages of TBI?
- How do family caregivers' characteristics, such as preinjury mental health, socioeconomic factors, and cultural beliefs, contribute to the effectiveness of interventions designed to support them?
- What are the predictors of physical health, mental health, and well-being in family caregivers?
- What naturally existing systems of support can facilitate family caregivers' coping with the daily demands of caring for someone with TBI?
- How can families be systematically engaged in post-acute rehabilitation? And what are the effects of this engagement on important outcomes for the person with TBI and family members?
- How can existing resources for family caregivers be disseminated widely in ways that make them available to caregivers at their time of need?

UNMET NEEDS IN THE CURRENT SYSTEM OF TBI REHABILITATION AND LONG-TERM CARE

Unfortunately, many factors interfere with an individual's ability to access an ideal care pathway after TBI, and these factors will have to be addressed if post-acute TBI care and outcomes are to be improved.

Barriers to rehabilitation and recovery include fragmented and variable care and the need for greater communication and continuity along the care continuum. Patients with TBI and their families need integrative, interdisciplinary treatment across the continuum of care and recovery, with care needs that may continue over a long period of time. In the military, continuity of care is improved by the fact that longer-term and rehabilitation care for service members and Veterans with TBI can be provided through the VA Polytrauma System of Care. As discussed in prior chapters, however, care systems in civilian populations are often fragmented. Moreover, as this chapter has laid out, the course of recovery can change, and challenges can arise after a person with TBI returns home; therefore, patients and families need pathways for accessing follow-up or additional support if needed.

Additional barriers to optimal rehabilitation and long-term care include difficulties in accessing the necessary expertise within one's geographic area, and other social determinants of health that significantly influence many health outcomes. A growing body of research has examined the relationship of these factors to rehabilitation access and utilization and to outcomes after TBI. As discussed in detail in Chapter 3, factors that affect TBI care and outcomes include not only geographic location, but also race and ethnicity and economic circumstances, such as unemployment, lack of health insurance, limitations in coverage, and high financial costs that are difficult for patients and families to bear on their own.

Finally, as this chapter has illustrated, while a range of clinical and other care practices are used to support post-TBI rehabilitation and recovery, which of these interventions are most effective for which individuals and at what stage of recovery remains largely unknown. Few well-controlled intervention trials have been carried out in the post-acute stage, and those that have been conducted have often been applied to exclusive samples and settings.

First identified by the 1998 National Institutes of Health (NIH) Rehabilitation of Persons with TBI Consensus Conference (NIH, 1999; Ragnarsson, 2002) and reiterated in subsequent systematic reviews through the Agency for Healthcare Research and Quality (Brasure et al., 2013) and the Institute of Medicine (IOM, 2011), rigorous research on the effectiveness of rehabilitation practices for persons with TBI continues to be sparse. These reviews identified the following difficulties with conducting RCTs in TBI rehabilitation:

- high population heterogeneity with associated differences in spontaneous recovery, requiring either large samples for stratification or strict inclusion criteria that reduce generalizability;
- difficulty or impossibility of blinding;
- extensive range of rehabilitation practices, making it difficult to identify, compare, and characterize interventions in a way that facilitates generalization; and
- ethical concerns with withholding treatment during a period when the patient is thought to reap the most benefit.

Research to date has also been hampered by limited follow-up, particularly for studies employing neuroimaging and biomarkers, and inconsistencies in definitions of injury severity. The simultaneous application of multiple treatments and interventions, a common aspect of TBI rehabilitation, also raises the question of whether it is more meaningful to attempt to define and evaluate the effects of individual rehabilitation components or of the service delivery system more holistically. New types of study approaches, such as a multiphase optimization strategy, may assist in evaluating the effectiveness of rehabilitation components and their interactions (Strayhorn et al., 2021). There also is an ongoing "need for evidence in TBI rehabilitation that delineates the extent that differences in outcomes are attributable to patients' characteristics such as age, severity, time since injury, and pre-injury factors, and how much outcomes can be attributed to the timing and dose of specific rehabilitation interventions" (Horn et al., 2015, p. S189). The documented impacts on TBI caregivers have also not been addressed through funding for research to develop and disseminate interventions and programs for caregivers.

FEATURES OF AN EFFECTIVE SYSTEM OF POST-ACUTE TBI CARE

Based on the literature, evidence-based guidelines, the committee's information-gathering sessions, and other sources, a best-practice care pathway for rehabilitation and recovery after TBI would need to include the following features:

- Clear communication between providers as the person with TBI moves along the care pathway from acute stabilization to post-acute, rehabilitation, and longer-term care. The purpose of such communication is to enable effective information sharing while minimizing the chances for patients and families to "fall through the cracks."
- Clear communication to the person with TBI and their family or caregiver to ensure that they are prepared for the TBI recovery trajectory.
- Development of a person-centered follow-up and rehabilitation plan with input from the person with TBI and their family and taking account of individual needs, goals, and interests. Given the diverse and multidisciplinary needs that accompany TBI, developing this plan would also require input from fields including physical medicine, occupational therapy, physical therapy, speech therapy, rehabilitation psychology, neuropsychology, nursing, and behavioral health.
- Access to and provision of high-quality inpatient and/or outpatient rehabilitation as soon as possible after injury, based on the person's injury and needs. Initiating TBI rehabilitation shortly after injury is beneficial unless precluded by the person's condition.
- Planning to ensure that a person can discharged to a safe environment after acute or inpatient care, including screening for risks from falls, driving, sports, or other activities.
- Use of integrated health services to address TBI comorbidities, including mental health difficulties and risky substance use.
- Development and maintenance of culturally competent materials, in multiple languages, providing information about TBI and recovery for patients and families and caregivers.
- Provision of TBI-informed community-based social services to reduce social and societal barriers to optimal recovery and long-term quality of life.
- Support for families and caregivers of persons with TBI, who play critical roles in the recovery process but often report significant stress and burden. Families and caregivers for persons with TBI need support to carry out their caregiving roles, as well as to sustain their own physical and mental health and well-being.

CONCLUSIONS

A variety of high-quality rehabilitation interventions and longer-term services and supports can be provided to people with TBI and their families. However, the current system for TBI care does not provide access to follow-up or rehabilitation for all who could benefit and is often difficult for patients, families, and caregivers to navigate, with no clear roadmap for support and for community-based services after injury. To address these gaps will require meeting the following needs:

- Clinical pathways need to exist for all persons who experience a TBI, of whatever initial severity, to maintain continuity of care and provide follow-up care for any TBI-related consequences that may arise. Multiple care and recovery pathways are needed to address the range of patient needs. Further research is needed as well to compare outcomes for persons with TBI who experience different types of interventions and different systems of care to determine the care pathways that lead to optimal outcomes for these varied scenarios.

- The criteria for authorization and insurance coverage of rehabilitation need to be revisited and to better align with when that rehabilitation is likely to be most effective, rather than being tied to arbitrary intervals with respect to the initial injury. For example, rehabilitation coverage is commonly denied if a person is unable to tolerate a trend toward 3 hours of therapy per day (or 15 hours per week), despite the lack of consistent evidence that the receipt of 3 hours of therapy per day is a significant driver of outcomes from inpatient rehabilitation for persons with TBI in the United States.
- The system needs to encompass the multiple elements of an optimal patient- and family-centered approach to TBI rehabilitation and recovery identified in this chapter.

REFERENCES

AAPM&R (American Academy of Physical Medicine and Rehabilitation). 2021. *Disorders of Consciousness.* https://www.aapmr.org/about-physiatry/conditions-treatments/rehabilitation-of-central-nervous-system-disorders/disorders-of-consciousness (accessed December 5, 2021).

Abraham, T., S. Ono, H. Moriarty, L. Winter, R. Bender. R. Facundo, and G. True. 2021. Revealing the invisible emotion work of caregivers: A photovoice exploration of informal care provided by family caregivers for post-9/11 veterans with traumatic brain injuries. *Journal of Head Trauma Rehabilitation* 36(1):25-33.

ACS (American College of Surgeons) Committee on Trauma. 2014. *Resources for optimal care of the injured patient.* 6th ed. https://www.facs.org/-/media/files/quality-programs/trauma/vrc-resources/resources-for-optimal-care.ashx (accessed November 10, 2021).

Anderson, J., N. Parr, and K. Vela. 2020. *Evidence brief: Transcranial magnetic stimulation (TMS) for chronic pain, PTSD, TBI, opioid addiction, and sexual trauma.* Washington, DC: Department of Veterans Affairs. https://www.ncbi.nlm.nih.gov/books/NBK566938 (accessed November 10, 2021).

Backhaus, S., S. Ibarra, D. Klyce, L. Trexler, and J. Malec. 2010. Brain injury coping skills group: A preventative intervention for patients with brain injury and their caregivers. *Archives of Physical Medicine and Rehabilitation* 91(6):840-848.

Bailey, C., J. Meyer, S. Briskin, C. Tangen, S. A. Hoffer, J. Dundr, B. Brennan, and P. Smith. 2019. Multidisciplinary concussion management: A model for outpatient concussion management in the acute and post-acute settings. *Journal of Head Trauma Rehabilitation* 34(6):375-384.

Baker, A., S. Barker, A. Sampson, and C. Martin. 2017. Caregiver outcomes and interventions: A systematic scoping review of the traumatic brain injury and spinal cord injury literature. *Clinical Rehabilitation* 31(1):45-60.

Bay, E. H., A. J. Blow, and X. Yan. 2012. Interpersonal relatedness and psychological functioning following traumatic brain injury: Implications for marital and family therapists. *Journal of Marital and Family Therapy* 38:556-567.

Bayley, M., R. Tate, J. M. Douglas, L. Turkstra, J. Ponsford, M. Stergiou-Kita, A. Kua, P. Bragge, and INCOG Expert Panel. 2014. INCOG guidelines for cognitive rehabilitation following traumatic brain injury. *Journal of Head Trauma Research* 29(4):290-386.

Beaulieu, C. L., J. Peng, E. M. Hade, J. D. Corrigan, R. T. Seel, M. P. Dijkers, F. M. Hammond, S. D. Horn, M. L. Timpson, M. Swan, and J. Bogner. 2019. Level of effort and 3 hour rule compliance. *Archives of Physical Medicine and Rehabilitation* 100(10):1827-1836.

Begemann, M., Leon, M., van der Horn, H. J., van der Naalt, J., and I. Sommer. 2020. Drugs with anti-inflammatory effects to improve outcome of traumatic brain injury: A meta-analysis. *Scientific Reports* 10(1):16179. https://doi.org/10.1038/s41598-020-73227-5.

Bell, J. M., C. L. Master, and M. R. Lionbarger. 2019. The clinical implications of youth sports concussion laws: A review. *American Journal of Lifestyle Medicine* 13(2):172-181.

BIAUSA (Brain Injury Association of America). *Adults: What to expect at home.* https://www.biausa.org/brain-injury/about-brain-injury/adults-what-to-expect/adults-what-to-expect-at-home (accessed December 5, 2021).

Biester, R. C., D. Krych, M. J. Schmidt, D. Parrott, D. I. Katz, M. Abate, and C. I. Hirshson. 2016. Individuals With Traumatic Brain Injury and Their Significant Others' Perceptions of Information Given About the Nature and Possible Consequences of Brain Injury: Analysis of a National Survey. *Professional case management* 21(1):22-E4. https://doi.org/10.1097/NCM.0000000000000121.

Bogner, J., E. Hade, J. Peng, C. Beaulieu, S. Horn, J. Corrigan, F. Hammond, M. Dijkers, E. Montgomery, K. Gilchrist, C. Giuffrida, A. Lash, and M. Timpson. 2019a. Family involvement in traumatic brain injury inpatient reha-bilitation: A propensity score analysis on effects on outcomes during the first year after discharge. *Archives of Physical Medicine and Rehabilitation* 100(10):1801-1809.

Bogner J., M. Dijkers, E. Hade, C. Beaulieu, E. Montgomery, C. Giuffrida, M. Timpson, J. Peng, K. Gilchrist. A. Lash, F. Hammond, S. Horn, and J. D. Corrigan. 2019b. Contextualized treatment in traumatic brain injury inpatient rehabilitation: Effects on outcomes during the first year after discharge. *Archives of Physical Medicine and Rehabilitation* 100(10):1810-1817.

Boschen, K., J. Gargaro, C. Gan, G. Gerber, and C. Brandys. 2007. Family interventions after acquired brain injury and other chronic conditions: A critical appraisal of the quality of the evidence. *NeuroRehabilitation* 22:19-41.

Boss, P. 2005. *Loss, trauma and resilience: Therapeutic work with ambiguous loss.* New York: Norton.

Brasure, M., G. J. Lamberty, N. A. Sayer, N. W. Nelson, R. Macdonald, J. Ouellette, and T. J. Wilt. 2013. Participa-tion after multidisciplinary rehabilitation for moderate to severe traumatic brain injury in adults: A systematic review. *Archives of Physical Medicine and Rehabilitation* 94(7):1398-1420.

CDC (Centers for Disease Control and Prevention). 2018. *Report to Congress on the management of traumatic brain injury in children: Opportunities for action.* Atlanta, GA: National Center for Injury Prevention and Control, Division of Unintentional Injury Prevention.

Cefalu, C. A. 2011. Theories and mechanisms of aging. *Clinics in Geriatric Medicine* 27(4):491-506.

Coleman, K., B. T. Austin, C. Brach and E. H. Wagner. 2009. Evidence on the chronic care model in the new mil-lennium. *Health Affairs* 28(1):75-85.

Corrigan, J. D., and F. M. Hammond. 2013. Traumatic brain injury as a chronic health condition. *Archives of Physi-cal Medicine and Rehabilitation* 94(6):1199-1201.

Corrigan, J. D., J. P. Cuthbert, G. G. Whiteneck, M. P. Dijkers, V. Coronado, A. W. Heinemann, C. Harrison-Felix, and J. E. Graham. 2012. Representativeness of the Traumatic Brain Injury Model Systems National Database. *Journal of Head Trauma Rehabilitation* 27(6):391-403.

Corrigan, J. D., M. Vuola, J. Bogner, A. Botticello, S. Pinto, and G. Whiteneck. 2021. Do state supports for persons with brain injury affect outcomes in the 5 years following acute rehabilitation? *Health & Place* 72:102674.

Cox, C. S., Jr. 2018. Cellular therapy for traumatic neurological injury. *Pediatric Research* 83(1-2):325-332.

Crowe, K. 2016, November 3. Private concussion clinics called a "wild west" of unregulated treatment. *CBC News.* https://www.cbc.ca/news/health/concussion-hotline-baseline-testing-treatment-industry-for-profit-unregulated-1.3833158 (accessed August 17, 2021).

Cuthbert, J. P., J. Corrigan, C. Harrison-Felix, V. Coronado, M. Dijkers, A. Heinemann, and G. Whiteneck. 2011. Factors that predict acute hospitalization discharge disposition for adults with moderate to severe traumatic brain injury. *Archives of Physical Medicine and Rehabilitation* 92(5):721-730.e3.

Dams-O'Connor, K., K. Sy, A. Landau, Y. Bodien, S. Dikmen, E. Felix, J. Giacino, L. Gibbons, F. Hammond, T. Hart, D. Johnson-Greene, J. Lengenfelder, A. Lequerica, J. Newman, T. Novack, T. O'Neil-Pirozzi, and G. Whiteneck. 2018. The feasibility of telephone-administered cognitive testing in individuals 1 and 2 years after inpatient rehabilitation for traumatic brain injury. *Journal of Neurotrauma* 35(10):1138-1145.

Darkins, A. 2006. Changing the location of care: Management of patients with chronic conditions in Veterans Health Administration using care coordination/home telehealth. *Journal of Rehabilitation Research & Development* 43(4):vii-xii.

Dausch, B. M., and S. Saliman. 2009. Use of family focused therapy in rehabilitation for veterans with traumatic brain injury. *Rehabilitation Psychology* 54(3):279-287.

DaVanzo, J. E., A. El-Gamil, J. Li, M. Shimer, N. Manolov, and A. Dobson. 2014. *Assessment of patient outcomes of rehabilitative care provided in inpatient rehabilitation facilities (IRFs) and after discharge.* Final report 13-127. Submitted to ARA Research Institute. https://amrpa.org/portals/0/dobson%20davanzo%20final%20report%20-%20patient%20outcomes%20of%20irf%20v_%20snf%20-%207_10_14%20redated.pdf (accessed November 10, 2021).

De Luca, R., M. Maggio, A. Naro, S. Portaro, A. Cannavò, and R. Calabrò. 2020. Can patients with severe traumatic brain injury be trained with cognitive telerehabilitation? An inpatient feasibility and usability study. *Journal of Clinical Neuroscience* 79:246-250.

Desai, N., D. Wiebe, D. J., Corwin, J., Lockyer, M. Grady, and C. L. Master. 2019. Factors affecting recovery trajec-tories in pediatric female concussion. *Clinical Journal of Sport Medicine* 29(5):361-367.

Dillahunt-Aspillaga, C., T. Jorgensen-Smith, S. Ehlke, M. Sosinki, D. Monroe, and J. Thor. 2013. Traumatic brain injury: Unmet support needs of caregivers and families in Florida. *PLoS One* 8(12):1-9.

Edlow, B., J. Claassen, N. Schiff, and D. Greer. 2021. Recovery from disorders of consciousness: Mechanisms, prognosis and emerging therapies. *Nature Reviews Neurology* 17:135-156.

Ellis, M. J., L. Ritchie, E. Selci, S. Grossi, S. Frost, P. J. McDonald, and K. Russell. 2017. Googling concussion care in the USA: A critical appraisal of online concussion healthcare providers. *Concussion* 2(2):CNC33. https://doi.org/10.2217/cnc-2016-0027.

Ellis, M. J., J. Leddy, D. Cordingley, and B. Willer. 2018. A physiological approach to assessment and rehabilitation of acute concussion in collegiate and professional athletes. *Frontiers in Neurology* 9:1115.

Ergh T. C., L. Rapport, R. Coleman, and R. D. Hanks. 2002. Predictors of caregiver and family functioning following traumatic brain injury: Social support moderates caregiver distress. *Journal of Head Trauma Rehabilitation* 17:155-174.

Ettel, D., A. E. Glang, B. Todis, and S. C. Davies. 2016. Traumatic brain injury: Persistent misconceptions and knowledge gaps among educators. *Exceptionality Education International* 26(1):1-18.

Fann, J. R., T. Hart, M. Ciol, M. Moore, J. Bogner, J. Corrigan, K. Dams-O'Connor, S. Driver, R. Dubiel, F. Hammond, M., Kajankova, T. Watanabe, and J. M. Hoffman. 2021. Improving transition from inpatient rehabilitation following traumatic brain injury: Protocol for the BRITE pragmatic comparative effectiveness trial. *Contemporary Clinical Trials* 104:106332.

Flanagan, S. R., M. R. Hibbard, and W. A. Gordon. 2005. The impact of age on traumatic brain injury. *Physical Medicine and Rehabilitation Clinics* 16(1):163-177.

Forrest, G., A. Reppel, M. Kodsi, and J. Smith. 2019. Inpatient rehabilitation facilities: The 3-hour rule. *Medicine* 98(37):e17096. https://doi.org/10.1097/MD.0000000000017096.

Foster, A., J. Armstrong, A. Buckley, J. Sherry, T. Young, S. Foliaki, T. M. James-Hohaia, A. Theadom, and K. McPherson. 2012. Encouraging family engagement in the rehabilitation process: A rehabilitation provider's development of support strategies for family members of people with traumatic brain injury. *Disability and Rehabilitation* 34(22):1855-1862.

Fuentes, M. M., S. Apkon, N. Jimenez, and F. P. Rivara. 2016. Association between facility type during pediatric inpatient rehabilitation and functional outcomes. *Archives of Physical Medicine and Rehabilitation* 97(9):1407-1412.

Fure, S., E. Howe, N. Andelic, C. Brunborg, U. Sveen, C. Røe, P. Rike, A. Olsen, Ø. Spjelkavik, H. Ugelstad, J. Lu, J. Ponsford, E. Twamley, T. Hellstrøm, and M. Løvstad. 2021. Cognitive and vocational rehabilitation after mild-to-moderate traumatic brain injury: A randomised controlled trial. *Annals of Physical and Rehabilitation Medicine* 64(5):101538.

Gardner, R. C., K. Dams-O'Connor, M. R. Morrissey, and G. T. Manley. 2018. Geriatric traumatic brain injury: Epidemiology, outcomes, knowledge gaps, and future directions. *Journal of Neurotrauma* 35:889-906.

Giacino, J. T., A. Christoforou, and M. J. G. Bergin. 2016. *Rehabilitation access and outcome after severe traumatic brain injury: A TBI Model System-Sponsored Stakeholder Summit.* https://mghcme.org/app/uploads/2020/07/TBI-Event-Summit-Briefing-book_05102016_Final.pdf (accessed September 24, 2021).

Giacino, J. T., D. I. Katz, N. D. Schiff, J. Whyte, E. J. Ashman, S. Ashwal, R. Barbano, F. Hammond, S. Laureys, G. Ling, R. Nakase-Richardson, R. T. Seel, S. Yablon, T. Getchius, G. S. Gronseth, and M. J. Armstrong. 2018. Practice guideline update recommendations summary: Disorders of consciousness: Report of the Guideline Development, Dissemination, and Implementation Subcommittee of the American Academy of Neurology; the American Congress of Rehabilitation Medicine; and the National Institute on Disability, Independent Living, and Rehabilitation Research. *Neurology* 91(10):450-460.

Giacino, J. T., M. Sherer, A. Christoforou, P. Maurer-Karattup, F. Hammond, D. Long, and E. Bagiella. 2020. Behavioral recovery and early decision making in patients with prolonged disturbance in consciousness after traumatic brain injury. *Journal of Neurotrauma* 37(2):357-365.

Gioia, G. A. 2016. Medical-school partnership in guiding return to school following mild traumatic brain injury in youth. *Journal of Child Neurology* 31(1):93-108.

Girard, P. 2007. Military and VA telemedicine systems for patients with traumatic brain injury. *Journal of Rehabilitation Research and Development* 44(7):1017-1026.

Glang, A., B. Todis, C. W. Thomas, D. Hood, G. Bedell, and J. Cockrell. 2008. Return to school following childhood TBI: Who gets services? *NeuroRehabilitation* 23(6):477-486.

Graff, H. J., U. Christensen, I. Poulsen, and I. Egerod. 2018. Patient perspectives on navigating the field of traumatic brain injury rehabilitation: A qualitative thematic analysis. *Disability and Rehabilitation* 40(8):926-934.

Greene, N. H., M. A. Kernic, M. S. Vavilala, and F. P. Rivara. 2014. Variation in pediatric traumatic brain injury outcomes in the United States. *Archives of Physical Medicine and Rehabilitation* 10(14):00180-00184.

Griesbach, G. S., B. Masel, R. E. Helvie, and M. J. Ashley. 2018. The impact of traumatic brain injury on later life: Effects on normal aging and neurodegenerative diseases. *Journal of Neurotrauma* 35(1):17-24.

Griffin, J. M., M. K. Lee, L. R. Bangerter, C. H. Van Houtven, G. Friedemann-Sánchez, S. M. Phelan, K. F. Carlson, and L. A. Meis. 2017. Burden and mental health among caregivers of veterans with traumatic brain injury/polytrauma. *American Journal of Orthopsychiatry* 87(2):139-148.

Groom, K. N., T. G. Shaw, M. E. O'Connor, N. I. Howard, and A. Pickens. 1998. Neurobehavioral symptoms and family functioning in traumatically brain-injured adults. *Archives of Clinical Neuropsychology* 13:695-711.

Haarbauer-Krupa, J. 2012. Schools as TBI service providers. *ASHA Leader* 17(8):10-13.

Haarbauer-Krupa, J., A. Ciccia, J. Dodd, D. Ettell, B. Kurowski, A. Lumba-Brown, and S. Suskauer. 2017. Service delivery in the healthcare and educational systems for children following traumatic brain injury: Gaps in care. *Journal of Head Trauma Rehabilitation* 32(6):367-377.

Halstead, M. E., K. McAvoy, C. D. Devore, R. Carl, M. Lee, and K. Logan. 2013. Returning to learning following a concussion. *Pediatrics* 132(5):948-957.

Hammond, F. M., S. Katta-Charles, M. B. Russell, R. D. Zafonte, J. Claassen, A. K. Wagner, L. Puybasset, S. Egawa, S. Laureys, M. Diringer, R. D. Stevens, and the Curing Coma Campaign and its Contributing Members. 2021. Research needs for prognostic modeling and trajectory analysis in patients with disorders of consciousness. *Neurocritical Care* 35(Suppl 1):55-67.

Hanks, R. A., L. J. Rapport, J. Wertheimer, and C. Koviak. 2012. Randomized controlled trial of peer mentoring for individuals with traumatic brain injury and their significant others. *Archives of Physical Medicine and Rehabilitation* 93(8):1297-1304.

Hart, T., J. Whyte, M. Dijkers, A. Packel, L. Turkstra, J. Zanca, M. Ferraro, C. Chen, and J. Van Stan. 2018. *Manual of rehabilitation treatment specification.* Version 6.2. https://acrm.org/manual-for-rehabilitation-treatment-specification (accessed November 23, 2021).

Hartman, L. R., A. Tibbles, A. Paniccia, and S. Lindsay. 2015. A qualitative synthesis of families' and students' hospital-to-school transition experiences following acquired brain injury. *Global Qualitative Nursing Research* 2:2333393615614307. https://doi.org/10.1177/2333393615614307.

Haskins, E. C., K. Cicerone, K. Eberle, K. Dam-O Connor, D. Langenbahn, A. Shapiro-Rosenbaum, and L. E. Trexler. 2012. *Cognitive Rehabilitation Manual: Translating Evidence-Based Recommendations into Practice.* Reston, VA: American Congress of Rehabilitation Medicine.

Hawley, L., C. Morey, M. Sevigny, J. Ketchum, G. Simpson, C. Harrison-Felix, and C. Tefertiller. 2021. Enhancing self-advocacy after traumatic brain injury: A randomized controlled trial. *Journal of Head Trauma Rehabilitation.* https://doi.org/10.1097/HTR.0000000000000689.

Heiden, S. M., and B. S. Caldwell. 2018. Considerations for developing chronic care system for traumatic brain injury based on comparisons of cancer survivorship and diabetes management care. *Ergonomics* 61(1):134-147.

Hofer, A-S., and M. Schwab. 2019. Enhancing rehabilitation and functional recovery after brain and spinal cord trauma with electrical neuromodulation. *Current Opinion in Neurology* 32(6):828-835.

Hoge, C., D. McGurk, J. Thomas, A. Cox, C. Engel, and C. Castro. 2008. Mild traumatic brain injury in U.S. soldiers returning from Iraq. *New England Journal of Medicine* 358(5):453-463.

Hong, I., J. Goodwin, T. Reistetter, Y. Kuo, T. Mallinson, A. Karmarkar, Y. Lin, and K. Ottenbacher. 2019. Comparison of functional status improvements among patients with stroke receiving postacute care in inpatient rehabilitation vs skilled nursing facilities. *JAMA Network Open* 2(12):e1916646.

Horn, S. D., J. D. Corrigan, J. Bogner, F. M. Hammond, R. T. Seel, R. J. Smout, R. S. Barrett, M. P. Dijkers, and G. G. Whiteneck. 2015. Traumatic brain injury-practice based evidence study: Design and patients, centers, treatments, and outcomes. *Archives of Physical Medicine and Rehabilitation* 96(8 Suppl):S178-196.

Howland, J., H. Hackman, A. Torres, J. Campbell, and J. Olshaker. 2021. It is time to rewrite state youth sports concussion laws. *BMJ Open Sport & Exercise Medicine* 7(1):e000959.

INESSS-ONF (Institut National d'Excellence en Santé et en Services Sociaux and Ontario Neurotrauma Foundation). 2015. Clinical Practice Guideline for the Rehabilitation of Adults with Moderate to Severe TBI. https://braininjuryguidelines.org/modtosevere (accessed December 8, 2021).

IOM (Institute of Medicine). 2011. *Cognitive rehabilitation therapy for traumatic brain injury: Evaluating the evidence.* Washington, DC: The National Academies Press.

Irvine, K. A., and J. D. Clark. 2018. Chronic pain after traumatic brain injury: Pathophysiology and pain mechanisms. *Pain Medicine* 19(7):1315-1333.

Jaglal, S. B., S. Guilcher, T. Bereket, M. Kwan, S. Munce, J. Conklin, J. Versnel, T. Packer, M. Verrier, C. Marras, K. Pitzul, and R. Riopelle. 2014. Development of a chronic care model for neurological conditions (CCM-NC). *BMC Health Services Research* 14:409.

Juengst, S. B., K. Graham, I. Pulantara, M. McCue, E. Whyte, B. Dicianno, B. Parmanto, P. Arenth, E. Skidmore, and A. Wagner. 2015. Pilot feasibility of an mHealth system for conducting ecological momentary assessment of mood-related symptoms following traumatic brain injury. *Brain Injury* 29(11):1351-1361.

Knight, R. G., R. Devereux, and H. P. D. Godfrey. 1998. Caring for a family member with a traumatic brain injury. *Brain Injury* 12:476-481.

Kolakowsky-Hayner, S. A., K. D. Miner, and J. S. Kreutzer. 2001. Long-term life quality and family needs after traumatic brain injury. *Journal of Head Trauma Rehabilitation* 16:374-385.

Kontos, A. P., K. Jorgensen-Wagers, A. Trbovich, N. Ernst, K. Emami, B. Gillie, J. French, C. Holland, R. Elbin, and M. W. Collins. 2020. Association of time since injury to the first clinic visit with recovery following concussion. *JAMA Neurology* 77(4):435-440.

Kornblith, E. S., K. Langa, K. Yaffe, and R. C. Gardner. 2020. Physical and functional impairment among older adults with a history of traumatic brain injury. *Journal of Head Trauma Rehabilitation* 35(4):e320-e329.

Kreitzer, N., G. G. Kurowksi, and T. Bakas. 2018. Systematic review of caregiver and dyad Interventions after adult traumatic brain injury. *Archives of Physical Medicine and Rehabilitation* 99:2342-2354

Kreutzer, J. S., A. H. Gervasio, and P. S. Camplair. 1994. Primary caregivers' psychological status and family functioning after traumatic brain injury. *Brain Injury* 8(3):197-210.

Kreutzer, J. S., T. Stejskal, J. M. Ketchum, J. H. Marwitz, L. A. Taylor, and J. C. Menzel. 2009. A preliminary investigation of the brain injury family intervention: Impact on family members. *Brain Injury* 23:535-547.

Landau, J., and J. L. Hissett. 2008. Mild traumatic brain injury: Impact on identity and ambiguous loss in the family. *Families, Systems, & Health* 26:69-85.

Leddy, J. J., M. Haider, M. Ellis, and B. S. Willer. 2018. Exercise is medicine for concussion. *Current Sports Medicine Reports* 17(8):262-270.

Li, M., and S. Sirko. 2018. Traumatic brain injury: At the crossroads of neuropathology and common metabolic endocrinopathies. *Journal of Clinical Medicine* 7(3):59.

Lishner, D. M., P. Levine, and D. Patrick. 1996. Access to primary health care among persons with disabilities in rural areas: A summary of the literature. *Journal of Rural Health* 12(1):45-53.

Malec, J. F., F. Hammond, S. Flanagan, J. Kean, A. Sander, M. Sherer, and B. E. Masel. 2013. Recommendations from the 2013 Galveston Brain Injury Conference for implementation of a chronic care model in brain injury. *Journal of Head Trauma Rehabilitation* 28(6):476-483.

Malec, J. F., C. H. Van Houtven, T. Tanielian, A. Atizado, and M. C. Dorn. 2017. Impact of TBI on caregivers of veterans with TBI: Burden and interventions. *Brain Injury* 31(9):1235-1245.

Marsh, N. V., D. A. Kersel, J. H. Havill, and J. W. Sleigh. 1998a. Caregiver burden at 6 months following severe traumatic brain injury. *Brain Injury* 12:225-238.

Marsh, N. V., D. A. Kersel, J. H. Havill, and J. W. Sleigh. 1998b. Caregiver burden at 1 year following traumatic brain injury. *Brain Injury* 12:1045-1059.

Marsh, N. V., D. A. Kersel, J. H. Havill, and J. W. Sleigh. 2002. Caregiver burden during the year following severe traumatic brain injury. *Journal of Clinical and Experimental Neuropsychology* 24:434-447.

Masel, B. E., and D. S. DeWitt. 2010. Traumatic brain injury: A disease process, not an event. *Journal of Neurotrauma* 27(8):1529-1540.

Mashima, P. A., and C. Doarn. 2008. Overview of telehealth activities in speech-language pathology. *Telemedicine and E-Health* 14(10):1101-1117.

Master, C. L., B. Katz, K. Arbogast, M. McCrea, T. McAllister, P. Pasquina, M. Lapradd, W. Zhou, S. Broglio, and CARE Consortium Investigators. 2020. Differences in sport-related concussion for female and male athletes in comparable collegiate sports: A study from the NCAA-DoD Concussion Assessment, Research and Education (CARE) Consortium. *British Journal of Sports Medicine* bjsports-2020-103316. https://doi.org/10.1136/bjsports-2020-103316.

Matsumoto, H., and Y. Ugawa. 2016. Adverse events of tDCS and tACS: A review. *Clinical Neurophysiology Practice* 2:19-25.

Matsumoto, M. E., G. C. Wilske, and R. Tapia. 2021. Innovative approaches to delivering telehealth. *Physical Medicine and Rehabilitation Clinics* 32(2):451-465.

McCrory, P., W. Meeuwisse, J. Dvorák, M. Aubry, J. Bailes, S. Broglio, R. Cantu, D. Cassidy, R. Echemendia, R. Castellani, G. Davis, R. Ellenbogen, C. Emery, L. Engebretsen, N. Feddermann-Demont, C. Giza, K. Guskiewicz, S. Herring, G. Iverson, K. Johnston, J. Kissick, J. Kutcher, J. Ledy, D. Maddocks, M. Makdissi, G. Manley, M. McCrea, W. Meehan, S. Nagahiro, J. Patricios, M. Putukian, K. Schneider, A. Sills, C. Tator, M. Turner, and P. Vos. 2017. Consensus statement on concussion in sport—The 5th International Conference on Concussion in Sport held in Berlin, October 2016. *British Journal of Sports Medicine* 51(11):838-847.

McPherson, K. M., B. Pentland, and H. K. McNaughton. 2000. Brain injury and the perceived health of carers. *Disability and Rehabilitation* 22:683-689.

Moriarty, H., L. Winter, K. Robinson, C. Verrier Piersol, T. Vause-Earland, D. Blazer Iacovone, B. Newhart, G. True, D. Fishman, N. Hodgson, and L. Gitlin. 2016. A randomized controlled trial to evaluate the Veterans' In-home Program (VIP) for military veterans with traumatic brain injury and their families: Report on impact for family members. *Physical Medicine and Rehabilitation* 8(6):495-509.

Moriarty, H., L. Winter, T. Short, and G. True. 2018. Exploration of factors related to depressive symptomatology in family members of military veterans with traumatic brain injury. *Journal of Family Nursing* 24 (2):184-216.

Mucha, A., Fedor, S., and D. DeMarco. 2018. Vestibular dysfunction and concussion. *Handbook of Clinical Neurology* 158:135-144.

Nabors, N., J. Seacat, and M. Rosenthal. 2002. Predictors of caregiver burden following traumatic brain injury. *Brain Injury* 16:1039-1050.

Nampiaparampil, D. 2008. Prevalence of chronic pain after traumatic brain injury. *Journal of the American Medical Association* 300(6):711-719.

Narapareddy, B. R., L. N. Richey, and M. E. Peters. 2019, April 30. The growing epidemic of TBI in older patients. *NeurologyLive.* https://www.neurologylive.com/view/growing-epidemic-tbi-older-patients (accessed January 18, 2021).

Nardone, R., L. Sebastianelli, V. Versace, F. Brigo, S. Golaszewski, P. Manganotti, L. Saltuari, and E. Trinka. 2020. Repetitive transcranial magnetic stimulation in traumatic brain injury: Evidence from animal and human studies. *Brain Research Bulletin* 159:44-52.

NASEM (National Academies of Sciences, Engineering, and Medicine). 2016. *A national trauma care system: Integrating military and civilian trauma systems to achieve zero preventable deaths after injury.* Washington, DC: The National Academies Press.

Nehra, D., Z. Nixon, C. Lengenfelder, E. Bulger, J. Cuschieri, R. Maier, and S. Arbabi. 2016. Acute rehabilitation after trauma: Does it really matter? *Journal of the American College of Surgeons* 223(6):755-763.

Ng, E. M. W., H. Polatajko, E. Marziali, A. Hunt, and D. Dawson. 2013. Telerehabilitation for addressing executive dysfunction after traumatic brain injury. *Brain Injury* 27(5):548-564.

NIH (National Institutes of Health) Consensus Development Panel on Rehabilitation of Persons with Traumatic Brain Injury. 1999. Rehabilitation of persons with traumatic brain injury. *Journal of the American Medical Association* 282(10):974-983.

Norup, A., P. B. Perrin, G. Cuberos-Urbano, A. Anke, N. Andelic, S. T. Doyle, M. Cristina Quijano, A. Caracuel, D. Mar, I. Guadalupe Espinosa Jove, and J. Carlos Arango-Lasprilla. 2015. Family needs after brain injury: A cross cultural study. *NeuroRehabilitation* 36(2):203-214.

Oberman, L. M., S. Exley, N. Philip, S. Siddiqi, M. Adamson, and D. L. Brody. 2020. Use of repetitive transcranial magnetic stimulation in the treatment of neuropsychiatric and neurocognitive symptoms associated with concussion in military populations. *Journal of Head Trauma Rehabilitation* 35(6):388-400.

ONC (Office of the National Coordinator for Health Information Technology). 2021. Department of Health and Human Services). *Telemedicine and telehealth.* https://www.healthit.gov/topic/health-it-health-care-settings/telemedicine-and-telehealth (accessed November 8, 2021).

ONF (Ontario Neurotrauma Foundation). 2017a. Standards for high quality post-concussion services and concussion clinics. *Concussions Ontario.* https://concussionsontario.org/healthcareprofessionals/standards/standards-for-high-quality-post-concussion-services-and-concussion-clinics (accessed August 17, 2021).

ONF. 2017b. Post-concussion care pathway. *Concussions Ontario.* https://concussionsontario.org/wp-content/uploads/2017/06/ONF-Standards-for-Post-Concussion-Care-June-8-2017.pdf (accessed August 17, 2021).

ONF. 2018. *Guideline for Concussion/Mild Traumatic Brain Injury & Prolonged Symptoms,* 3rd Edition, For Adults over 18 Years of Age. Toronto, Canada: ONF. https://braininjuryguidelines.org/concussion/fileadmin/pdf/Concussion_guideline_3rd_edition_final.pdf (accessed December 8, 2021).

ONF. 2020. *Living Guideline for Diagnosing and Managing Pediatric Concussion.* https://braininjuryguidelines.org/pediatricconcussion (accessed December 8, 2021).

Opeyemi, O., M. Rogers, B. Firek, K. Janesko-Feldman, V. Vagni, S. Mullett, S. Wendell, B. Nelson, L. New, E. Mariño, P. Kochanek, H. Bayir, R. Clark, M. Morowitz, and D. Simon. 2021. Sustained dysbiosis and decreased fecal short-chain fatty acids after traumatic brain injury and impact on neurologic outcome. *Journal of Neurotrauma.* https://doi.org/10.1089/neu.2020.7506.

Ownsworth, T., U. Arnautovska, E. Beadle, D. Shum, and W. Moyle. 2018. Efficacy of telerehabilitation for adults with traumatic brain injury: A systematic review. *Journal of Head Trauma Rehabilitation* 33(4):E33–E46.

Peters, L. C., M. Stambrook, A. D. Moore, and L. Esses. 1990. Psychosocial sequelae of closed head injury: Effects on the marital relationship. *Brain Injury* 4:39-47.

Peters, M. E. 2016. Traumatic brain injury (TBI) in older adults: Aging with a TBI versus incident TBI in the aged. *International Psychogeriatrics* 28(12):1931-1934.

Peters, M. E. 2020. Traumatic brain injury in older adults: Shining light on a growing public health crisis. *International Review of Psychiatry* 32(1):1-2.

Peters, M. E., and R. C. Gardner. 2018. Traumatic brain injury in older adults: Do we need a different approach? *Concussion* 3:CNC56.

Ponsford J., J. P. Olver, M. Ponsford, and R. Nelms. 2003. Long-term adjustment of families following traumatic brain injury where comprehensive rehabilitation has been provided. Brain Injury 17:453-468.

Possin, K., J. Merrilees, S. Dulaney, S. Bonasera, W. Chiong, K. Lee, S. Hooper, I. Allen, T. Braley, A. Bernstein, T. Rosa, K. Harrison, H. Begert-Hellings, J. Kornak, J. Kahn, G. Naasan, S. Lanata, A. Clark, A. Chodos, R. Gearhart, C. Ritchie, and B. Miller. 2019. Effect of collaborative dementia care via telephone and internet on quality of life, caregiver well-being, and health care use: The Care Ecosystem Randomized Clinical Trial. *JAMA Internal Medicine* 179(12):1658-1667.

Postupna, N., S. Rose, L. Gibbons, N. Coleman, L. Hellstern, K. Ritchie, A. Wilson, E. Cudaback, X. Li, E. Melief, A. Beller, J. Miller, A. Nolan, D. Marshall, R. Walker, T. Montine, E. Larson, P. Crane, R. Ellenbogen, E. Lein, K. Dams-O'Connor, and C. D. Keene. 2021. The delayed neuropathological consequences of traumatic brain injury in a community-based sample. *Frontiers in Neurology* 12:624696.

Potoka, D. A., L. C. Schall, M. J. Gardner, P. W. Stafford, A. B. Peitzman, and H. R. Ford. 2000. Impact of pediatric trauma centers on mortality in a statewide system. *Journal of Trauma* 49(2):237-245.

Powell, J. M., R. Fraser, J. A. Brockway, N. Temkin, and K. R. Bell. 2016. A telehealth approach to caregiver self-management following traumatic brain injury: A randomized controlled trial. *Journal of Head Trauma Rehabilitation* 31(3):180-190.

Provencio, J. J., J. Claassen, B. Edlow, and J. C. Hemphill. 2020. The Curing Coma Campaign: Framing initial scientific challenges—Proceedings of the first Curing Coma Campaign scientific advisory council meeting. *Neurocritical Care* 33(4). https://doi.org/10.1007/s12028-020-01028-9.

Ragnarsson, K. T. 2002. Results of the NIH consensus conference on "Rehabilitation of persons with traumatic brain injury." *Restorative Neurology and Neuroscience* 20(3-4):103-108.

Ramchand, R., T. Tanielian, M. P. Fisher, C. A. Vaughan, T. E. Trail, C. Epley, P. Voorhies, M. W. Robbins, E. Robinson, and B. Ghosh-Dastidarb. 2014. *Hidden heroes: American's military caregivers.* Santa Monica, CA: RAND Corporation.

Reinard, S., A. Houser, K. Ujvari, and C. Gaultieri. 2020. Long-term Services and Supports State Scorecard, 2020 Edition. *Advancing action: A state scorecard on long-term services and supports for older adults, people with physical disabilities, and family caregivers.* http://longtermscorecard.org (accessed September 16, 2021).

Rietdijk, R., E. Power, M. Brunner, and L. Togher. 2020. The reliability of evaluating conversations between people with traumatic brain injury and their communication partners via videoconferencing. *Neuropsychological Rehabilitation* 30(6):1074-1091.

Riley, G. A. 2007. Stress and depression in family carers following traumatic brain injury: the influence of beliefs about difficult behaviours. *Clinical Rehabilitation* 21(1):82-88.

Rivera, P., T. Elliott, J. Berry, and J. Grant. 2008. Problem-solving training for family caregivers of persons with traumatic brain injuries: A randomized controlled trial. *Archives of Physical Medicine and Rehabilitation* 89(5):931-941.

Romano, M. D. 1974. Family response to traumatic brain injury. *Scandinavian Journal of Rehabilitation Medicine* 6:1-4.

Rose, S. C., McNally, K. A., and G. L. Heyer. 2015. Returning the student to school after concussion: what do clinicians need to know? *Concussion* 1(1):CNC4.

Schimmel, S. J., S. Acosta, and D. Lozano. 2017. Neuroinflammation in traumatic brain injury: A chronic response to an acute injury. *Brain Circulation* 3(3):135-142.

Shepherd-Banigan, M. E., J. R. McDuffie, A. Shapiro, M. Brancu, N. Sperber, N. Mehta, C. van Houtven, and J. Williams Jr. 2018. *Interventions to support caregivers or families of patients with TBI, PTSD, or polytrauma: A systematic review.* VA ESP Project #09-009. https://www.hsrd.research.va.gov/publications/esp/informal-caregiving.pdf (accessed August 17, 2021).

Smith, D. H., J. Dollé, K. Ameen-Ali, A. Bretzin, E. Cortes, J. Crary, K. Dams-O'Connor, et al. 2021. COllaborative Neuropathology NEtwork Characterizing ouTcomes of TBI (CONNECT-TBI). *Acta Neuropatholologica Communications* 9:32. https://doi.org/10.1186/s40478-021-01122-9.

Stein, D. M., R. A. Kozar, H. Livingston, F. Luchette, S. D. Adams, V. Agrawal, S. Arbabi, J. Ballou, R. Barraco, A. Bernard, W. Biffl, P. Bosarge, K. Brasel, Z. Cooper, P. Efron, S. Fakhry, C. Hartline, F. Hwang, B. Joseph, S. Kurek, F. Moore, A. Mosenthal, A. Pathak, M. Truitt, J. Yelon, and AAST Geriatric Trauma/ACS Committee. 2018. Geriatric traumatic brain injury—What we know and what we don't. *Journal of Trauma and Acute Care Surgery* 85(4):788-798.

Stejskal, T. M. 2012. Removing barriers to rehabilitation: Theory-based family intervention in community settings after brain injury. *NeuroRehabilitation* 31(1):75-83.

Stevens, L. F., J. C. Arango-Lasprilla, X. Deng, K. W. Schaaf, C. J. de los Reyes Aragón, M. C. Quijano, and J. Kreutzer. 2012. Factors associated with depression and burden in Spanish speaking caregivers of individuals with traumatic brain injury. *NeuroRehabilitation* 31:443-452.

Stevens, L. F., Y. Lapis, X. Tang, A. M. Sander, L. E. Dreer, F. M. Hammond, J. S. Kreutzer, T. M. O'Neil-Pirozzi, and R. Nakase-Richardson. 2017. Relationship stability after traumatic brain injury among veterans and service members: A VA TBI Model Systems study. *Journal of Head Trauma Rehabilitation* 32(4):234-244.

Strayhorn, J. C., L. M. Collins, T. R. Brick, S. H. Marchese, A, F. Pfammatter, C. Pellegrini, and B. Spring. 2021. Using factorial mediation analysis to better understand the effects of interventions. *Translational Behavioral Medicine* 12(1):ibab137.

Stultz, D. J., S. Osburn, T. Burns, S. Pawlowska-Wajswol, and R. Walton. 2020. Transcranial magnetic stimulation (TMS) safety with respect to seizures: A literature review. *Neuropsychiatric Disease and Treatment* 16:2989-3000.

Tanielian, T., L. Jaycox, D. Adamson, and K. Metscher. 2008. Introduction. In T. Tanielian and L. Jaycox (Eds.), *Invisible wounds of war: Psychological and Cognitive injuries, their consequences, and services to assist recovery* (pp. 3-17). Santa Monica, CA: RAND.

Thompson, L. L., V. H. Lyons, M. McCart, S. A. Herring, F. P. Rivara, and M. S. Vavilala. 2016. Variations in state laws governing school reintegration following concussion. *Pediatrics* 138(6):e20162151.

Trexler, L.E., L. Trexler, J. Malec, D. Klyce, and D. Parrott. 2010. Prospective randomized controlled trial of resource facilitation on community participation and vocational outcome following brain injury. *Journal of Head Trauma Rehabilitation* 25(6):440-446.

Tsaousides, T., E. D'Antonio, V. Varbanova, and L. Spielman. 2014. Delivering group treatment via videoconference to individuals with traumatic brain injury: A feasibility study. *Neuropsychological Rehabilitation* 24(5):784-803.

Turkstra, L. S., M. Quinn-Padron, J. Johnson, M. Workinger, and N. Antoniotti. 2012. In-person versus telehealth assessment of discourse ability in adults with traumatic brain injury. *Journal of Head Trauma Rehabilitation* 27(6):424-432.

Tyerman A. and J. Booth. 2001. Family intervention after traumatic brain injury: A service example. *NeuroRehabilitation* 16:59-66.

VA (Department of Veterans Affairs). 2021. *VA/DoD Clinical Practice Guideline for the Management and Rehabilitation of Post-Acute Mild Traumatic Brain Injury.* https://www.healthquality.va.gov/guidelines/Rehab/mtbi (accessed December 8, 2021).

Vaughn, S. 2018. *State programs and services for individuals with traumatic brain injury (TBI) and their families.* Washington, DC: National Association of State Head Injury Administrators.

Verhaeghe, S., T. Defloor, and M. Grypdonck. 2005. Stress and coping among families of patients with traumatic brain injury: A review of the literature. *Journal of Clinical Nursing* 14:1004-1012.

Viola-Saltzman, M., and N. Watson. 2012. Traumatic brain injury and sleep disorders. *Neurologic Clinics* 30(4):1299-1312.

Wagner, E. H., C. Davis, J. Schaefer, M. Von Korff, and B. Austin. 1999. Survey of leading chronic disease management programs: Are they consistent with the literature? *Managed Care Quarterly* 7(3):56-66.

Wells, M. J, P. Dukarm, and A. Mills. 2021. Telehealth in rehabilitation psychology and neuropsychology. *Physical Medicine & Rehabilitation Clinics of North America* 32(2):405-18.

Whiteneck, G., C. B. Eagye, J. Cuthbert, J. Corrigan, J. Bell, J. Haarbauer-Krupa, A. C. Miller, J. Ketchum, F. Hammond, K. Dams-O'Connor, and C. Harrison-Felix. 2018. *One and five year outcomes after moderate-to-severe traumatic brain injury requiring inpatient rehabilitation: Traumatic brain injury report.* Centers for Disease Control and Prevention. https://www.cdc.gov/traumaticbraininjury/pdf/CDC-NIDILRR-Self-Report-508.pdf (accessed August 17, 2021).

WHO (World Health Organization). 2015. *WHO Global Disability Action Plan 2014-2021.* Geneva, Switzerland: World Health Organization.

Whyte, J., R. Nakase-Richardson, F. Hammond, S. McNamee, J. Giacino, K. Kalmar, B. Greenwald, S. Yablon, and L. Horn. 2013. Functional outcomes in traumatic disorders of consciousness: 5-year outcomes from the National Institute on Disability and Rehabilitation Research Traumatic Brain Injury Model Systems. *Archives of Physical Medicine and Rehabilitation* 94(10):1855-1860.

Wilson, L., W. Stewart, K. Dams-O'Connor, R. Diaz-Arrastia, L. Horton, D. Menon, and S. Polinder. 2017. The chronic and evolving neurological consequences of traumatic brain injury. *Lancet Neurology* 16(10):813-825.

Winter, L., and H. J. Moriarty. 2017. Quality of relationship between veterans with traumatic brain injury and their family members. *Brain Injury* 31(4):493-501.

Winter, L., H. Moriarty, C. Piersol, T. Vause-Earland, K. Robinson, and B. Newhart. 2016a. Patient- and family-identified problems of traumatic brain injury: Value and utility of a target outcome approach to identifying the worst problems. *Journal of Patient-Centered Research and Reviews* 3(1):30-39.

Winter, L., H. Moriarty, K. E. Robinson, C. V. Piersol, T. Vause-Earland, D. B. Iacovone, L. Holbert, B. Newhart, D. Fishman, N. Hodgson, and L. N. Gitlin. 2016b. Efficacy and acceptability of a home-based, family-inclusive intervention for veterans with TBI: A randomized controlled trial. *Brain Injury* 30(4):373-387.

Yue, J. K., P. S. Upadhyayula, L. N. Avalos, and T. A. Cage. 2020. Pediatric traumatic brain injury in the United States: Rural-urban disparities and considerations. *Brain Sciences* 10(3):135.

Zaninotto, A. L., M. El-Hagrassy, J. Green, M. Babo, V. Paglioni, G. Benute, and W. S. Paiva. 2019. Transcranial direct current stimulation (tDCS) effects on traumatic brain injury (TBI) recovery: A systematic review. *Dementia & Neuropsychologia* 13(2):172-179.

7

Gaps, Challenges, and Opportunities

rior chapters have described the knowledge gaps and clinical care challenges that constrain the ability of providers to meet the needs of TBI patients and their families. This chapter recaps those gaps and challenges and details opportunities for addressing them. The discussion is framed within the bio-psycho-socio-ecological view of TBI (Chapter 3), as leveraging these opportunities will require addressing gaps and overcoming challenges associated with all of these dimensions to advance care and improve outcomes for persons with TBI.

GAPS AND CHALLENGES IN CURRENT TBI CARE AND RESEARCH

People who experience TBI and their families need to receive the best possible medical care, be prepared for the nature of the injury and the likely course of recovery, and receive rehabilitation services that address postinjury symptoms and enable a return to the greatest possible level of preinjury function. To meet these needs, health care providers must be able to identify accurately whether a person has experienced a TBI (diagnosis), and have access to, and impart to patients and their families in an accurate and caring manner, the best possible information on the expected course of recovery, the potential for changes in symptoms, and the patient's future quality of life (prognosis). Also essential is for providers to deliver across the full care continuum care that is both evidence-based and tailored to the individual's unique characteristics and needs. Yet, major gaps and challenges exist in all these aspects of TBI care, as well as in the research enterprise that supports it. These gaps and challenges fall into the seven key areas detailed below.

1. The high degree of heterogeneity and variability of symptoms among people who experience TBI; the many types of brain injuries they experience; and the suite of biological, psychological, social, and ecological factors that influence outcomes

Understanding of the natural history of recovery after TBI and the factors that predict outcomes remains relatively rudimentary. While a combination of injury severity and premorbid factors influences outcomes after TBI, a granular understanding of how these factors interact is currently lacking. This knowledge gap is attributable to the vast heterogeneity that characterizes TBI along dimensions that include injury setting (military, civilian, sport), and characteristics (fragment or projectile, blunt trauma, blast overpressure injury), severity (concussion to coma), and neuropathology (neuronal, axonal, vascular damage; focal versus diffuse trauma). Preinjury factors—who is injured—and postinjury factors—such as the individual's response to the injury and social environment—also influence TBI outcomes. Conventional approaches to data analysis have proven inadequate to overcome the complexities of TBI and its multivariate nature, falling short of fully interrogating and integrating data on injury mechanisms, effects, and recovery. Specific gaps and challenges in this area include those described below.

Lack of sufficiently precise criteria and terminology for classifying TBI. There are no universally accepted criteria for classifying TBI, and the current classification scheme of mild, moderate, and severe, based on Glasgow Coma Scale (GCS) summative scores, is imprecise and can lead to biases in care. Variability also exists around a definition of so-called "mild TBI," which has at least 38 possible definitions, many based on overlapping criteria (Carroll et al., 2004). Varying significantly as well is the terminology used to refer to this condition among clinicians from different medical specialties (e.g., "mild TBI," "concussion," "minor head injury").

Need for greater understanding of the factors that affect outcomes after TBI. The current health care system is designed around making early predictions of a patient's trajectory after injury.[1] However, the ability to predict outcomes after TBI is limited, and as discussed in Chapter 6, an individual's condition often evolves. Clinicians are generally unable to predict who will do well and who will do poorly, regardless of acute injury characteristics and initial GCS score. Better understanding of what factors predict outcomes, along with identification and validation of additional outcome metrics, would help improve both care and management. Unmet needs and open questions include the following:

- Better understanding of the effects of biological sex. Sex-based differences in TBI remain poorly understood (Levin et al., 2021). Research has identified differences in inflammation, neuroplasticity, mitochondrial function, and other characteristics of brain injury and recovery associated with biological sex, but "sex differences in mechanistic measures of neuropathology or physiology are not always associated with differences in functional or neurocognitive outcome" (Gupte et al., 2019, pp. 3079–3080). The biological basis for and implications of observed differences, as well as how they should translate to improved care for patients, remain under investigation. There is also limited knowledge on how certain types of interventions, such as neuromodulation, are affected by biological sex (Phillips et al., 2020).
- Better understanding of TBI in older adults. Relative to younger individuals, older adults are more likely to have preinjury comorbidities that complicate treatment, and tools used to measure TBI severity and predict outcomes may be compromised

---

[1] Hammond, F. 2021. TBI Care Gaps and Opportunities: Provider Perspectives on the Post-Acute Continuum of Care. Panel discussion during virtual workshop for the Committee on Accelerating Progress in Traumatic Brain Injury Research and Care, March 18, 2021.

by age-related cognitive decline. Further research is needed to inform case management of this population (Stein et al., 2018). In addition, the aging population includes people who experienced TBI at younger ages, highlighting the need to understand how prior TBI intersects with the experience of aging and with neurodegenerative processes that may manifest in later years (Griesbach et al., 2018). Research conducted over longer periods to examine later effects could help elucidate connections between acute and long-term outcomes (such as mortality, risk of dementia, risk of sleep disorder, or risk of Parkinson's disease), as well as the underlying mechanisms behind these connections.

- Study of TBI outcomes in subgroups that reflect the diversity of the populations who experience TBI—for example, groups stratified by biological factors (such as age or biological sex) and by social constructs (such as race or ethnicity, location [rural, urban], or military service). Trial exclusion criteria may be exacerbating disparities in TBI outcomes by failing to include key groups.[2] During its information gathering for this study, the committee heard about the need to reflect social determinants of health in study populations and to include information on such social determinants in electronic medical records, as well as a need to go beyond a reliance on demographic covariates conveniently collected in studies to pinpoint sources of disparities. Rather, to be truly informative on these issues, research needs to incorporate empirically and theoretically based variables, particularly those that might be amenable to change, such as perceived cultural competence of providers, racial or ethnic identity, disability identity, and endorsement of traditional gender-role ideologies.[3] Studies need also to identify and connect results to implementation strategies aimed at reducing disparities in TBI care and outcomes.

Lack of tools for precision diagnosis, prognosis, and monitoring. No validated tools are currently available for predicting acute or chronic outcomes of TBI or for identifying which patients will have a favorable recovery and which will remain at risk of poor long-term outcomes. It is generally accepted that patients with seemingly equivalent injuries can experience a wide range of recovery trajectories and functional outcomes. As of this writing, no Food and Drug Administration (FDA)-approved biomarker is available that can accurately predict outcomes after TBI. Even serial computed tomography (CT) scanning has only limited predictive ability unless it demonstrates a nonsurvivable injury. More sophisticated imaging, such as magnetic resonance imaging (MRI), may have a role, but although MRI provides additional information, it, too, is incapable of accurately predicting long-term outcomes. Monitoring the evolution of TBI as a condition over time remains a major challenge, and additional research is needed to understand whether or which biomarkers can be most useful for monitoring a patient's progress and potential responses to treatments. Unmet needs and open questions include the following:

- Identifying and validating new types of biomarkers and incorporating those shown to add value into clinical care. A number of the biomarkers currently available for use and those in development are summarized in Appendix B.
- Ensuring that validation of candidate biomarkers is conducted across diverse patient populations.

---

[2] Thompson, H. 2021. Research to Fill Identified TBI Care Gaps. Panel discussion during virtual workshop for the Committee on Accelerating Progress in Traumatic Brain Injury Research and Care, March 18, 2021.

[3] Perrin, P., and J. Iyasere. 2021. Social Determinants of Health. Presentations and panel discussion during virtual workshop for the Committee on Accelerating Progress in Traumatic Brain Injury Research and Care, April 1, 2021.

- Studying the ability of multimodal biomarkers to improve outcome prediction and incorporating them into enhanced prognostic tools.
- Leveraging large datasets to analyze risk factors and develop tools capable of better predicting outcomes based on patient characteristics.

2. **Fragmented care systems with multiple handoffs, during which information can be lost and people can fall out of the system, and the lack of a clear health care lead for addressing TBI over time**

A person with TBI can experience multiple handoffs from the site of injury and pre-hospital care, to care locations within a hospital, to post-acute and rehabilitation care, to community-level services and supports. TBI care and recovery also involve multidisciplinary teams, diverse rehabilitation and community interactions during recovery, and needs that can evolve over long time scales. Handoffs can easily turn into gaps, and coordination is challenging across the many phases of care, specialties, types of providers, and community environments. Unmet needs and open questions include the following:

- Ensuring continuity of care from the point of injury to acute care, post-acute care, rehabilitation, and life-course outcomes. As noted, TBI can have lifelong implications. Yet TBI care is currently episodic, and care transitions represent an opportunity for mistakes to be made. Patients and families often are left to navigate specialized services that are confusing and difficult to find and do not share data with other services. As discussed in Chapter 6, many patients with TBI lack access to the types or amount of rehabilitation care and supportive services they may need over time. Families and caregivers of people with TBI continue to report significant burdens and unmet needs.
- Addressing the need for expanded prehospital research and guidance on the management and triaging of TBI patients, along with an effective handoff process from prehospital environments to hospital emergency departments (EDs). Questions include whether blood biomarkers and/or mobile head CT scanners could be used to improve prehospital triaging; what strategies could enable easier identification of severe TBI that requires surgery, so that patients could be brought directly into surgery from a prehospital setting; and what neurocognitive and neuropsychiatric assessment tools can be developed and used effectively in prehospital settings and EDs.
- Meeting the need for enhanced communication and connections between the care and research communities. The breadth of research issues that touch TBI makes it difficult to communicate about TBI among and between researchers. Researchers also need to understand what new or expanded capabilities are most needed by patients, families, and care providers. However, bidirectional communication between the care and research communities—particularly the basic science and preclinical research communities—remains challenging.
- Enhancing data integration, which remains a key issue. While multiple national, state, and organizational registries, databanks, and databases capture clinical and research data on TBI, there is no national TBI registry. Data cannot be integrated across the care continuum from prehospital care environments to hospital-based care, rehabilitation settings, and community services. And while many care environments use electronic health records (EHRs), neither these systems nor the ways in which patients' TBI information is entered into them are standardized. This lack of

standardized TBI information in EHRs limits the ability to conduct certain types of research, such as comparative effectiveness trials using causal inference methods.

3. **Unwarranted variability in the care patients receive and the failure of available evidence-based guidelines to cover all aspects of TBI care**

The quality of care received by a TBI patient is provider- and facility-dependent. Absent established and agreed-upon treatment algorithms and endpoints, variation in care increases. In some areas, the best practices for managing brain and patient health are not fully understood, and more research is needed to fill these knowledge gaps (see below). In other areas, the need is to implement more consistently what is already known and increase adherence to clinical practice guidelines. Variability is seen, for example, in adherence to existing decision rules for identifying patients who warrant head CT evaluation. In addition, the TBI care available to patients is variable based on such factors as geographic location and socioeconomic factors, with limited providers or services available in rural and underserved areas.

4. **Insufficient access to care, often because of insurance preapproval or reimbursement issues**

Access to rehabilitation care remains a key issue for many people with TBI and their families. The rehabilitation and long-term needs of many TBI patients are not sufficiently provided for by current health and insurance systems. It is important that insurance payment for post-acute and long-term TBI care and rehabilitation align better with the evidence on what care helps and when. In particular, current payment guidelines often appear to be inadequate, too restrictive, and poorly timed. For example, windows for effective rehabilitation may lie well downstream of the end of current benefit designs. Lack of access to care, particularly inequitable access to care, may also impede the ability to conduct clinical research by limiting or skewing who can be recruited into studies aimed at understanding and improving outcomes.

5. **Lack of evidence-guided therapies for treating TBI**

Despite significant efforts, preclinical and clinical research has been difficult to translate into improvements in clinical care. No FDA-approved therapy yet exists for treating underlying damage resulting from TBI, and treatments for acute TBI have failed to demonstrate effectiveness in promoting recovery in large randomized controlled trials with global outcomes.[4] Both the development of effective treatments and information on when and to whom to administer them are needed. Therapies aimed at reducing TBI morbidity and mortality are actively being tested in large animal models and in clinical trials. Selected examples of acute-stage interventions assessed in recent studies include use of the anticonvulsant drug valproic acid to reduce neurologic impairment after TBI (Dekker et al., 2021; Wakam et al., 2021), use of prehospital plasma transfusion to improve survival of severely injured TBI patients at risk of hemorrhagic shock (Sperry et al., 2018; Gruen et al., 2020), and prehospital or ED administration of tranexamic acid to improve survival and post-TBI outcomes (Brenner et al., 2020; Rowell et al., 2020). The studies illustrate the need to identify the most effective interventions given the heterogeneity of TBI and the many circumstances under which it occurs, as well as the impor-

---

[4] Brody, D. 2021. Research to Fill Identified TBI Care Gaps. Panel discussion during virtual workshop for the Committee on Accelerating Progress in Traumatic Brain Injury Research and Care, March 18, 2021.

tance of and challenges inherent in conducting prehospital research. Continued efforts to identify those patients at higher risk for various adverse outcomes (such as intracranial bleeding) and those most likely to benefit from various interventions will be needed, along with further studies on these and other TBI treatments. Ongoing advances in assessment tools, such as the expanded incorporation of blood-based biomarker tests, may also help refine study designs and clinical decision making on which patients should receive which treatments.

Unmet needs and open questions in preclinical research include the following:

- Understanding longer-term risks and outcomes after TBI. While difficult, there is a continuing need to explore how preclinical research can represent the clinical reality past acute-stage TBI, including whether or what animal models might be developed to better capture long-term effects. In addition, there is a need to conduct preclinical studies over longer times and to make greater use of longitudinal study designs.
- Enhancing preclinical models to be more representative of the human populations who experience TBI. These questions are difficult and may not be possible to address, since different preclinical models are more or less representative of different human attributes, use of the models (e.g., certain types of animal models) may have ethical and cost implications, and no model can fully represent the broad range of human TBI experiences. Moreover, such factors as social determinants of health and quality-of-life issues are difficult to measure in preclinical models. However, experimental injury models have used predominantly male rodents (Gupte et al., 2019), and ensuring greater inclusion of female animals may be one straightforward improvement. It may be possible as well to consider such issues as whether and how preclinical models can incorporate the effects of comorbidities and preexisting medical conditions or multiple injuries (such as polytrauma), and whether and how preclinical models can incorporate other elements, including biological sex, age, time to treatment, and prior history of TBI, associated with differences in outcomes after TBI.

Unmet needs and open questions in clinical research include the following:

- Undertaking clinical research that is more representative of the diverse populations that experience TBI (see also the above discussion on research outcomes). This might include conducting additional studies involving older adults and those with preexisting conditions. It might also include recruiting more women with TBI into trials to advance the limited knowledge of sex and gender differences in symptoms, treatment responses, rehabilitation outcomes, and recovery.
- Conducting clinical research over longer periods to illuminate clinical trajectories beyond the acute period.
- Using study designs that incorporate multiple outcome measures, including mechanistic and functional outcomes; using outcome measures that better capture the full burden of disability; and/or using measures that can better capture outcomes identified as being most relevant to patients and families.

6. Gaps in the knowledge base informing best practices and evidence-based acute care

As described in Chapter 5, further evidence and clinical guidance are needed on aspects of acute TBI care, especially when a patient has concomitant injuries or confounding comorbidities. Unmet needs and open questions include the following:

- Determination of more exact treatment thresholds, including development of additional clinical decision tools to guide acute care of TBI patients. Areas of identified knowledge gaps include (1) use of hypertonic saline, mannitol, and nutrition provision; (2) indications for and timing of intracranial pressure monitoring; (3) indications for and timing of decompressive craniectomy, despite recent guidance on this issue in patients with severe TBI; (4) which vasoactive agent should be used to augment cerebral perfusion pressure; (5) lack of a clear definition for hypotension in pediatric and geriatric populations; and (6) transfusion thresholds studied in sufficient numbers of patients to allow stratification by sex and TBI severity.
- Roles and indications for emerging therapies, such as superoxide radicals, deep brain stimulators to awaken patients in minimally conscious states, vagal nerve stimulators, or use of stimulating devices to treat post-TBI depression.
- Cost/benefit evaluation and translation to clinical practice of advanced imaging technologies, such as MRI. Evidence-based guidelines for when and in whom to use MRI or other newer imaging modalities are currently lacking, and there is a need for decision aids to identify patients who warrant further evaluation with brain MRI imaging. Improved informatics are also needed for consistent interpretation of brain imaging results.
- Effects of multisystem trauma on TBI and uncertainty regarding optimal management of such patients to improve outcomes. The optimal interventions and their timing for TBI patients experiencing life-threatening hemorrhage is one significant concern, with unknowns including blood pressure target, use of resuscitation fluids, and the priority order of surgical interventions. The timing of non-life-threatening, noncranial surgeries in the setting of TBI also remains unclear (Wang et al., 2007). The contribution of medical comorbidities and preexisting risk factors, such as hypertension, diabetes, hypercholesterolemia, and prior cardiovascular disease, to clinical outcomes after TBI needs further research.
- Understanding of how multimodal data can be integrated to enhance clinical decisions, including optimizing diagnosis, informing transport to the appropriate level of care, and informing appropriate use of neuroimaging. For example:
  - Could blood-based biomarker tests be incorporated into decision guidance on when to conduct brain CT imaging? Could imaging or blood-based biomarkers further aid decision making on surgical timing for intracranial bleeding?
  - Would equipping ambulances with mobile CT scanners so paramedics could perform CT scans at the injury scene or en route to the hospital be useful and cost-effective?
  - Would incorporating point-of-care testing for approved blood biomarkers, such as glial fibrillary acidic protein (GFAP, a structural protein found in astrocytes) and ubiquitin carboxy-terminal hydrolase L1 (UCH-L1, a highly abundant enzyme found in neuronal cell bodies), into prehospital guidelines improve triaging of patients to the appropriate level of care?
  - Would widely implementing neurocognitive and neuropsychiatric TBI assessment tools in hospital EDs be effective at enhancing diagnosis and management of TBI?

7. Gaps in the knowledge base informing rehabilitation interventions

The evidence base for the effectiveness of many rehabilitation interventions is limited, which also complicates obtaining insurance coverage for such therapies. Few well-controlled intervention trials have been conducted in the post-acute stage, and many of those trials that have been conducted were applied to exclusive samples and settings. Research in this area has been hampered by limited follow-up, particularly for studies employing neuroimaging and biomarkers, and by the inconsistencies in definitions of injury severity noted earlier. Thus the availability of systematic, evidence-based interventions—therapies that are also culturally resonant and patient-centered—is limited. Unmet needs and open questions include the following:

- Development and evaluation of rehabilitation interventions that are tailored to individual and family needs and strengths. As part of such efforts, stakeholder engagement will be needed to identify and refine research questions of greatest interest and impact for patients, families, and caregivers (Winter et al., 2016).
- A general lack of efficacy, effectiveness, pragmatic, causal inference/comparative effectiveness, and implementation studies on comprehensive TBI rehabilitation. As noted above, the evidence base also remains limited on how best to tailor and deliver rehabilitation care for older adults with TBI.
- A need to evaluate the most effective and practical methods for providing follow-up to patients and families once they return to their communities, including through community-based services, interactions with primary care providers, self-management, and/or case management. As one example, a pragmatic trial is currently under way on optimized follow-up for persons with moderate to severe TBI who received inpatient rehabilitation (Fann et al., 2021).

OPPORTUNITIES

Learning from and Connecting Existing Care Systems and Networks

The TBI landscape is not a blank canvas. Connections can be strengthened among existing networks and models of care and research, and best practices further disseminated, to help build an optimized TBI system. As reported in prior chapters, there remains a general disconnect between acute hospital-based care and rehabilitation and community reintegration systems, including a need for greater connections among smaller trauma centers and rehabilitation services.[5] In addition, many patients who experience "mild TBI" are assessed by and referred from primary care practices rather than being seen in trauma systems.

Continuing efforts are needed to connect prehospital care and research and to connect primary care practices with other TBI care system elements. Better linkages and stronger connections among components of the TBI care system would benefit patients and families. At the rehabilitation stage, periodic reassessment of a person's progress and needs could better inform decision making about interventions that could help them and their families regain function and recover to the greatest extent possible. Selected examples of existing TBI care and research efforts that can be integrated into such a TBI system are described below. Learning from and leveraging the success of such efforts can provide an important foundation for the development of an integrated TBI system.

---

[5] Wright, D. 2021. TBI Care Gaps and Opportunities: Provider Perspectives on the Acute-Stage Continuum of Care; and Moore, M. 2021. Disparities in TBI Outcomes. Presentations and panel discussion during virtual workshop for the Committee on Accelerating Progress in Traumatic Brain Injury Research and Care, March 16 and March 18, 2021.

Department of Defense (DoD) and Department of Veterans Affairs (VA) care systems. DoD's military health system is a $50 billion enterprise that comprises 51 hospitals, 424 clinics, and 248 dental clinics. It supports 9.5 million beneficiaries and encounters between 12,000 and 14,000 TBI-related cases each month.[6] The DoD Intrepid Network for TBI, including the National Intrepid Center of Excellence and a network of Intrepid Spirit Centers, provides comprehensive outpatient services for military service members with TBI, particularly concussion (Lee et al., 2019). In addition, eligible service members and Veterans with TBI may receive care through the VA's Polytrauma System of Care (PSC), which was established in coordination with DoD to provide a cadre of specialized clinicians to address the rehabilitation needs of this TBI/polytrauma cohort. The PSC operates as a hub-and-spoke model, with five regional Polytrauma Rehabilitation Centers. The centers provide specialized inpatient rehabilitation and coordinate with numerous network sites to offer comprehensive and sustained care from the stage of acute rehabilitation to transition back to the person's community and ongoing outpatient care (Chung et al., 2015).[7] Additional programs, including programs focused on assistive technology, amputation needs, case management, and vision rehabilitation, work in concert to support care.[8] The DoD/VA system casts a wide net to identify TBI among service members and Veterans, and because it is an encompassing system, it aids in reducing some of the variability in and barriers to care that may be encountered in current civilian health systems.

Civilian trauma care systems. Trauma care in the United States involves state, local, and regional systems for injury response, from emergency medical services (EMS) to designated trauma centers. The American College of Surgeons (ACS) provides a voluntary process for verification of Level I, II, and III trauma centers as having the resources and capabilities outlined in Resources for Optimal Care of the Injured Patient:

> Level I centers, which are often university-based teaching hospitals, provide care for every aspect of injury and have responsibility for leading trauma education, research, and system planning. Level II centers offer many of the same clinical services as Level I centers, but may not provide the same level of comprehensive care or care for the most complex injuries. Level III, IV, and V centers serve patients in communities that lack immediate access to Level I or II centers, and provide emergency assessment, resuscitation, and stabilization before possible transfer to a higher-level trauma center. (NASEM, 2016, p. 83)

Movement toward a national trauma care system. Many trauma health systems are strong but disjointed, and there are a reported "50 million Americans unable to reach a level I and II center within 60 min" (Soto et al., 2018, p. 78). Efforts are under way to foster the creation of a better-integrated, national trauma care system, building on recommendations made in the National Academies report A National Trauma System: Integrating Military and Civilian Trauma Systems to Achieve Zero Preventable Deaths After Injury (NASEM, 2016). The Mission Zero Act of 2019[9] incorporated military trauma care providers into civilian trauma systems. Significant efforts to advance this concept are also under way through such

---

[6] Lee, K. 2021. System Challenges for TBI Care. Panel discussion during virtual workshop for the Committee on Accelerating Progress in Traumatic Brain Injury Research and Care, March 30, 2021.

[7] See also https://www.polytrauma.va.gov/system-of-care/index.asp (accessed August 31, 2021).

[8] See, for example VA Assistive Technology: https://www.prosthetics.va.gov/AssistiveTechnology/index.asp; Regional Amputation Centers: https://www.prosthetics.va.gov/asoc/Regional_Amputation_Centers.asp; Care Management for Post 9/11 Veterans: https://www.oefoif.va.gov/; and Blind Rehabilitation Centers: https://www.rehab.va.gov/PROSTHETICS/blindrehab/locations.asp (all accessed August 31, 2021).

[9] Part of Public Law No. 116-22: Pandemic and All Hazards Preparedness and Advancing Innovation Act.

organizations as the ACS. Fostering relationships and feedback between larger and smaller trauma centers is one area of opportunity for system development.

Civilian and VA Longitudinal Research on TBI Outcomes. The National Institute on Disability, Independent Living, and Rehabilitation Research (NIDILRR) within the Administration for Community Living has established a network of TBI Model Systems (TBIMS) sites that focus on rehabilitation research and knowledge translation. Currently, 16 sites distributed throughout the United States are funded. To be part of the network, centers must provide comprehensive multidisciplinary rehabilitation, conduct clinical research studies, share results though the Model Systems Knowledge Translation Center (MSKTC), and submit longitudinal data for inclusion in the TBIMS National Database. The TBIMS National Database is currently the largest multisite longitudinal TBI resource with information from preinjury through acute care and long-term outcomes among patients who received inpatient rehabilitation (Tso et al., 2021). As of this writing, the TBIMS centers were collecting data on outcomes up to 30 years postinjury. In 2008, the VA and NIDILRR collaborated to establish a VA TBIMS among the five Polytrauma Rehabilitation Centers that address TBI rehabilitation in Veterans. The VA TBIMS includes data on Veterans and service members who experienced TBI of any severity. The TBIMS network enables essential research that informs best practices in care for people with TBI to optimize functional outcomes, particularly in rehabilitation.

Care organization accreditors.[10] Many trauma centers participate in the ACS verification program, while the Commission on Accreditation of Rehabilitation Facilities (CARF) accredits a number of programs providing rehabilitation services. The Joint Commission is the largest accreditor of health care organizations in the United States. Other organizations, such as the National Commission on Correctional Health Care, play roles in accrediting components of the U.S. health care system. The organizations have quality standards and metrics on which accreditation is based. Studies have generally found that adopting quality standards and achieving accreditation contribute to the delivery of quality care for patients and families, including providing recommended care, applying evidence-based practices, and enhancing efficiency, safety, effectiveness, timeliness, and patient-centeredness (Araujo et al., 2020; Bogh et al., 2016; Devkaran et al., 2019; Falstie-Jensen et al., 2017; Hussein et al., 2021). For example, a study of 3,891 U.S. hospitals found that those that were Joint Commission-accredited in 2004 and 2008 performed better than nonaccredited hospitals on most of 16 performance measures (Schmaltz et al., 2011), while a study of 246 CARF-accredited nursing homes showed better outcomes on short-stay quality measures relative to 15,393 non-CARF-accredited nursing homes (Wagner et al., 2013). Although not all studies report consistent impacts from accreditation, the process represents an opportunity to encourage diverse care settings to incorporate current clinical guidance and best practices in care delivery to support positive outcomes after TBI. Engaging relevant accreditation organizations thus provides an additional opportunity to help create and establish an improved TBI system across the full care continuum.

Approaches to conducting out-of-hospital research. The ability to conduct research outside of acute inpatient settings remains challenging, but is essential to advancing TBI care and research. Relevant settings include prehospital environments, EDs, and outpatient rehabilitation and home and community services locations. The Resuscitation Outcomes Consortium (ROC) is an example of an effort to improve out-of-hospital cardiac arrest and trauma

---

[10] See https://www.facs.org/quality-programs/trauma/tqp/center-programs/vrc; http://www.carf.org/Accreditation (both accessed March 2, 2022).

outcomes. The ROC, funded by the National Institutes of Health (NIH), DoD, the American Heart Association, and organizations in Canada, encompassed 10 regions in North America. Research was initiated in the field with a waiver from informed consent. The effort continued for more than 10 years and demonstrated that out-of-hospital research could be performed on a large scale and over diverse geographic regions. The ROC completed two major TBI studies—one on the efficacy of a bolus of hypertonic saline and the other on the efficacy of tranexamic dosing regimens (Bulger et al., 2010; Rowell et al., 2020). Although the studies did not find significant differences in outcomes, they proved that research and 6-month follow-up could be assessed in 85 percent of patients (Rowell et al., 2020).

Box 7-1 describes features within the VA system that can serve the specialized needs of patients with TBI. A nationally integrated health care system for the provision of coordinated rehabilitation services does not exist in the private sector. In addition, the demographics of the patient population served by the VA are skewed toward a greater percentage of male versus female patients, and possibly toward an older patient population, compared with private-sector rehabilitation providers. Although the rehabilitation care provided by the VA is unique relative to what is available in many civilian care settings, these practices can serve as a benchmark for rehabilitation care and provides examples of strategies that may be adaptable to other settings.

BOX 7-1 FEATURES OF VA REHABILITATION SERVICES FOR TBI

- A full continuum of coordinated rehabilitation services within the national VA health care system. Patients with a diagnosis of TBI have access to a national network of providers specialized in TBI rehabilitation.
- Decisions to provide rehabilitation services driven by identification of clinical need, without regard for discharge disposition or financial constraints. VA rehabilitation service providers can therefore meet the needs of those who may be disadvantaged psychosocially or financially.
- A model of team-based interdisciplinary care, as opposed to a model of multidisciplinary care. Patient goals can be addressed across disciplines in a coordinated manner. For example, co-treatment sessions with the patient are conducted concurrently by the physical therapist and the occupational therapist to address the impact of vestibular system deficits on activities of daily living, and the speech-language pathologist and the psychologist work concurrently with the patient to address cognitive rehabilitation needs.
- Access to rehabilitation professionals beyond the traditional therapies (physical, occupational, and speech-language), addressing the mind–body connection as well as holistic and alternative medicine, and providing access to services not typically available in private-sector rehabilitation. For example, services may be provided by chaplains, vision rehabilitation specialists, recreational therapists, family counseling therapists, and art therapists.
- Access to specialized programs and professionals with expertise to meet the specific needs of the individual, including the Emerging Consciousness Program (ECP), Headache Center of Excellence (HCoE), Assistive Technology Center (ATC), Spinal Cord Injury/Disorders (SCI/D) system of care, Polytrauma System of Care (PSC), Traumatic Brain Injury Center of Excellence (TBI CoE), Regional Amputation Center (RAC), Intensive Evaluation and Treatment Program (IETP), Epilepsy Center of Excellence, and Adaptive Sports Program.
- A system able to address the long-term needs of patients served through the established supporting programs. For example, the Military 2 Veterans Affairs (M2VA) program provides case management services on a long-term basis. Long-term case management services are often not available to patients served by private-sector rehabilitation providers.

continued

BOX 7-1   CONTINUED

- The nation's largest teaching health care organization. VA medical centers are affiliated with leading universities, connections that are instrumental in advancing medicine and providing access to evolving evidence, research opportunities, and services to meet the rehabilitation needs of medically complex patients in an efficient and effective manner. For example, the PSC can meet the needs of a person with diagnoses of severe TBI, spinal cord injury, burns, vision loss, and multiple limb loss through access to specialized, coordinated care within one health care system.
- Rehabilitation services with setting, duration, and intensity driven by the clinical needs of the patient, without the constraints of a third-party payer, providing optimal clinical outcomes. Although length of stay may be longer than in the private sector, outcomes achieved are often superior to those achieved by private-sector rehabilitation providers because VA providers are able to fully rehabilitate patients before transitioning them to the next level of care or discharge (i.e., the percentage of patients discharged to the community is higher within the VA compared with private-sector rehabilitation service providers).
- Availability through the national VA health care system of seed funding for the development of specialty programming, which can subsequently be integrated on a national level.

Enhancing and Connecting Existing Data Systems

Multiple registries, databanks, and information systems capture aspects of TBI care and research. Two issues—data integration to improve the capability to collate and analyze patient TBI information, and the ability to tie patient outcomes back to clinical care—remain, given the varied settings in which TBI occurs, the multiple phases of care and recovery, the heterogeneity of injury and diversity of people affected by TBI, and the active base of preclinical and clinical research. This issue starts with the need to link prehospital data to in-hospital or posthospital registries, connecting data across the continuum of care and services. The need for trauma information systems and access to patient-level data was also noted in the *Zero Preventable Deaths* report (NASEM, 2016); efforts to advance and integrate data systems as part of developing a national trauma system may provide valuable building blocks applicable to TBI as well.

Selected examples of databanks and registries relevant to TBI include the National EMS database, NEMSIS, supported by the National Highway Traffic Safety Administration (NHTSA); the ACS's National Trauma Databank (NTDB), a voluntary aggregation of U.S. trauma registry data; and multiple state trauma registries. DoD's Trauma Registry (DoDTR) was established in 2005, modeled after the NTDB; it incorporates subregistries, including one for TBI. The VA's Traumatic Brain Injury Veterans Health Registry collects information on Veterans with a TBI-related diagnostic code who served in Iraq or Afghanistan, applied for VA disability benefits, and/or screened positive for TBI on the screening assessment administered when a Veteran seeks VA health care. In addition, the NIDILRR and VA TBI Model Systems databases contain information on long-term outcomes and rehabilitation.

Although there is no U.S. national TBI registry, efforts to connect or crosslink data sources provide an opportunity to better harness the wealth of collected TBI information. Potential areas of study that might be aided by analyzing registry data include optimization and timing of patient transport, indications for intracranial pressure monitoring and novel monitoring methods, optimal ventilation strategies, and development of point-of-care biomarkers.

Care providers and hospitals have also widely implemented EHRs. Large EHR providers such as EPIC, Cerner, and Meditech are estimated to provide software to almost three-quarters of the hospital market.[11] In addition, the VA is in the process of a large-scale EHR modernization effort,[12] due to be completed by 2028, whose purpose is to create a connected EHR across DoD and VA medical centers and facilitate connections with community care providers. These efforts provide valuable opportunities to establish within EHR systems the collection of standardized patient information needed to support research on TBI care and outcomes. For example, data on social determinants of health are missing from many systems, but greater collection of such information could be encouraged by including relevant EHR fields. The VA, for instance, includes primary care screening questions on housing instability and refers at-risk Veterans for services (Montgomery et al., 2013). And a project to implement the Centers for Disease Control and Prevention's (CDC's) Stopping Elderly Accidents, Deaths, and Injuries (STEADI) program for older adults at risk of falls identified the incorporation of screening tools into the clinic's workflows and EHR system as key components of the effort (Casey et al., 2017). This issue may represent an opportunity for lessons learned and further public–private dialogue and partnership efforts.

In the research community, investigators are required to enter data from federally funded TBI research into the Federal Informatics System for Research Data (FITBIR), used by both NIH and DoD. Entered information includes Common Data Elements (CDEs) encompassing information from clinical studies, and now being extended to include preclinical research. Although entering the information into the system can reportedly be time-consuming, the system enables valuable access to DoD- and NIH-funded data in a common place.

Collectively, crosslinking or finding improved ways to share and connect information from these valuable resources provides an opportunity to advance an integrated TBI system.

Analyzing Data from Recent Large-Scale and Long-Term Research Efforts

Large-scale and longitudinal TBI studies, such as those highlighted throughout this report and in Appendix A, are providing a wealth of data to enable better understanding of TBI. It has been a challenge to apply a precision medicine approach to TBI treatment, in which management strategies are targeted to the right patient at the right time and in the right setting. The lack of predictive tools also inhibits rational initiation and timing of interventions to reduce overall disability associated with TBI. There is an opportunity to leverage the information being obtained from the past decade of TBI efforts to better understand how multiple individual biological, psychological, social, and ecological factors affect outcomes after TBI, and to identify and validate new imaging, blood-based, and other types of biomarkers that can contribute now and in the future, as research advances.

Significant efforts have been devoted to discovery, validation, and optimization of objective TBI biomarkers that can supplement such injury information as physiological measures and vital signs. A biomarker is an indicator of the presence of a condition, such as TBI, and

---

[11] See https://klasresearch.com/blog/top-trends-in-emr-market-share/856 and https://www.beckershospitalreview.com/ehrs/ehr-market-share-2021-10-things-to-know-about-major-players-epic-cerner-meditech-allscripts.html (both accessed March 2, 2022).

[12] See https://www.ehrm.va.gov (accessed March 2, 2022).

can also be measured or monitored for changes in the condition over time. The primary TBI biomarker types are

- neuroimaging, such as CT and MRI;
- biofluid-based, such as those from cerebrospinal fluid (CSF), saliva, urine, or blood; and
- neurophysiological, such as electroencephalography (EEG) and eye tracking.

These biomarkers are being studied to identify such features as the nature, location, and extent of injuries—such as bleeding and swelling in the brain; disruption of the blood–brain barrier; inflammation; changes in cellular metabolism; and damage to brain cells, such as changes in brain cell signaling and markers of neurodegeneration—to identify and track the effects of TBI. During the past decade, candidate biomarkers have emerged that may provide insight into the mechanisms and dynamic course of TBI (Agoston et al., 2017; Di Battista et al., 2015; Diaz-Arrastia et al., 2014; McCrea et al., 2020; Zetterberg et al., 2013). Appendix B reviews progress in TBI biomarkers in greater detail.

The lack of demonstrated effectiveness for TBI therapies in randomized controlled trials supports the need for more precise recruitment of participants into trials designed to test the efficacy of these therapies. Lumping heterogeneous patient populations together for recruitment into clinical trials and evaluation of trial results has made it challenging to demonstrate effectiveness. It is difficult, for example, to target a drug to the ill-defined category of "mild" TBI. It is also challenging to target a drug to "patients who have in common a 'severe' injury phenotype who may vary widely in other injury classification schemes, such as those based on pathoanatomic or pathophysiological features, which may be more relevant to the neuroprotectant action of a particular intervention" (Saatman et al., 2008, p. 722). In today's world of precision medicine, no one would imagine conducting a drug trial for mild, moderate, or severe cancer.

Analyzing information from recent studies has provided a basis for identifying and refining TBI "phenotypes" that can aid in more standardized and precise stratification. Ongoing efforts to identify and validate multiple biomarkers are also contributing to these efforts. For example, Gravesteijn and colleagues (2020) conducted a cluster analysis of the European CENTER-TBI database and identified four patient clusters "defined by injury mechanism, presence of major extracranial injury and GCS" (p. 1002). A recent paper from Pugh and colleagues (2021) describes a machine learning–based tool and data repository for identifying TBI patient phenotypes and enhancing precision care. In addition to aiding in patient stratification for trials, predictive and pharmacodynamics biomarkers may be able to serve as secondary endpoints in trials evaluating new therapies, providing more objective means of assessing response to treatment at the neurobiological or mechanistic level. Ideally, advances in biomarkers and other tools for phenotyping TBI will increase the likelihood of success in developing novel treatments to improve outcomes.

Developing and Disseminating an Improved Classification System for TBI Diagnosis, Prognosis, Monitoring, and Research

As noted earlier, current methods for classification of acute TBI are based primarily on the GCS score (GCS 3–8: severe, GCS 9–12: moderate, GCS 13–15: mild). Some operational definitions incorporate acute injury characteristics (e.g., loss of consciousness or post-traumatic amnesia) into the classification of mild, moderate, or severe TBI. The construct of "complicated mild TBI" is often applied in reference to patients with GCS 13–15 and abnormal radiologic findings (e.g., positive head CT or MRI). Still, in most clinical settings, the universal TBI taxonomy is broadly reduced to "mild, moderate, or severe." Knowledge gained from the past decade of TBI studies has yielded clinical, imaging, and blood-based biomarker elements with diagnostic and prognostic value that can be incorporated to improve on traditional TBI classification. As new biomarkers are developed and validated, it will be important to reevaluate periodically the TBI classification system and how it can be refined and further improved.

Establishing a more accurate framework for characterizing and classifying TBI would help achieve the goals of precision medicine models for individualized treatment, improved prognostic models for predicting a patient's trajectory of recovery and outcome, and more precise selection of subjects for clinical trials (e.g., phenotyping).

A multidimensional "basic TBI classification" system could be adopted now. It would include

- GCS sum, or total, score (not mild, moderate, or severe);
- clinical neuroimaging results (head CT scan and brain MRI, when available and clinically indicated); and
- blood biomarker results (acute GFAP and UCH-L1 levels, when available and clinically indicated).

This basic system would provide a more precise and objective description of the injury, and while more complex than the current system, would be feasible in the acute care arena.

An "advanced TBI classification" system could be developed to extend the basic system by including additional information that could be obtained in the acute and sub-acute settings, fully characterizing the patient based on factors now known to affect recovery and outcomes after TBI. This information would include

- mechanism of injury;
- GCS score with each of the three components described (e.g., eye, verbal, and motor responses);
- acute injury characteristics, including duration of unconsciousness, duration of post-traumatic amnesia, and duration of altered mental status;
- clinical neuroimaging results;
- blood biomarker results;
- premorbid factors, including history of prior TBI or neurologic disorder, psychiatric or substance use disorder, and major health conditions;
- social factors, such as family support, living situation, and employment status; and
- health care disparities, such as inability to access follow-up care.

Because a single point assessment is insufficient for a dynamic and complex condition such as TBI, which is affected by many factors, repeated measures will be needed as the person's condition evolves. Implementing improved, multimodal approaches for classifying patients could provide the opportunity for more precise targeting and monitoring of care, as well as more successful translation of therapies from the bench to the bedside.

Making Greater Use of All Types of Study Designs

The TBI field will need to use multiple research design tools, beyond randomized controlled trials, to improve the evidence base in a manner that also allows for implementation in the real world. Using the full range of clinical trial designs and engaging the voices of those living with TBI would provide important opportunities to advance the evidence base across the continuum of care and recovery.

A variety of clinical trial methods are needed to address the complexities of TBI. Measuring longitudinal outcomes with simple trials is unsustainably inefficient.[13] Evaluation needs to focus not on time points but on trajectories of recovery from TBI (e.g., using such approaches as recovery progression models), and to use such methods as Bayesian adaptive design. A "one bite at a time" approach has been proposed for tackling TBI as well, in which studies would address specific symptoms and deficits in particular TBI subpopulations (Brody et al., 2019).

Establishing a platform approach to clinical trials would also be valuable for enhancing the efficiency of discovery and tackling the complexity of TBI. A first step in such an approach is often to build the initial structure of the platform so that the cost of conducting trials using the platform is lower than that of not using it.[14] An example of such a platform is the Strategies to Innovate Emergency Care Clinical Trial Network (SIREN),[15] funded by the National Institute of Neurological Disorders and Stroke (NINDS) and the National Heart, Lung, and Blood Institute (NHLBI), which consists of centers with neurological and cardiac emergency and critical care expertise. Investigator-initiated, funded grants are executed through the trial network and have included Brain Oxygen Optimization in Severe TBI Phase 3 (BOOST-3: NCT03754114), Hyperbaric Oxygen Brain Injury Treatment Trial (HOBIT: NCT02407028), and ancillary studies. An aim of establishing trial platforms is to reduce the overall time and cost investment for individual trials by using a network of partner clinical trial sites, flexible Bayesian adaptive designs, and streamlined regulatory processes.

The simultaneous application of multiple treatments and interventions, a common aspect of TBI rehabilitation, further raises the question of whether it is meaningful to try to define the effects of individual rehabilitation components rather than the services and delivery system more holistically. Conducting trials in which interventions are tailored to the needs of individual patients and families rather than being standardized is a challenge, but certain research design methods can aid in achieving the goals of both tailoring and flexibility (e.g., pragmatic trials can be designed to allow for some tailoring to the individual and flexibility in application while yielding evidence that can be applied to a larger proportion of the population who receive care outside the controlled environments often required by randomized controlled trials). There is also an ongoing need for "evidence in TBI rehabilitation that delineates the extent that differences in outcomes are attributable to patients' characteristics such as age, severity, time since injury, and pre-injury factors, and how much outcomes can be attributed to the timing and dose of specific rehabilitation interventions" (Horn et al., 2015, p. S189). Further research will be needed to compare outcomes of persons who receive different types of interventions and different systems of care. The use of ecological momentary assessments may be one feasible method for measuring outcomes, such as mental health, that can change over time (Juengst et al., 2021).

In addition, using participatory research approaches strengthens the voice of people and families living with TBI in the research process and can help ensure that issues of greatest interest to these communities are being addressed. The use of such approaches also promotes translation of findings to the community (Frank et al., 2014; Winter et al., 2016).

---

[13] Lewis, R. 2021. Research to Fill Identified TBI Care Gaps. Panel discussion during virtual workshop for the Committee on Accelerating Progress in Traumatic Brain Injury Research and Care, March 18, 2021.

[14] Ibid.

[15] Yaffe, K. 2021. Research to Fill Identified TBI Care Gaps. Panel discussion during virtual workshop for the Committee on Accelerating Progress in Traumatic Brain Injury Research and Care, March 18, 2021.

Expanding Consensus Processes for Guidance on TBI Care

As discussed in Chapters 5 and 6, multiple guidelines inform aspects of TBI care. Because there are so many types of TBI in so many populations and involving so many clinical specialties and care providers, there is a need to systematically review and coordinate the content of clinical guidance to promote consistent access to high-quality care and reduce unwarranted variability. Guideline development processes consider the strength of the evidence available to support recommendations, often ranking evidence on a scale in which Level 1 evidence has been obtained through randomized controlled trials, evidence obtained through other types of studies is considered Level 2, and practices based on expert opinion are considered Level 3 (VA, 2019). Guidelines differ in how they treat different types of evidence and which types they include in the guidance development process.

It has been a significant challenge to obtain evidence from randomized controlled trials to inform all relevant aspects of TBI care and recovery. In some cases, such a trial may not yet have been conducted on a specific question. In other cases, such as for many rehabilitation interventions, evidence has been difficult to obtain through randomized controlled trials, and using an expanded toolkit of study designs could better address salient research questions. As a result, guidelines to inform TBI care, and reimbursement for care, have gaps if they rely only on evidence from such trials.

Consensus-based processes represent an important mechanism for collating and disseminating best-practice guidance. One example in which this approach has been successful is the work of the Concussion in Sport group. Over six cycles since 2001, the group has developed and iterated an influential Consensus Statement on Concussion and has successfully disseminated standardized recommendations for the identification and management of this type of TBI in sports. The process for developing the statement incorporates both the latest high-quality evidence and best clinical practices, and can serve as an exemplar for the development of clinical guidelines for TBI more broadly.

The committee believes that multiple types of evidence remain important for informing TBI care. Thus there are opportunities for further rigorously conducted, consensus-based processes to guide care across the phases of TBI, including by providing practical information on current best practices in areas in which evidence is still being gathered.

Harnessing Insights from Implementation Science

Implementation science is the study of methods for promoting the "systematic uptake of proven clinical treatments, practices, organizational, management interventions into routine practice, and hence to improve health."[16] Clinical research is needed to identify "what works," while implementation research is needed to identify "how to make it work" (Forrest et al., 2014, p. 1172). To maximize practical impact, specific, concrete aims and implementation strategies must be married to the generation of new knowledge. Both considering in advance what can go wrong through initial planning and "premortem analysis" and learning afterward from study limitations or failures are valuable.

Incorporating insights from implementation science into TBI study design and planning for more effective translation of research results to practice represents an important opportunity to accelerate progress in TBI care. Taking advantage of this opportunity would likely require greater awareness of the role of implementation science among researchers and

---

[16] Beidas, R. 2021. "Lessons from Implementation Science." Presentations and panel discussion during virtual workshop for the Committee on Accelerating Progress in Traumatic Brain Injury Research and Care, April 1, 2021, and quoting from Eccles et al., 2012, p. 2.

clinicians and closer engagement with experts in this field. In particular, widespread adoption of improvements in TBI care will depend on close and ongoing relationships among researchers, active clinicians, and other community stakeholders, and between centers of excellence in TBI care and community-based hospitals and clinicians. Given the extent of the TBI burden and the opportunities for improvement, TBI may indeed be an ideal topic for expanded implementation science research.

CONCLUSIONS

Despite ongoing gaps and challenges, there are a number of opportunities for advancing TBI care and research. These opportunities build on prior efforts and investments made to advance the understanding of TBI and to develop needed care and research infrastructures. Collectively, these opportunities can help the field strengthen and create an optimized system for TBI.

REFERENCES

Agoston, D. V., A. Shutes-David, and E. R. Peskind. 2017. Biofluid biomarkers of traumatic brain injury. *Brain Injury* 31(9):1195-1203.

Araujo, C. A. S., M. M. Siqueira, and A. M. Malik. 2020. Hospital accreditation impact on healthcare quality dimensions: a systematic review. *International Journal for Quality Health Care* 32(8):531-544.

Brenner, A., A. Belli, R. Chaudhri, T. Coats, L. Frimley, S. F. Jamaluddin, R. Jooma, R. Mansukhani, P. Sandercock, H. Shakur-Still, T. Shokunbi, I. Roberts, and CRASH-3 trial collaborators. 2020. Understanding the neuroprotective effect of tranexamic acid: An exploratory analysis of the CRASH-3 randomised trial. *Critical Care* 24(1):560.

Bogh, S. B., A. M. Falstie-Jensen, E. Hollnagel, R. Holst, J. Braithwaite, and S. P. Johnsen. 2016. Improvement in quality of hospital care during accreditation: A nationwide stepped-wedge study. *International Journal for Quality in Health Care* 28(6):715-720.

Brody, D., L. Chan, and G. Cizza. 2019. How do you treat traumatic brain injury? One symptom at a time. *Annals of Neurology* 86(3):329-331.

Bulger, E. M., S. May, K. J. Brasel, M. Schreiber, J. D. Kerby, S. A. Tisherman, C. Newgard, A. Slutsky, R. Coimbra, S. Emerson, J. P. Minei, B. Bardarson, P. Kudenchuk, A. Baker, J. Christenson, A. Idris, D. Davis, T. C. Fabian, T. P. Aufderheide, C. Callaway, C. Williams, J. Banek, C. Vaillancourt, R. van Heest, G. Sopko, J. S. Hata, and D. Hoyt, for the ROC Investigators. 2010. Out-of-hospital hypertonic resuscitation following severe traumatic brain injury: A randomized controlled trial. *Journal of the American Medical Association* 304(13):1455-1464.

Carroll, L., J. D. Cassidy, L. Holm, J. Kraus, V. Coronado, and WHO Collaborating Centre Task Force on Mild Traumatic Brain Injury. 2004. Methodological issues and research recommendations for mild traumatic brain injury: The WHO Collaborating Centre Task Force on Mild Traumatic Brain Injury. *Journal of Rehabilitation Medicine* 43(Suppl):113-125.

Casey, C. M., E. M. Parker, G. Winkler, X. Liu, G. H. Lambert, and E. Eckstrom. 2017. Lessons learned from implementing CDC's STEADI falls prevention algorithm in primary care. *Gerontologist* 57(4):787-796.

Chung, J., F. Aguila, and O. Harris. 2015. Validity assessment of referral decisions at a VA health care system polytrauma system of care. *Cureus* 7(1):e240. https://doi.org/10.7759/cureus.240.

Dekker, S. E., B. E. Biesterveld, T. Bambakidis, A. M. Williams, R. Tagett, C. N. Johnson, M. Sillesen, B. Liu, Y. Li, and H. B. Alam. 2021. Modulation of brain transcriptome by combined histone deacetylase inhibition and plasma treatment following traumatic brain injury and hemorrhagic shock. *Shock* 55(1):110-120.

Devkaran, S., P. N. O'Farrell, S. Ellahham, and R. Arcangel. 2019. Impact of repeated hospital accreditation surveys on quality and reliability, an 8-year interrupted time series analysis. *BMJ Open* 9(2):e024514.

Di Battista, A. P., J. E. Buonora, S. G. Rhind, M. G. Hutchison, A. J. Baker, S. B. Rizoli, R. Diaz-Arrastia, and G. P. Mueller. 2015. Blood Biomarkers in moderate-to-severe traumatic brain injury: Potential utility of a multi-marker approach in characterizing outcome. *Frontiers in Neurology* 6:110. https://doi.org/10.3389/fneur.2015.00110.

Diaz-Arrastia, R., K. K. Wang, L. Papa, M. D. Sorani, J. K. Yue, A. M. Puccio, P. J. McMahon, T. Inoue, E. L. Yuh, H. F. Lingsma, A. I. Maas, A. B. Valadka, D. O. Okonkwo, G. T. Manley, and TRACK-TBI Investigators. 2014. Acute biomarkers of traumatic brain injury: Relationship between plasma levels of ubiquitin C-terminal hydrolase-L1 and glial fibrillary acidic protein. *Journal of Neurotrauma* 31(1):19-25.

Eccles, M. P., R. Foy, A. Sales, M. Wensing, and B. Mittman. 2012. Implementation science six years on—Our evolving scope and common reasons for rejection without review. *Implementation Science* 7:71 https://doi.org/10.1186/1748-5908-7-71.

Falstie-Jensen, A. M., S. B. Bogh, E. Hollnagel, and S. P. Johnsen. 2017. Compliance with accreditation and recommended hospital care-a Danish nationwide population-based study. *International Journal for Quality in Health Care* 29(5):625-633.

Fann, J. R., T. Hart, M. A. Ciol, M. Moore, J. Bogner, J. D. Corrigan, K. Dams-O'Connor, S. Driver, R. Dubiel, F. M. Hammond, M. Kajankova, T. K. Watanabe, and J. M. Hoffman. 2021. Improving transition from inpatient rehabilitation following traumatic brain injury: Protocol for the BRITE pragmatic comparative effectiveness trial. *Contemporary Clinical Trials* 104:106332. https://doi.org/10.1016/j.cct.2021.106332.

Forrest, C. B., P. Margolis, M. Seid, and R. B. Colletti. 2014. PEDSnet: How a prototype pediatric learning health system is being expanded into a national network. *Health Affairs (Project Hope)* 33(7):1171-1177.

Frank, L., E. Basch, J. V. Selby; and Patient-Centered Outcomes Research Institute. 2014. The PCORI perspective on patient-centered outcomes research. *Journal of the American Medical Association* 312:1513-1514.

Gravesteijn, B., C. Sewalt, A. Ercole, C. Akerlund, D. Nelson, A. Maas, D. Menon, H. Lingsma, E. Stseyerberg, and the Collaborative European NeuroTrauma Effectiveness Research for Traumatic Brain Injury Collaborators. 2020. Toward a new multi-dimensional classification of traumatic brain injury: A collaborative European NeuroTrauma Effectiveness Research for Traumatic Brain Injury Study. *Journal of Neurotrauma* 37(7):1002-1010.

Griesbach, G. S., B. Masel, R. E. Helvie, and M. J. Ashley. 2018. The impact of traumatic brain injury on later life: Effects on normal aging and neurodegenerative diseases. *Journal of Neurotrauma* 35(1):17-24.

Gruen, D. S., F. X. Guyette, J. B. Brown, D. O. Okonkwo, A. M. Puccio, I. K. Campwala, M. T. Tessmer, B. J. Daley, R. S. Miller, B. G. Harbrecht, J. A. Claridge, H. A. Phelan, M. D. Neal, B. S. Zuckerbraun, M. H. Yazer, T. R. Billiar, and J. L Sperry. 2020. Association of prehospital plasma with survival in patients with traumatic brain injury: A secondary analysis of the PAMPer cluster randomized clinical trial. *JAMA Network Open* 3(10):e2016869.

Gupte, R., W. Brooks, R. Vukas, J. Pierce, and J. Harris. 2019. Sex differences in traumatic brain injury: What we know and what we should know. *Journal of Neurotrauma* 36(22):3063-3091.

Horn, S., J. Corrigan, J. Bogner, F. Hammond, R. Seel, R. Smout, R. Barrett, M. Dijkers, and G. Whiteneck. 2015. Traumatic brain injury practice-based evidence study: Design and patients, centers, treatments, and outcomes. *Archives of Physical Medicine and Rehabilitation* 96(8):S178-S196.

Hussein, M., M. Pavlova, M. Ghalwash, and W. Groot. 2021. The impact of hospital accreditation on the quality of healthcare: A systematic literature review. *BMC Health Services Research* 21(1):1057.

Juengst, S. B., L. Terhorst, A. Nabasny, T. Wallace, J. A. Weaver, C. L. Osborne, S. P. Burns, B. Wright, P. S. Wen, C. N. Kew, and J. Morris. 2021. Use of mHealth technology for patient-reported outcomes in community-dwelling adults with acquired brain injuries: A scoping review. *International Journal of Environmental Research and Public Health* 18(4):2173.

Lee, K. M., W. Greenhalgh, P. Sargent, H. Chae, S. Klimp, S. Engel, B. Merritt, T. Kretzmer, L. Bajor, S. Scott, and S. Pyne. 2019. Unique features of the US Department of Defense Multidisciplinary Concussion Clinics. *Journal of Head Trauma Rehabilitation* 34(6):402-408.

Levin, H., N. Temkin, J. Barber, L. Nelson, C. Robertson, J. Brennan, M. Stein, et al. 2021. Association of sex and age with mild traumatic brain injury—Related symptoms: A TRACK-TBI study. *JAMA Network Open* 4(4):e213046. https://doi.org/10.1001/jamanetworkopen.2021.3046.

McCrea, M., S. Broglio, T. McAllister, J. Gill, C. Giza, D. Huber, J. Harezlak, K. Cameron, M. Houston, G. McGinty, J. Jackson, K. Guskiewicz, J. Mihalik, M. A. Brooks, S. Duma, S. Rowson, L. Nelson, P. Pasquina, T. Meier, and the CARE Consortium Investigators. 2020. Association of blood biomarkers with acute sport-related concussion in collegiate athletes: Findings from the NCAA and Department of Defense CARE Consortium. *JAMA Network Open* 3(1):e1919771. https://doi.org/10.1001/jamanetworkopen.2019.19771.

Montgomery, A. E., J. D. Fargo, T. H. Byrne, V. R. Kane, and D. P. Culhane. 2013. Universal screening for homelessness and risk for homelessness in the Veterans Health Administration. *American Journal of Public Health* 103(Suppl 2):S210-S211.

NASEM (National Academies of Sciences, Engineering, and Medicine). 2016. *A national trauma care system: Integrating military and civilian trauma systems to achieve zero preventable deaths after injury.* Washington, DC: The National Academies Press.

Phillips, A., S. Sami, and M. Adamson. 2020. Sex differences in neuromodulation treatment approaches for traumatic brain injury: A scoping review. *Journal of Head Trauma Rehabilitation* 35(6):412-429.

Pugh, M. J., E. Kennedy, E. Prager, J. Humpherys, K. Dams-O'Connor, D. Hack, M. K. McCafferty, J. Wolfe, K. Yaffe, M. McCrea, A. Ferguson, L. Lancashire, J. Ghajar, and A. Lumba-Brown. 2021. Phenotyping the spectrum of traumatic brain injury: A review and pathway to standardization. *Journal of Neurotrauma.* https://doi.org/10.1089/neu2021.0059.

Rowell, S. E., E. Meier, B. McKnight, D. Kannas, S. May, K. Sheehan, E. Bulger, A. Idris, J. Christenson, L. Morrison, R. Frascone, P. Bosarge, M. R. Colella, J. Johannigman, B. Cotton, J. Callum, J. McMullan, D. Dries, B. Tibbs, N. Richmond, M Weisfeldt, J. Tallon, J. Garrett, M. Zielinski, T. Aufderheide, R. Gandhi, R. Schlamp, B. Robinson, J. Jui, L. Klein, S. Rizoli, M. Gamber, M. Fleming, J. Hwang, L. Vincent, C. Williams, A. Hendrickson, R. Simonson, P. Klotz, G. Sopko, W. Witham, M. Ferrara, and M. Schreiber. 2020. Effect of out-of-hospital tranexamic acid vs placebo on 6-month functional neurologic outcomes in patients with moderate or severe traumatic brain injury. *Journal of the American Medical Association* 324(10):961-974.

Saatman, K., A-C. Duhaime, R. Bullock, A. Maas, A. Valadka, G. Manley, and Workshop Scientific Team and Advisory Panel Members. 2008. Classification of traumatic brain injury for targeted therapies. *Journal of Neurotrauma* 25:719-738.

Schmaltz, S. P., S. C. Williams, M. R. Chassin, J. M. Loeb, and R. M. Wachter. 2011. Hospital performance trends on national quality measures and the association with Joint Commission accreditation. *Journal of Hospital Medicine* 6(8):454-461.

Soto, J. M., Y. Zhang, J. H. Huang, and D. X. Feng. 2018. An overview of the American trauma system. *Chinese Journal of Traumatology* 21(2):77-79.

Sperry, J. L., F. X. Guyette, J. B. Brown, M. H. Yazer, D. J. Triulzi, B. J. Early-Young, P. W. Adams, B. J. Daley, R. S. Miller, B. G. Harbrecht, J. A. Claridge, H. A. Phelan, W. R. Witham, A. T. Putnam, T. M. Duane, L. H. Alarcon, C. W. Callaway, B. S. Zuckerbraun, M. D. Neal, M. R. Rosengart, R. M. Forsythe, T. R. Billiar, D. M. Yealy, A. B. Peitzman, M. S. Zenati, and PAMPer Study Group. 2018. Prehospital plasma during air medical transport in trauma patients at risk for hemorrhagic shock. *New England Journal of Medicine* 379(4):315-326.

Stein, D. M., R. A. Kozar, H. Livingston, F. Luchette, S. D. Adams, V. Agrawal, S. Arbabi, J. Ballou, R. Barraco, A. Bernard, W. Biffl, P. Bosarge, K. Brasel, Z. Cooper, P. Efron, S. Fakhry, C. Hartline, F. Hwang, B. Joseph, S. Kurek, F. Moore, A. Mosenthal, A. Pathak, M. Truitt, J. Yelon, and AAST Geriatric Trauma/ACS Committee. 2018. Geriatric traumatic brain injury—what we know and what we don't. *Journal of Trauma and Acute Care Surgery* 85(4):788-798.

Tso, S., A. Saha, and M. D. Cusimano. 2021. The Traumatic Brain Injury Model Systems National Database: A review of published research. *Neurotrauma Reports* 2(1):149-164.

VA (Department of Veteran Affairs). 2019. *Guideline for guidelines.* Department of Defense. Revised January 29, 2019. https://www.healthquality.va.gov/documents/GuidelinesForGuidelinesRevised013019.pdf (accessed August 3, 2021).

Wagner, L. M., S. M. McDonald, and N. G. Castle. 2013. Impact of voluntary accreditation on short-stay rehabilitative measures in U.S. nursing homes. *Rehabilitation Nursing* 38(4):167-177.

Wakam, G. K., B. E. Biesterveld, M. P. Pai, M. T. Kemp, R. L. O'Connell, A. M. Williams, A. Srinivasan, K. Chtraklin, A. Z. Siddiqui, U. F. Bhatti, C. A. Vercruysse, and H. B. Alam. 2021. Administration of valproic acid in clinically approved dose improves neurologic recovery and decreases brain lesion size in swine subjected to hemorrhagic shock and traumatic brain injury. *Journal of Trauma and Acute Care Surgery* 90(2):346-352.

Wang, M. C., N. R. Temkin, R. A. Deyo, G. J. Jurkovich, J. Barber, and S. Dikmen. 2007. Timing of surgery after multisystem injury with traumatic brain injury: Effect on neuropsychological and functional outcome. *Journal of Trauma: Injury, Infection, and Critical Care* 62(5):1250-1258.

Winter, L., H. J. Moriarty, C. V. Piersol, T. Vause-Earland, K. Robinson, and B. Newhart. 2016. Patient- and family-identified problems of traumatic brain injury: Value and utility of a target outcome approach to identifying the worst problems. *Journal of Patient-Centered Research and Reviews* 3:30-39.

Zetterberg, H., D. H. Smith, and K. Blennow. 2013. Biomarkers of mild traumatic brain injury in cerebrospinal fluid and blood. *Nature Reviews Neurology* 9(4):201-210.

8

Roadmap and Recommendations: Creating an Optimized System for TBI

The physical, psychological, and social effects of traumatic brain injury (TBI) along the full range of severity and with time horizons longer than the acute phase of management can have significant impacts on a person's function, relationships, and quality of life. The evidence and testimony reviewed by the committee suggest that many persons with TBI and their families find themselves without continuity of care or the full support needed downstream from an acute brain injury. In addition, as in almost all aspects of U.S. health care, TBI care and outcomes show evidence of racial, geographic, and socioeconomic inequities. Achieving high-quality care for all persons with TBI will depend on careful redesign of TBI care and research as an integrated system and as a "learning system" capable of continual progress toward ideal TBI care everywhere and for everyone.

These findings led the committee to draw four overarching conclusions that informed its recommendations for creating an optimized system for TBI care:

Conclusion: TBI care in the United States often fails to meet the needs of individuals, families, and communities affected by this condition. TBI is an ongoing condition that poses significant burdens over time, including substantial financial and social costs. For the most part, the nation has no mechanism in place for long-term follow-up and care of adults or children with TBI. The results of this gap include needless death, squandered human potential, family stress, and soaring social costs. Because of this gap, the true morbidity, mortality, and cost attributable to TBI, though undoubtedly vast, are unknown.

Conclusion: High-quality care for TBI requires that it be managed as a condition with both acute and long-term phases. Helping people with TBI and their families effectively requires that clinicians and community services address and improve the factors that affect care and recovery. After acute treatment, many people living with TBI drop into a black hole, lost to follow-up and without clear pathways to providers. Millions of people, especially in marginalized groups, face inequitable challenges that could have been avoided. In this black hole, there are no mechanisms for collecting data with which to document and improve these shortfalls in TBI care.

Conclusion: Public and professional misunderstandings are widespread with respect to the frequency; manifestations; long-term consequences; and proper detection, treatment, and rehabilitation of TBI.

Conclusion: The United States lacks a comprehensive framework for addressing TBI. A barrier to dramatic improvement in TBI care and research is the absence of a strategic framework and a lead agency or organization with a systemic view, responsibility for articulating goals and overseeing progress, the capacity to foster change, and the ability to convene the many stakeholders required to address the necessary multiple lines of effort. Absent a leadership entity, no one owns the problem, and major progress is unlikely.

AN OPTIMIZED SYSTEM FOR TBI

An optimized system for TBI needs to embody a number of key features, including integration across the phases of care and recovery and between the health care system and the research enterprise. Moreover, comprehensive and personalized care for TBI requires considering bio-psycho-socio-ecological (BPSE) dimensions beyond the injury itself. BPSE factors influence the recognition, initial management, and even immediate survival from TBI, as well as recovery; rehabilitation; and reintegration into employment, family, and social life. Research over the past decade has demonstrated that BPSE factors should help inform all phases of care. However, TBI care and management currently focus on acute presentation and the biological nature of the injury, and these factors are not adequately addressed by the current system. BPSE factors are also elements of disparities in risks, access to care, and outcomes after TBI that are associated with racial, ethnic, socioeconomic, geographic, and other subsets of the population. Continued failure to address the roles of these factors in care and outcomes is no longer tenable. The importance of BPSE dimensions also requires that a team-based approach be taken to managing TBI care and undertaking research aimed at achieving optimal clinical outcomes. Given the scope, scale, and heterogeneity of TBI, the optimized TBI system envisioned by the committee needs to incorporate a broad range of stakeholders and partners. Essential features of a truly optimized system for TBI include those described below.

Incorporates prevention, along with care and research. An optimized system for TBI starts with prevention. Efforts to prevent the occurrence or mitigate the severity of brain injuries make care necessary for as few individuals as possible.

Is person- and family-centered.[1] An optimized system takes a holistic approach to patient needs. At the core of the system is an understanding of and appreciation for the needs and perspectives of the people, families, and communities affected by TBI. Such a system engages persons with TBI and their families in both research and clinical care and considers the needs of all patients, with particular attention to those most vulnerable to poor outcomes.

---

[1] Person-centered care is "the experience (to the extent the informed, individual patient desires it) of transparency, individualization, recognition, respect, dignity and choice in all matters, without exception, related to one's person, circumstances, and relationships in health care" (Berwick, 2009, p. w560).

Uses a precise classification system. An optimized system relies on an accurate framework to characterize and classify TBI, contributing to more accurate and precise diagnosis, prognostication, monitoring, and research.

Provides the best possible care for everyone. An optimized system uses results of research conducted in real-world care settings to inform clinical practice, while at the same time, results and needs gleaned from clinical practice inform research efforts. The knowledge and understanding thus acquired make it possible to develop and disseminate evidence-based guidelines on best practices for care while supporting care that is personalized to both individuals and families. A system that provides the best possible care also strives to identify and address sources of disparities in access to high-quality TBI care and outcomes, including racial and ethnic, geographic, socioeconomic, and other sources of inequities.

Provides seamless transitions across the continuum of care. An optimized system supports connections among all components of the TBI landscape, building awareness of the interdependencies and promoting communication and collaboration.

Builds accountability and quality improvement into the system. An optimized system incorporates the capacity to identify and implement metrics of quality and to harness the resulting information to better meet patient and family needs.

Is transformed into an integrated learning system. Establishing a system is necessary but not sufficient; an optimized system for TBI is a learning system. The attributes of a learning health system have been defined in prior reports from the National Academies (IOM, 2007; NASEM, 2016). Such a system "is predicated on the active collaboration of all members of the system, from patients to clinicians to health system leaders, and success is defined by the impact of the system on the health and lives of patients."[2] A learning system for TBI enhances the ability to identify which gaps and challenges impede improved care and to work collectively across the system to address them. Table 8-1 summarizes essential components of a learning system and their application to TBI.

Incorporates leadership invested in making change happen. An optimized, learning system for TBI includes leaders and champions who embrace the system's mission and vision. These leaders support, implement, and sustain effective change.

RECOMMENDATIONS

Achieving the optimized TBI system described above will require addressing the current gaps and challenges in TBI care and research detailed in this report. For many people with TBI and their families, a "continuum of care" does not exist. Their journey is more aptly characterized as a fragmented series of silos (prehospital assessment, potential emergency department or hospital-based acute care, perhaps inpatient or outpatient rehabilitation, and possibly additional community or long-term services and supports) that is also insufficiently connected to fundamental and translational research. To effect the changes required to realize an optimized TBI system, it will be necessary to leverage the collaborative opportunities laid

---

[2] Remarks by Mate, K. 2021. "Introduction to a Learning Health System." Presentation and discussion during virtual workshop for the Committee on Accelerating Progress in Traumatic Brain Injury Research and Care, March 30, 2021.

TABLE 8-1 Components of a Learning Health System and Their Implications for an Optimized TBI System

Characteristic*	Implications for TBI
Science and Informatics	A Learning System for TBI…
Real-time access to knowledge	• Prepares care providers with up-to-date, evidence-based guidance to inform care, and incorporates processes for reviewing and coordinating information presented in care guidelines and for updating guidance regularly as information emerges. • Provides the best possible diagnostic, prognostic, and decision support tools for identifying and managing TBI. • Integrates and connects preclinical and clinical research and care and takes advantage of tools and methods for sharing and evaluating evidence to inform care and research efforts.
Digital capture of the care experience	• Captures data from population-based surveillance as well as patient data generated during all phases of TBI care, such as through electronic health records and TBI registries. • Uses the data obtained to support continuous improvement of prevention, care, and research.
Patient–Clinician Partnerships	
Engaged, empowered patients	• Provides patients and families with tailored, person-centered information and resources that support them and help them understand and navigate their process of recovery from TBI. • Partners with patients and families to identify and refine research questions and clinical outcomes of greatest interest.
Incentives	
Incentives aligned for value	• Aligns provider and organizational incentives with best practices in evidence-based care, including by authorizing acute and post-acute care and community-based services in accordance with the needs of the patient and family.
Full transparency	• Incorporates quality improvement processes and metrics, and regularly reviews these metrics. • Enables widespread access to the information used to derive evidence-based care guidelines and tools.
Continuous Learning Culture	
Leadership-instilled culture of learning	• Involves national, regional, and organizational leadership in driving continuous learning and striving to improve outcomes for patients with TBI and their families. • Connects prevention, care, and research in "one system for learning and doing." • Incorporates leadership and insights beyond the medical system, involving key stakeholders and partners across the broad TBI ecosystem.
Supportive system competencies	• Raises awareness of TBI among the public and care providers as a chronic condition influenced by bio-psycho-socio-ecological factors. • Incorporates training for those who assess TBI at the point of injury and those who provide care across the full continuum from acute care through recovery. • Establishes infrastructure for systematic learning and improvement, including enhanced and cross-connected data systems and the incorporation of TBI in efforts to improve the national trauma care system, • Establishes demonstration projects on providing effective continuity of care for persons with TBI.

* From NASEM, 2016.

out in Chapter 7 through evidence-based actions by all stakeholders and through research efforts aimed at addressing issues for which the evidence base is currently insufficient. The following sections present the committee's recommendations for actions to advance the TBI field toward an optimized system and for a research agenda to produce the evidence needed to support additional actions. Collectively, these recommendations and this research agenda constitute the committee's roadmap for advancing TBI care and research.

TBI Classification

The currently used classification of TBI as "mild, moderate, or severe" and reliance on the Glasgow Coma Scale to determine which of these categories applies to an individual patient are insufficiently nuanced and discriminating to support TBI treatment and prognosis utilizing the best available knowledge. Initial assessment of a TBI often does not predict the evolution of a person's condition over time or ultimate outcome. The care system therefore needs to support more precise diagnosis, prognostication, monitoring, and research. A TBI classification workshop was held by the National Institutes of Health's National Institute of Neurological Disorders and Stroke (NINDS) in 2007. The years since then have seen progress in imaging, blood-based, and other biologic markers and their relationship to understanding TBI pathophysiology and outcome that can be reviewed for incorporation in an improved classification scheme. Such discussions will need to consider the utility of the various markers across different TBI populations and injury severities and in different care environments.

> **Recommendation 1. Create and implement an updated classification system for TBI. The current clinical classification scheme for TBI should be updated to be more accurate and informative for care and research:**
>
> a. The National Institutes of Health (NIH) should convene a TBI Classification Workgroup to review data from recent large-scale clinical studies and determine which elements should be incorporated into a more descriptive, evidence-based, and precise classification system for clinical care and research. In this effort, NIH should engage professional communities that routinely diagnose and classify TBI.
> b. Relevant professional societies, including but not limited to those in emergency medicine, trauma care, and rehabilitation, should advise and train clinicians caring for people with TBI to classify patients based on their actual Glasgow Coma Scale (GCS) sum score (e.g., GCS 14) rather than the inaccurate and misleading three-category shorthand mild, moderate, or severe. Optimally, clinicians should also use results from neuroimaging and blood-based biomarkers, when available and clinically indicated, to classify patients. Clinicians should update the TBI classification for each patient as the person's condition evolves.

TBI as a Complex Acute and Chronic Condition

It is essential to recognize that TBI often has both acute and long-term physical, social, and psychological consequences, and that a person with TBI may experience ongoing, new, or worsening symptoms after discharge. Thus, individuals experiencing TBI frequently need long-term, person-centered support that may require months, years, or even a lifetime of care and adjustment. Accordingly, continuity of TBI care is crucial to quality. Also crucial is for TBI care to take into account the social determinants of health.

Recommendation 2. Integrate acute and long-term person- and family-centered management of TBI. All people with TBI should have reliable and timely access to integrated, multidisciplinary, and specialized care to address physical, cognitive, and behavioral sequelae of TBI and comorbidities that influence quality of life.

a. Relevant professional societies should encourage clinicians to recommend that all patients at discharge from inpatient and outpatient acute care settings have an opportunity for follow-up with a clinician experienced in managing TBI. Guidance to clinicians should also emphasize the need to connect patients and family caregivers with care navigation resources as needed.
b. In their intake processes, health care and social services organizations should be aware of lifetime TBI exposure so they can identify those needing accommodations, as well as those at increased risk for TBI-related symptoms or declining trajectories in health and function. These organizations should also give providers guidance on practical strategies and accommodations that can help patients and families cope with TBI-related symptoms, and on resources that can increase reliable and timely access to and appropriateness of care for persons with TBI.
c. Organizations that oversee or provide long-term care should consider the needs of families and caregivers for education and support as key components of long-term care plans.

Ensuring quality and continuity of care for all people with TBI is essential. Making progress toward a system that rewards a linked and coordinated continuum of care and supports optimal longer-term outcomes can also help address some of the inequities that exist around access to post-acute and rehabilitation care. Incorporating family and caregiver needs is critical as well, since many persons with TBI live with family and are dependent on family members and other caregivers to address their needs, navigate health care and community services, and facilitate community integration.

Quality of Care

TBI care in the United States too often deviates from known best practices in both the acute and chronic phases of care. Stronger commitment to and strategies for ensuring quality and continuity of care for all TBI patients, regardless of sex, age, race/ethnicity, socioeconomic status, geographic location, and other individual characteristics, are essential so that who you are and where you live do not determine whether and how you live. To this end, it will be necessary to address variability and gaps in available care guidance and in the implementation of existing guidelines, including their use to guide reimbursement practices (see also Recommendation 6). The evidence base informing acute and longer-term TBI care and rehabilitation needs to be expanded. In so doing, the evidence to inform TBI care decisions will need to be based on a range of rigorous methodologies for generating knowledge and include evidence obtained not only from randomized controlled trials but also from observational cohort and other study designs and from expert consensus on best practices.

Recommendation 3. Reduce unwarranted variability and gaps in administrative and clinical care guidance to ensure high-quality care for TBI. The federal agencies that lead the development of clinical practice guidelines for TBI, including the Department of Veterans Affairs, the Department of Defense, the Agency for Healthcare Research and Quality, and the Centers for Disease Control and Prevention, should convene at

regular intervals an expert panel to undertake the actions below in collaboration with clinical and patient community stakeholders. The Centers for Medicare & Medicaid Services (CMS) should be engaged in this effort to ensure alignment of coverage with clinical guidelines:

a. Survey the landscape of existing clinical care guidelines for all elements of TBI care, during all phases of care, and involving all salient specialties. Synthesize best current clinical practice and evidence to develop consensus-based guidelines where evidence is currently limited, using rigorous methods for such consensus processes. Guidelines should be sensitive to local contexts and potential sources of inequity, such as race/ethnicity, rurality, and limited access to health care resources.
b. Identify and resolve problems of inconsistency among current clinical care guidelines.
c. Identify guidelines and practices that are contraindicated by current evidence, and issue guidance on their deimplementation.
d. Identify common criteria for the inclusion of studies used to inform the development of guidelines and for how topics are covered for which limited evidence from randomized controlled trials or other rigorous study designs is available (see Recommendation 7).
e. Identify gaps in the evidence base informing current clinical care guidelines, and recommend research to develop the necessary evidence (see also gaps identified in the research agenda presented later).
f. Develop evidence-guided and consensus-based criteria for identifying patients who should be referred to inpatient and outpatient TBI rehabilitation (see Recommendation 5).
g. Identify avenues for emerging best practices to guide third-party coverage of care, regardless of payer source and type of medical facility.

Relevant clinical organizations that have been active in TBI guideline development and can be engaged in this effort include the Brain Trauma Foundation, Concussion in Sport Group, American College of Surgeons, American Academy of Neurology, American College of Emergency Physicians, American Congress of Rehabilitation Medicine, Neurocritical Care Society, and others.

Awareness and Understanding

Too large a fraction of TBI is unrecognized as such, either at the time of injury or as symptoms and signs develop after injury. Both the public at large and clinicians need better understanding of the condition and information on types of supports or accommodations persons with TBI may need in their daily lives.

Recommendation 4. Enhance awareness and identification of TBI by health care providers and the public. Education and awareness are essential for achieving high-quality care and improving outcomes, and are particularly important in the following areas:

a. *Public awareness.* The Centers for Disease Control and Prevention, working with organizations in TBI prevention, care, and rehabilitation and those that work with at-risk groups, should enhance efforts to raise awareness among the public on the context, causes, and long-term effects of TBI; the importance of follow-up; and resources that may be available to the person with TBI.

b. *Professional awareness, education, and training.* Education and training programs for health care professions should include information on the burden, risk factors, and signs and symptoms of TBI and should correct misconceptions about the condition. Materials should emphasize adherence to evidence-based guidelines where they exist to bring greater consistency to TBI care across the United States, while taking into account patient characteristics and preferences in order to provide personalized care. Guidance should also emphasize eliminating practices that are contraindicated by current evidence and reducing inequities in care and outcomes.

c. *Patient and family empowerment.* National- and state-level patient and family organizations should work with clinical communities in primary care, acute care, and rehabilitation to ensure that all TBI patients and families receive anticipatory guidance on expected symptoms and trajectory, steps to decrease the risk of delayed recovery, and available TBI resources.

Multiple professionals across the health care enterprise, including emergency medical technicians, physicians, nurses, psychologists, and rehabilitation professionals, need sufficient training and guidance on TBI; however, few clinical training curricula address TBI risk factors, diagnosis, and management in any depth. Organizations working closely with communities at particular risk of experiencing a TBI or at risk of poorer outcomes after TBI should be part of efforts to develop and disseminate practical information. Given the complexities of the care systems for conditions such as TBI, engaging investigators with complementary expertise in such areas as social sciences, implementation science, and cost analysis and health economics is also an important part of the roadmap for advancing TBI care and research.

The Care System

Challenges and unmet needs in TBI care and recovery illustrate systemic issues in U.S. health care. As is the case with many chronic illnesses in the United States, care for TBI can be fragmented; interrupted; and unresponsive to the evolving medical, psychological, and social support needs of TBI patients and their families. At present, no entity is "in charge" of ensuring continuity of care or follow-up for TBI patients, and as a result, many patients feel lost and even abandoned as their condition evolves. Inequities in TBI outcomes also become magnified when only some patients and families have access to high-quality care across the full continuum or have insurance coverage or financial resources to pay for such care, particularly for rehabilitation and longer-term services. To address this gap, professional societies should confront and mitigate the problems of care discontinuity; government and private philanthropy should invest in developing prototypes of integrated TBI care, including regional system designs; and public and private payers should ensure that benefit structures accord with the evidence for proper TBI care across all phases and environments of care.

Recommendation 5. Establish and reinforce local and regional integrated care delivery systems for TBI. The Secretary of Health and Human Services should work to establish geographically based, integrated care delivery systems for TBI, emphasizing the continuum of care across the acute, rehabilitation, and recovery phases and all severities. The effort should build on the nation's success with regional trauma systems and incorporate practices and lessons learned from the Department of Defense (DoD) and the Department of Veterans Affairs (VA). Specifically:

a. The American College of Surgeons (ACS) and other trauma verification systems should incorporate comprehensive standards for TBI care in trauma center verification processes and data systems and as a national trauma system evolves. As part of this effort, ACS should expand efforts to foster communication between acute care and rehabilitation care providers and expand outreach on the signs and management of TBI to the public, first responders, and acute care providers.

b. Settings that provide TBI care across the post-acute rehabilitation continuum should meet standards for integrated, evidence-based, and individualized brain injury care, such as those required by the Commission on Accreditation of Rehabilitation Facilities for the Brain Injury Specialty. The Joint Commission should review and promulgate standards for high-quality TBI care in the broader spectrum of care settings that treat people with TBI, such as primary care, community hospitals, and concussion programs.

c. The Department of Health and Human Services and the Center for Medicare and Medicaid Innovation should support local and regional pilot demonstration projects to create prototype civilian care infrastructures focused on providing continuity of care for follow-up, rehabilitation, and longer-term care and recovery from TBI. The demonstration projects should document best practices and effects on patient outcomes, and identify the components of a chronic care management model that are most effective for persons with TBI. Prototype systems should address the needs of TBI across the spectrum of severity and venues of care, including community-based services.

d. The Centers for Medicare & Medicaid Services (CMS) and commercial health care insurers should align coverage for TBI care with clinical guidelines to ensure equity in access to, affordability of, and quality of care. For example, payers should use criteria identified under Recommendation 3 when authorizing inpatient and outpatient rehabilitation services, including for long-term TBI sequelae. CMS, the VA, and DoD should test alternative benefit structures for TBI rehabilitation care instead of relying on the current time-based metric (e.g., the "3-hour rule") or preset benefits.

These types of activities support the delivery of high-quality care, and the actions identified in this recommendation are aimed at multiple parts of the TBI care system. Although not every trauma center participates, ACS and other organizations operate programs that verify the presence of components identified as being part of optimal trauma care. ACS also operates a consultation process for trauma systems interested in obtaining guidance.[3] The CARF Brain Injury Specialty Program designation or demonstration of equivalent standards operates for provision of integrated and specialized rehabilitation care, while the Joint Commission is the largest accreditor of health care organizations in the United States.

A Learning System

As discussed above, multiple reports from the National Academies have described the ideal properties of a learning health care system, and TBI care should have those properties. In addition to care and research, such a learning system encompasses processes for quality improvement and education. A full learning system for TBI also involves public health agencies and community organizations across the phases of prevention, care, and recovery.

---

[3] See https://www.facs.org/quality-programs/trauma/tqp/systems-programs/tscp.

To support a learning health care system, high-quality, comprehensive data spanning pre-hospital, acute, rehabilitation, and longer-term care for TBI need to be available. Although a number of relevant databases and components of such a data enterprise exist, they currently do not form a connected system, making it difficult to define the full scope and burden of TBI and improve its management. Relevant databases are owned by multiple federal agencies and organizations, which will need to work together to address this challenge. For example, the Department of Transportation's National Highway Traffic Safety Administration manages the National Emergency Medical Services Information System (NEMSIS). ACS maintains a National Trauma Databank and Trauma Quality Improvement Program, and individual state trauma registries exist as well. The National Institute on Disability, Independent Living, and Rehabilitation Research (NIDILRR) TBI Model Systems network, operated under the Department of Health and Human Services' Administration for Community Living, maintains longitudinal data, which are especially relevant to rehabilitation care. DoD has a Trauma Registry, and the VA similarly operates registries containing information on TBI. Better linking these data sources across sites and through time can provide one of the foundations for a learning system capable of continual analysis and improvement.

> **Recommendation 6. Integrate the TBI system of care and TBI research into a learning health care system. Reducing the burden of TBI will require a learning system capable of continual improvement. Important elements are thorough surveillance, standardized and longitudinal patient information, and accessibility of data. The Secretary of Health and Human Services (HHS) should therefore work to establish an integrated TBI data system, taking the following actions:**
>
> a. *Conduct thorough surveillance.* The Centers for Disease Control and Prevention should expand efforts to track TBI mortality, morbidity, and long-term outcomes more completely and accurately, including by adding validated, standardized TBI questions to population-based and weighted surveys and working to ensure consistency of information across states and surveys. The Agency for Healthcare Research and Quality should modify and expand the Healthcare Cost and Utilization Project to enable improved analysis of TBI care patterns, costs, and outcomes, both acute and long-term.
> b. *Standardize the capture of patient-level data.* HHS should work with health care systems and electronic health record vendors to bring data infrastructure into line with the state of the science by investing in and developing the ability to capture high-quality, TBI-relevant data in medical records. This data infrastructure will help in identifying causal factors and longitudinal outcomes, enabling comparative effectiveness, implementation, and translation studies across health care systems.
> c. *Emphasize longitudinal data, and integrate information across the continuum of care.* HHS should work with the owners of national and regional TBI registries and databanks to crosslink patient-level data across sites and through time. In addition, data systems should collect clinical information in alignment with the refined TBI classification system proposed in Recommendation 1.

Research

Further research efforts are needed to address gaps and challenges where the evidence base to support action toward more effective TBI prevention, care, and recovery is currently inadequate.

Recommendation 7. Improve the quality and expand the range of TBI studies and study designs. TBI research and investment by the National Institutes of Health, the Department of Defense, the Department of Veterans Affairs, and private-sector funders should be commensurate with the public health burden of the condition. The research agenda proposed herein identifies eight areas for further progress and additional attention. When identifying research priorities and requests for applications, the above funders should take the following actions:

a. Significantly expand financial support and research efforts to address the priorities identified in the research agenda.
b. Establish translational research and implementation science centers to undertake collaborative efforts toward improved standardization and clinical care for TBI throughout the continuum of care. These centers should use insights from implementation science to enable effective translation of study results from the laboratory to clinical trials and from clinical trials to practice.
c. Encourage multidisciplinary and multistakeholder research efforts to strengthen the evidence base informing care. These efforts should:
   1. Use the TBI classification system called for in Recommendation 1 to better stratify participants in clinical trials of novel interventions for TBI.
   2. Engage patient and family voices early in study design by using stakeholder engagement (i.e., community-based participatory research) to identify unmet needs and refine research questions.
   3. Recruit diverse study participants to ensure that research is broadly representative of the people who experience TBI.
   4. Use all forms of rigorous study designs when appropriate to answer research questions. Study methods should be eclectic and adaptive, and should include not only randomized controlled trials for efficacy but also pragmatic trials, adaptive designs, comparative effectiveness trials, observational studies (including those using statistical control for causal inference), and mixed methods, as appropriate to the research questions.
   5. Engage laboratory scientists and clinicians to ensure better research translation, including rigorous parallels across animal and human injury models, therapeutic targets, comorbidities, and study design outcome metrics and endpoints.

Leadership

The nation needs but currently lacks leadership to provide a locus for innovation and improvement in TBI care and research, as well as a mechanism for convening stakeholders to better organize TBI care as a system. Federal leadership is needed to establish a strategic framework for dramatically improving TBI care. Because this framework will require the efforts of multiple partners and substantial resources, it will also be essential early on to develop a clear plan for implementation that includes a timeline and metrics of progress and is curated thereafter as circumstances change. This coordinated approach will support innovation and improvement in TBI research and care, and will align the expansive range of partners and stakeholders whose efforts are critical to establishing an optimized system that aims to achieve high-quality care and health equity among all groups and across the lifespan.

Recommendation 8. Create and promulgate a national framework and implementation plan for improving TBI care. The Secretary of Health and Human Services (HHS)

should, under the aegis of the Assistant Secretary for Health, create, promulgate, and curate a strategic national framework and implementation plan for improving TBI care:

a. To this end, the Secretary of HHS should establish, for a period of 10 years, a national Traumatic Brain Injury Task Force as a successor to the National Research Action Plan. The TBI Task Force should move beyond an emphasis solely on research coordination to encompass a focus on research implementation and application of the evidence in support of better treatment and systems of care delivery, engaging an expanded group of federal, private-sector, and philanthropic partners. It should enlist and help coordinate TBI-related care improvements among HHS components (such as the Centers for Medicare & Medicaid Services, the National Institutes of Health, the Centers for Disease Control and Prevention, the Administration for Community Living, the Agency for Healthcare Research and Quality, and the Health Resources and Services Administration, among others) and should include participation from other relevant departments, such as the Department of Veterans Affairs, the Department of Defense, the Social Security Administration, and the Department of Transportation.
b. The TBI Task Force's first actions should be to develop a strategic framework addressing the issues reflected in the committee's recommendations and within 2 years, to release a specific implementation plan to guide and coordinate efforts within that framework. This plan should be curated and updated over time.
c. The TBI Task Force should engage a multistakeholder public–private coalition to continually advance and accelerate implementation of the national framework and plan. Stakeholders in this coalition should include, but not be limited to, the federal agencies that provide funding for TBI research and clinical care, relevant patient and family advocacy organizations, Veterans service organizations, relevant professional societies, youth and adult sports associations, health payment organizations, philanthropic foundations, and companies developing new tools and treatments for TBI.

A wide range of partners and stakeholders need to be involved in efforts to effect the improvements necessary to transform TBI care and research. DoD and the VA are focused on the delivery of TBI care to military service members and Veterans, as well as on relevant research. Multiple agencies under HHS, including ACL, AHRQ, NIH, CDC, CMS, HRSA, the Food and Drug Administration (FDA), and the Substance Abuse and Mental Health Services Administration (SAMSHA), also play important roles in TBI-related health care delivery, quality, reimbursement, research, regulation, and surveillance. HRSA oversees the Federally Qualified Health Centers, which provide community-based health care services such as those that may be needed by people with TBI. ACL houses NIDILRR's TBI Models Systems program enabling data collection and research, while AHRQ operates the Healthcare Cost and Utilization Project (HCUP) health care databases, including longitudinal data on hospital-based care.

Numerous professional societies are relevant to TBI care and recovery as well.[4] The proposed TBI coalition will also need to include and work closely with patient and family

---

[4] These societies include, but are not limited to, Academy of Rehabilitation Psychology, American Academy of Clinical Neuropsychology, American Academy of Family Physicians, American Academy of Neurology, American Academy of Nursing, American Academy of Pediatrics, American Academy of Physical Medicine and Rehabilitation, American Association of Critical Care Nurses, American Association of Neurological Surgeons, American College of Emergency Medicine, American College of Sports Medicine, American College of Surgeons, American Congress of Rehabilitation Medicine, American Medical Association, American Medical Rehabilitation Providers Association, American Nurses Association, American Occupational Therapy Association, American Physical Therapy Association, American Psychological Association, American Speech-Language-Hearing Association, American Therapeutic Recreation Association, Association for Behavioral and Cognitive Therapies, Association of Rehabilitation Nurses, National Medical Association, and National Association of State Head Injury Administrators.

advocacy and Veterans' service organizations. These types of organizations are often financially constrained, further highlighting the fact that to make substantial progress in advancing TBI care and research will take a commitment of financial resources.

A process that engages a broad coalition of stakeholders in TBI care and research is critical to enabling the consideration of diverse opinions on necessary actions and metrics, and for ensuring that lessons from impactful research and from efforts that advance infrastructure and improve clinical care are discussed and disseminated.

A RESEARCH AGENDA TO ACCELERATE THE EXPANSION OF KNOWLEDGE

The following eight areas are among the most urgent priorities for continued and expanded research to address existing gaps in the evidence base for action to improve TBI prevention, care, and recovery.

A. **Conduct national and international epidemiological studies to better understand the scope and burden of TBI and inform prevention efforts.**

Every segment of the population can experience TBI. Population-based surveillance for TBI relies largely on analysis of hospital diagnostic codes and information collected from such sources as death certificates, incidents recorded in trauma databanks, and the U.S. National Vital Statistics System. Currently available data underestimate the incidence, prevalence, and burden of TBI. In particular, there is currently no good way to estimate the many milder-spectrum injuries in which acute medical care may not have been sought or care was provided in non–trauma care settings, such as outpatient clinics or sports medicine centers. These cases represent the base of a "TBI iceberg" that cannot be identified today through any of the current TBI surveillance approaches.

B. **Understand the economic impact of TBI both within health care and within the family and broader community.**

Health economics research is necessary to better understand the full costs of TBI, particularly the burden of indirect costs associated with longer-term symptoms, and to undertake cost/benefit analyses of TBI interventions. For example, teleconsultation may provide one potential opportunity for cost-effective follow-up with patients in resource-poor areas, but may not be feasible or effective in all circumstances or for all patients.

C. **Understand how combinations of injury characteristics, individual factors, and social-environmental variables affect short- and long-term care and outcomes after TBI.**

Differential outcomes after TBI are associated with a broad range of factors, including preinjury status and comorbidities, as well as such personal, social, and environmental factors as age, biological sex and gender, race, ethnicity, socioeconomic status, insurance status, employment status, and geographic location. Significant gaps remain in understanding why and how these factors act and interact to affect TBI symptoms and recovery. Involving the social sciences as well as clinical and economic disciplines will be important in understanding and addressing how social determinants of health impact TBI outcomes.

D. **Enhance research to understand and reduce disparities in TBI incidence, diagnosis, care, and outcomes.**

Information obtained from studies addressing item C above would yield important insights that could help identify approaches for overcoming inequities and disparities associated with TBI. Establishing a TBI system that can meet the needs of all patients and families will require designing, evaluating, and implementing such strategies while at the same time deimplementing practices that are that are contraindicated by the evidence or exacerbate disparities.

E. **Expand the number and breadth of validated tools for measuring TBI risk factors and improving diagnosis, classification, monitoring, short- to long-term outcome assessment, and prognostication.**

The heterogeneous nature of TBI requires multimodal information, including clinical assessments, imaging results, and results from blood-based biomarker tests. New types of neuroimaging, biofluid-based, and physiological biomarkers are in development, and if validated, will be able to provide further information that could be collected from patients. Approaches that synthesize multimodal data and incorporate the resulting information into clinical practice guidelines and decision support tools will improve diagnosis and classification of TBI, aid in prognosis of a person's anticipated recovery trajectory, and enable more effective monitoring of the response to care.

F. **Develop evidence-guided therapies for treating TBI and improving outcomes.**

Despite the progress made over the past several decades in understanding the molecular and cellular mechanisms of TBI, these advances have yet to be translated to a single successful Phase 3 clinical trial or treatment for the brain in healing from TBI during acute-stage care. An array of shortcomings has contributed to this record of failure in TBI clinical trials. Novel therapies are needed, and achieving this goal will likely require a variety of efforts to improve the translation of research to practice.

G. **Innovate and disseminate improved designs for coordinated TBI care in organizations and regions, with special attention to patients' and families' long-term needs and follow-up.**

Further research conducted in pragmatic environments is needed to understand how to improve outcomes of TBI in real-world settings of assessment, care, recovery, and reintegration—especially research conducted in environments other than inpatient hospital settings. In addition, pilot testing is needed to develop, evaluate, and establish strategies for better integrating the diverse components and stakeholders that make up the TBI system.

H. **Expand TBI research in areas with a weak history of TBI focus, including health care quality, health economics, and implementation science research.**

Better understanding is needed of the scope and economic impact of TBI within health care and within families and the broader community. Existing data sources for population-based surveillance have limitations, and there are challenges in calculating the full costs associated with TBI. Those who study health care quality can help the TBI field study, identify, and develop new knowledge of ways to make care safer, more effective, more timely, more efficient, more patient- and family-centered, and more equitable. The field of implementation science, including planning for implementation in study designs, can support the effective translation of new knowledge into practice, as well as deimplementation of ineffective or contraindicated practices. Further engaging and collaborating with those from such key fields would broaden the scope of expertise brought to bear on addressing the challenges of TBI.

REFERENCES

Berwick, D. M. 2009. What "patient-centered" should mean: Confessions of an extremist. *Health Affairs* 28(4):w555-w565.
IOM (Institute of Medicine). 2007. *The learning healthcare system: Workshop summary.* Washington, DC: The National Academies Press.
NASEM (National Academies of Sciences, Engineering, and Medicine). 2016. *A national trauma care system: Integrating military and civilian trauma systems to achieve zero preventable deaths after injury.* Washington, DC: The National Academies Press.

Appendix A

Highlights of Selected Recent TBI Research Efforts

The landscape of recent of traumatic brain injury (TBI) research is dynamic and diverse. Over the past decade, various government agencies, academic institutions, nonprofit organizations, and other stakeholders have sought to study, diagnose, treat, classify, measure, and track TBI. This appendix provides selected highlights of some of these recent efforts.

Efforts to study TBI can be broadly categorized in terms of purpose, funding source (e.g., government, academic, private, public–private partnership), target populations (e.g., civilian, military, pediatric, athletes), or type of effort (e.g., consortia, research networks, guideline creation, studies). However, the landscape of TBI research may be best understood as a constellation of efforts working within their respective settings and scopes to meet specific—and often overlapping—research aims to better understand TBI.

RESEARCH PRIORITY-SETTING EFFORTS

The diversity of the TBI research landscape mirrors the diversity of populations impacted by TBI, from military personnel (Veterans, active duty military personnel, cadets and military trainees), to athletes (professional, collegiate, student, youth), to patients across the entire lifespan. The Department of Defense (DoD) and the Department of Veterans Affairs (VA) are heavily involved in the TBI research and care landscape across the gamut from funding to implementation. From enlistment, to active duty, to Veteran status, many military personnel are impacted by TBI throughout their career and beyond. Military personnel and Veterans also make up a large and unique population that can be studied to better understand long-term impacts of TBI. Athletes face a heightened risk of TBI, and their lives and livelihoods are impacted by TBI in unique ways. The National Football League (NFL), the National Collegiate Athletic Association (NCAA), and other athletic institutions have supported athlete-focused research to explore the effects of TBI on athletes during and after their athletic careers.

Because of the complexity and breadth of TBI, the research needed to diagnose, treat, and improve outcomes can vary according to the setting in which TBI occurs, the individual,

179

the setting where TBI is being diagnosed or treated, and numerous other factors. Thus, funders and organizing bodies that support and advocate for TBI research often have needs that are connected to specific populations and settings. Other TBI initiatives address cross-cutting issues and include all or more than one of these population groups. For instance, the needs of athletes and their coaches to assess potential TBI in high-pressure scenarios share some similarities with the needs of military medical staff assessing potential TBI in combat; the challenges of mild TBI are of similar significance in civilian and military settings; the study of TBI among aging Veterans may offer insights into the impacts of TBI among aging civilians; and novel advances in classification and measurement could improve the sensitivity of all TBI research, while efforts to promote data interoperability similarly affect all research settings.

National Research Action Plan

The current TBI landscape has been fundamentally shaped by the National Research Action Plan (NRAP) (DoD et al., 2013; White House, 2012). Mandated by Executive Order 13625 (August 31, 2012), NRAP was created to promote

> strategies to establish surrogate and clinically actionable biomarkers for early diagnosis and treatment effectiveness; develop improved diagnostic criteria for TBI; enhance our understanding of the mechanisms responsible for PTSD [posttraumatic stress disorder], related injuries, and neurological disorders following TBI; foster development of new treatments for these conditions based on a better understanding of the underlying mechanisms; improve data sharing between agencies and academic and industry researchers to accelerate progress and reduce redundant efforts without compromising privacy; and make better use of electronic health records to gain insight into the risk and mitigation of PTSD, TBI, and related injuries. (sec. 5b)

NRAP called for interagency collaboration to promote new research and innovations in PTSD, TBI, and related conditions. The major funders of TBI research under the current iteration of NRAP have been the National Institutes of Health (NIH), DoD, the VA, and the Centers for Disease Control and Prevention (CDC). NRAP's original 10-year mandate is now coming to a close. During this period, it has served as a launching pad for a host of research efforts of various sizes and scopes. Since its launch in 2012, the landscape of TBI research has advanced, and new challenges, research needs, and questions have emerged in the field.

Brain Trauma Blueprint

The Brain Trauma Blueprint, launched by the nonprofit Cohen Veterans Bioscience, aims to provide a coordinated framework to "identify unmet patient needs, associated research priorities, landscape state of the science, identify research gaps and barriers and provide recommendations for progress" (Brain Trauma Blueprint, 2021). A 2-day State of the Science Summit was held in 2019 on "Pathways to Effective Treatments for Traumatic Brain Injuries," focusing on chronic effects of TBI and the need to develop precision therapeutics (Cohen Veterans Bioscience, 2019). Building on the summit discussions, a six-part series is currently in development and is being published in the *Journal of Neurotrauma*[1]:

---

[1] See https://www.braintraumablueprint.org/soss2019 (accessed January 10, 2022) for "outcomes currently under development from the summit."

- "Roadmap for Advancing Preclinical Science in Traumatic Brain Injury" (Smith et al. 2021b)
- "Epidemiology of Chronic Effects of Mild Traumatic Brain Injury" (Haarbauer-Krupa et al., 2021)
- "Phenotyping the Spectrum of Traumatic Brain Injury: A Review and Pathway to Standardization" (Pugh et al., 2021)
- "Biomarker Development to Advance Diagnosis and Treatment of Traumatic Brain Injury"
- "Designing Successful Clinical Trials for Traumatic Brain Injury"
- "A Review of Implementation Concepts and Strategies Surrounding Traumatic Brain Injury Clinical Care Guidelines" (Lumba-Brown et al., 2021).

Congressionally Directed Medical Research Program on TBI and Psychological Health

The Congressionally Directed Medical Research Program (CDMRP) on TBI and Psychological Health[2] was established in fiscal year 2007. Funds provided by Congress through the Defense Appropriations Act support research addressing key medical issues affecting military service members, Veterans, and other military health system beneficiaries. In April 2021, the CDMRP office held a stakeholders meeting to identify potential areas of impact for its program of peer-reviewed TBI awards. The 2021 funding priorities were subsequently announced, with the following core program areas:

Understand: Research will address knowledge gaps in foundational science, epidemiology, and etiology of TBI and psychological health.

Prevent: Research will address the prevention or progression of TBI or psychological health conditions through population, selective, and indicated prevention approaches. Efforts that focus on primary prevention (including protection), screening, diagnosis, and prognosis are within scope.

Treat: Research will address immediate and long-term treatments and improvements in systems of care, including access to and delivery of healthcare services. Treatment topics may include novel treatments and interventions, personalized medicine approaches, length and durability of treatment, rehabilitation, relapse, and relapse prevention. (*FY21 TBIPHRP Focus Areas*, https://cdmrp.army.mil/tbiphrp/pdfs/FY21-TBIPHRP-FOCUS-AREAS.pdf [accessed December 14, 2021])

ENABLING RESEARCH INFRASTRUCTURE

Several efforts have focused on developing standards for research data and establishing systems for collecting TBI-related data to inform future research (see Table A-1).

Common Data Elements (CDE)[3] standards were first published in 2010 through efforts funded by NIH and the Department of Health and Human Services (HHS). CDE Version 2

[2] See https://cdmrp.army.mil/tbiphrp (accessed January 10, 2022) and https://cdmrp.army.mil/tbiphrp/pdfs/FY21-TBIPHRP-FOCUS-AREAS.pdf (accessed January 10, 2022).
[3] More information about CDE is available at https://www.commondataelements.ninds.nih.gov/Traumatic%20Brain%20Injury (accessed July 2, 2021).

was published in 2012, and the guidelines have been continually updated since. CDE established data standards for TBI clinical research that are relevant to patients of all ages in all populations, along with common definitions and metadata protocols to ensure that data are captured and recorded consistently in studies throughout the TBI landscape. Pediatric Common Data Elements (PED-CDE)[4] was first established in 2013, with the goal of enhancing the ability to conduct multicenter research and provide evidence-based care across Canada to assist in the diagnosis and treatment of pediatric mild TBI.

In 2011, the Federal Interagency TBI Research (FITBIR) informatics system[5] was created through joint funding from DoD, the VA, and NIH. FITBIR offers a secure, centralized database for TBI clinical research and serves as a data repository, allowing for comparison of new and existing data. FITBIR includes data collected from more than 80,000 individuals from both military and civilian populations. Federal grants for TBI research typically stipulate that research data be shared via FITBIR.

In 2018, the National Concussion Surveillance System (NCSS)[6] was created by CDC, with the aim of measuring the number and causes of concussions, the prevalence of brain injury, and the impacts of prevention measures. NCSS deals with civilian population data, with a focus on youth sports.

RESEARCH NETWORKS, CONSORTIA, AND STUDIES

As a diverse and interdisciplinary field, TBI research is often conducted through collaboration. The establishment of TBI research networks has aided collaboration and connected experts throughout the field (see Table A-2). A number of TBI networks have been formed, with an emphasis on improving patient outcomes; consolidating data and biological samples;

---

[4] More information about PED-CDE is available at https://www.ctrc-ccrt.ca/projects/ped-cde-pediatric-common-data-elements-mtbi-concussion (accessed July 2, 2021) and https://www.thechildren.com/canada-pediatric-mild-traumatic-brain-injury-common-data-elements-study-mtbi-cde (accessed July 2, 2021).

[5] More information about FITBIR is available at https://fitbir.nih.gov (accessed July 2, 2021).

[6] More information about NCSS is available at https://www.cdc.gov/traumaticbraininjury/research-programs/ncss/index.html (accessed July 2, 2021).

TABLE A-1 TBI Research Infrastructure

Effort	Key Funders	Year(s)	Target Population(s)	Description
Common Data Elements (CDE)	NIH, HHS	2010–present		Effort to create data standards for TBI clinical research
Pediatric Common Data Elements (PED-CDE)	CIHR	2013–2018	Pediatric TBI patients	Effort to create an assessment battery to advance clinical TBI
Federal Interagency TBI Research (FITBIR) informatics system	DoD, VA, NIH	2011–Present	Military personnel and civilians	Centralized TBI research database for clinical research
National Concussion Surveillance System (NCSS)	CDC	2018	Civilians and youth athletes	Database created to investigate the incidence of TBI and the efficacy of prevention efforts

NOTE: CDC = Centers for Disease Control and Prevention; CIHR = Canadian Institutes of Health Research; DoD = Department of Defense; HHS = Department of Health and Human Services; NIH = National Institutes of Health; TBI = traumatic brain injury; VA = Department of Veterans Affairs.

accelerating research in specific areas, such as concussions research; and connecting clinicians to improve clinical standards of care.

COllaborative Neuropathology NEtwork Characterizing OuTcomes of TBI (CONNECT-TBI)[7] was established in 2020 among more than 10 universities in the United States, the United Kingdom, and Canada (Smith et al., 2021a). CONNECT-TBI is a network of brain banks and research institutions that share tissues and clinical datasets to support TBI research, investigate the pathologies of TBI, and explore the connections between TBI and neurodegenerative disease. CONNECT-TBI includes datasets from military, civilian, and athlete populations.

The Strategies to Innovate Emergency Clinical Care Trials Network (SIREN)[8] was established in 2016 by NIH in collaboration with clinical centers at U.S. academic institutions. SIREN supports clinical trials with the aim of improving the outcomes of patients with neurologic, cardiac, respiratory, and hematologic emergencies by identifying effective treatments that can be provided in the earlier stages of TBI care. SIREN is associated with three noteworthy clinical studies:

- ProTECT (Progesterone for the Treatment of TBI III)[9]—failed clinical progesterone trial for moderate to severe TBI
- BOOST3 (Brain Oxygen Optimization in Severe TBI, Phase 3)[10]—study for severely injured intensive care unit (ICU) patients over the age of 14
- HOBIT (Hyberbaric Oxygen Brain Injury Treatment Trial)[11]—study for adults aged 16–65 years with severe TBI

The Big Ten-Ivy League Concussion Taskforce[12] is a network and database established in 2012 to improve understanding of sport-related concussion and TBI. Studies conducted within the network are aimed at informing biomedical and behavioral sciences, enhancing clinical practice, and benefiting civilian and military populations through innovative TBI research (Putukian et al., 2019). The network's efforts are focused on student athlete TBI cases.

The Collaborative European NeuroTrauma Effectiveness Research in TBI (CENTER-TBI)[13] project arose from a workshop held to promote international TBI research. The CENTER-TBI prospective longitudinal observational study included 4,500 patients with 6-month patient follow-up, and the CENTER-TBI registry includes observational data from more than 15,000 patients. CENTER-TBI's aims are to better characterize TBI as a disease; to identify effective interventions; to develop an open-source database that is compatible with FITBIR; to validate CDE for international settings; and to translate research outputs into practical information and guidelines for patients, clinicians, and policy makers.

Linking Investigations in Trauma and Emergency Services (LITES)[14] was established in 2018 through collaboration between DoD and the University of Pittsburgh. The project

---

[7] More information about CONNECT-TBI is available at http://connect-tbi.med.upenn.edu/team (accessed July 2, 2021) and https://gbirg.inp.gla.ac.uk/connect-tbi (accessed July 2, 2021).

[8] More information about SIREN is available at https://siren.network/about-siren (accessed July 2, 2021).

[9] More information about ProTECT is available at https://clinicaltrials.gov/ct2/show/NCT00822900?term=ProTECT&cond=TBI+%28Traumatic+Brain+Injury%29&draw=2&rank=2 (accessed July 2, 2021).

[10] More information about BOOST3 is available at https://clinicaltrials.gov/ct2/show/NCT03754114?term=BOOST-3&cond=TBI+%28Traumatic+Brain+Injury%29&draw=2&rank=2 (accessed July 2, 2021).

[11] More information about HOBIT is available at https://clinicaltrials.gov/ct2/show/NCT02407028?term=HOBIT&cond=TBI+%28Traumatic+Brain+Injury%29&draw=2&rank=1 (accessed July 2, 2021).

[12] More information about Big Ten-Ivy League Concussion Taskforce is available at https://www.btaa.org/research/traumatic-brain-injury-research-collaboration (accessed July 2, 2021).

[13] More information about CENTER-TBI is available at https://www.center-tbi.eu (accessed July 2, 2021).

[14] More information about LITES is available at https://www.litesnetwork.org (accessed July 2, 2021).

created a network of medical professionals, prehospital providers, and emergency medical services providers to provide injury care and conduct outcomes research. The project's goal is to inform clinical practice guidelines and update existing standards of care for traumatic injuries. The network is focused on adults with TBI who have hemorrhagic shock (SWAT [Shock, Whole Blood and Assessment of TBI] Trial)[15] or need platelet transfusion (CriSP [Cold Stored Platelet Early Intervention in TBI] Trial).[16]

The DoD TBI Center of Excellence (TBICoE)[17] (originally called the Defense and Veterans Brain Injury Center) was established in 1992 to support a network of military treatment facilities and VA medical centers with TBI education and research initiatives (Jaffee and Martin, 2010).

The International Initiative for Traumatic Brain Injury Research (InTBIR)[18] coalition, supported by the European Commission, NIH's National Institute of Neurological Disorders and Stroke, the Canadian Institutes of Health Research, One Mind, DoD, and the Ontario Brain Institute, coordinates and leverages clinical research activities on TBI research to improve care and lessen the global burden of TBI. InTBIR is focused on investigating the causal relationship between TBI treatments and clinical outcomes. InTBIR investigates TBI among civilian, military, athlete, and pediatric populations.

TBI Model Systems (TBIMS)[19] was first established in 1987 as a demonstration project and expanded by HHS through the Administration for Community Living (Dijkers et al., 2010). A network of 16 TBIMS sites distributed throughout the United States focus on rehabilitation research and knowledge translation. The TBIMS National Database is currently the largest multisite longitudinal TBI study with information from preinjury through acute care and long-term outcomes among patients who received inpatient rehabilitation (Tso et al., 2021). In 2008, the VA and the National Institute on Disability, Independent Living, and Rehabilitation Research (NIDILRR) collaborated to establish a VA TBIMS among the five Polytrauma Rehabilitation Centers that address TBI rehabilitation in Veterans.

TBI research is also driven by individual studies and the efforts of dedicated clinicians and researchers working day by day to generate evidence and improve TBI patient outcomes. Many studies have been conducted and consortia created, efforts that often are conducted in parallel with other initiatives, such as the creation of guidelines or the development of a new database.

The Injury and Traumatic Stress Clinical Consortium (INTRuST)[20] was established in 2016 through DoD funding. The consortium aims to combine research efforts by PTSD and TBI experts to develop innovative treatments. INTRuST maintains an imaging data repository, which includes only data from military patients with TBI severe enough to have required inpatient rehabilitation.

Operation Brain Trauma Therapy (OBTT) is a multicenter, preclinical drug and biomarker screening consortium that began in 2010 (Kochanek et al., 2018). Its aim is to define therapies that show efficacy and have promise for randomized controlled trials (RCTs), including

---

[15] More information about SWAT Trial is available at https://clinicaltrials.gov/ct2/show/NCT03402035?term=SWAT&cond=TBI+%28Traumatic+Brain+Injury%29&draw=2&rank=1 (accessed July 2, 2021).

[16] More information about CriSP Trial is available at https://clinicaltrials.gov/ct2/show/NCT04726410?term=CRiSP&cond=TBI+%28Traumatic+Brain+Injury%29&draw=2&rank=1 (accessed July 2, 2021).

[17] More information about TBICoE is available at https://health.mil/About-MHS/OASDHA/Defense-Health-Agency/Research-and-Development/Traumatic-Brain-Injury-Center-of-Excellence (accessed July 2, 2021).

[18] More information about InTBIR is available at https://intbir.nih.gov (accessed July 2, 2021).

[19] More information about TBIMS is available at https://msktc.org/tbi/model-system-centers (accessed July 2, 2021).

[20] More information about INTRuST is available at https://cdmrp.army.mil/phtbi/research_highlights/16_Dec_intrust_highlight (accessed July 2, 2021).

TBI protein biomarker responses. OBTT has evaluated 10 therapeutics and assessed several blood biomarkers.

Warfighter Brain Health (WBH)[21] was chartered in 2011 by the U.S. Army Medical Research and Development Command to lead the development and acquisition of material products to warfighters suffering from brain injuries and psychological health issues. The project aims to advance knowledge, technology prototypes, training, tools, and practice guidelines for TBI assessment. Notably, the project has resulted in the development of a blood test to detect brain injury.

Approaches and Decisions in Acute Pediatric TBI Trial (ADAPT)[22] was conducted between 2014 and 2018 (final results not yet published). This international trial, supported by NIH and the University of Pittsburgh, was designed to evaluate the impact of interventions on severe TBI in children.

Army Study to Assess Risk and Resilience in Service members (ARMY STARRS) was a "multicomponent epidemiological and neurobiological study designed to generate actionable evidence-based recommendations to reduce army suicides and increase knowledge about risk and resilience factors for suicidality and its psychopathological correlates" (Ursano et al., 2014, p. 107). The study included a pre/post deployment component and a longitudinal study component.

Chronic Effects of Neurotrauma Consortium (CENC)[23] was conducted between 2013 and 2019. The largest study of TBI among Veterans, it aimed to address the long-term effects of mild TBI (mTBI) among military service personnel and Veterans. In 2019, CENC was succeeded by Long-term Impact of Military-relevant Brain Injury Consortium (LIMBIC),[24] which extended the research and has often been called LIMBIC-CENC to acknowledge those connections. LIMBIC aims to fill the gaps in basic science knowledge about mTBI and determine the effects on late-life outcomes and neurodegeneration. It also aims to identify service members most susceptible to the effects of mTBI and the most effective treatment strategies for these individuals. LIMBIC is funded by DoD and the VA in partnership with universities, research institutes, and health care organizations.

The Concussion Assessment, Research and Education Consortium (CARE)[25] began in 2014 with support from the NCAA and DoD. The largest mTBI study to date, it focuses on understanding the neurobiopsychosocial nature of concussive injury and recovery among student athletes and cadets in order to enhance the safety and health of youth athletes, service members, and civilian populations. Phase I is complete, and Phase II is ongoing.

Evaluation of Biomarkers of Traumatic Brain Injury (ALERT-TBI)[26] was conducted between 2012 and 2017 with funding from Banyan Biomarkers and DoD. It aimed to evaluate the utility of the Banyan UCH-L1/GFAP (ubiquitin carboxy-terminal hydrolase-L1/glial fibrillary acidic protein) Detection Assay as an aid in the evaluation of suspected TBI.

---

[21] More information about WBH is available at https://www.usammda.army.mil/index.cfm/project_management/neuro_psychological (accessed July 2, 2021).

[22] More information about ADAPT is available at https://www.adapttrial.org (accessed July 2, 2021) and https://clinicaltrials.gov/ct2/show/NCT04077411?term=ADAPT&cond=TBI+%28Traumatic+Brain+Injury%29&draw=2&rank=1 (accessed July 2, 2021).

[23] More information about CENC is available at https://vcurrtc.org/projects/viewPartner.cfm/13 (accessed July 2, 2021).

[24] More information about LIMBIC is available at https://www.limbic-cenc.org/index.php/about (accessed July 2, 2021).

[25] More information about CARE is available at http://careconsortium.net (accessed July 2, 2021).

[26] More information about ALERT-TBI is available at https://clinicaltrials.gov/ct2/show/NCT01426919 (accessed July 2, 2021).

TABLE A-2 TBI Consortia and Networks

Effort	Key Funders	Year(s)	
COllaborative Neuropathology NEtwork Characterizing OuTcomes of TBI (CONNECT-TBI)	NINDS, University of Pennsylvania	2020–present	
Strategies to Innovate Emergency Clinical Care Trials Network (SIREN)	NIH, academic institutions	2016–present	
Big Ten-Ivy League Concussion Taskforce	Academic institutions	2012–present	
Collaborative European NeuroTrauma Effectiveness Research in TBI (CENTER-TBI)	20 European universities	2013–present	
Linking Investigations in Trauma and Emergency Services (LITES)	DoD, University of Pittsburgh	2018–present	
TBI Center of Excellence (TBICoE), formerly Defense and Veterans Brain Injury Center (DVBIC)	DoD	1992–present	
International Initiative for Traumatic Brain Injury Research (InTBIR)	NIH, European Commission, Canadian Institutes of Health Research	2011–2019	
TBI Model Systems (TBIMS)	NIDILRR, Administration for Community Living, HHS	1987–present	
VA TBMIS Research Program	VA, NIDILRR (HHS)	2008–present	
Operation Brain Trauma Therapy (OBTT)	DoD and academic institutions	2010–present	
Warfighter Brain Health (WBH)	DoD, USAMMDA	2011–present	
Approaches and Decisions in Acute Pediatric TBI Trial (ADAPT)	NIH, University of Pittsburgh	2014–2019	
Army Study to Assess Risk and Resilience in Servicemembers (ARMY STARRS) and STARRS Longitudinal Study (STARRS-LS)	DoD, NIMH, Uniformed Services University, UCSD, Harvard, Univ. of Michigan	2009–present	
Chronic Effects of Neurotrauma Consortium (CENC)	DoD, VA	2013–2019	
Long-term Impact of Military-relevant Brain Injury Consortium (LIMBIC)	DoD, VA, universities, private research institutions	2019–present	
Concussion Assessment, Research and Education Consortium (CARE)	NCAA, DoD	2014–present	
Evaluation of Biomarkers of Traumatic Brain Injury (ALERT-TBI)	Banyan Biomarkers, DoD	2012–2017	
NCAA concussion study	NCAA	1999–2001	
Predicting and Preventing Post-concussive Problems in Pediatrics (5P)	CHEO research institute	2013–2015	
Transforming Research and Clinical Knowledge in TBI (TRACK-TBI)	NIH, DoD, OneMind, NeuroTruama Sciences LLC, Abbott Laboratories	2009–present	
TBI Endpoint Development Initiative (TED)	DoD, FDA, PPPs	2014–present	

NOTE: CENC = Chronic Effects of Neurotrauma Consortium; CHEO = Children's Hospital of Eastern Ontario; DoD = Department of Defense; FDA = Food and Drug Administration; GFAP = glial fibrillary acidic protein; HHS = Department of Health and Human Services; NCAA = National Collegiate Athletic Association; NIDILRR = National Institute on Disability, Independent Living, and Rehabilitation Research; NIH = National Institutes of Health; NIMH = National Institute of Mental Health; NINDS = National Institute of Neurological Disorders and Stroke; PPP = public–private partnership; TBI = traumatic brain injury; UCH-L1 = ubiquitin carboxy-terminal hydrolase-L1; UCSD = University of California, San Diego; USAMMDA = U.S. Army Medical Materiel Development Activity; VA = Department of Veterans Affairs.

Target Population(s)	Description
Athletes, military personnel, and civilians	Network to promote the sharing of tissue and datasets
Civilians	Network created to improve patient outcomes by identifying emergency treatments
Student athletes	Efforts to understand the causes and effects of sports-related concussion
European civilians	Various efforts to study TBI, develop TBI databases, and translate research to policy
Adults with TBI	Investigation of TBI care to inform guidelines for clinical practice
Military personnel	Effort to support a multicenter network of military TBI treatment facilities
Civilians, military personnel, athletes, and pediatric populations	International effort to reduce TBI burden by leveraging and coordinating TBI research
Civilians	Longitudinal study of long-term outcomes of individuals with moderate to severe TBI who received inpatient rehabilitation.
Military service members and Veterans	Longitudinal study of outcomes after inpatient rehabilitation at 5 VA Polytrauma Rehabilitation Centers
Preclinical	Studies to explore TBI drugs and biomarker screening
Military personnel	Studies and database to support development of comprehensive TBI strategies
Pediatric populations	International efforts to study the impact of server mild TBI (mTBI) interventions
Military personnel	Multicomponent studies to generate evidence-based recommendations
Military Veterans	Study to investigate the long-term effects of mTBI among military service personnel and Veterans
Military Veterans	Further research for TBI military personnel and Veterans; newest iteration of CENC
Student athletes and cadets	Study to explore concussive injury and recovery
Adults with moderate to mild TBI	Study to evaluate the utility of Banyan UCH-L1/GFAP detection assay
College football players	Prospective cohort study to evaluate concussions among college football players
Pediatric populations	Study to develop indicators for pediatric persistent postconcussive symptoms
Civilians	Largest-scale initiative to analyze clinical TBI data and TBI outcomes
Civilians, athletes, military personnel	Efforts to identify/validate measures of TBI and recovery

The NCAA concussion study was conducted between 1999 and 2001 (Guskiewicz et al., 2003). The seminal prospective cohort study evaluated 2,905 college football players to explore how common concussions are among college football players, average recovery time, and whether concussions occur more frequently among players who have previously experienced concussion.

Predicting and Preventing Post-concussive Problems in Pediatrics (5P)[27] was conducted between 2013 and 2015 by the Children's Hospital of Eastern Ontario (CHEO) research institute in Canada (Zemek et al., 2013). This prospective, multicenter cohort study aimed to derive and validate easy-to-use prognosticators that would enable clinicians to identify children and youth at risk of persistent postconcussive symptoms. The study focused on pediatric patients aged 5–18 years who were evaluated within the first 48 hours after a TBI.

Transforming Research and Clinical Knowledge in TBI (TRACK-TBI),[28] which began in 2009, is the largest, most comprehensive civilian TBI initiative. The study is funded by NIH, DoD, and industry and philanthropic partners. Its aim is to collect and analyze detailed clinical data on subjects across the TBI spectrum, including computed tomography (CT) and magnetic resonance imaging (MRI) data, blood biospecimens, and detailed clinical outcomes. The study also aims to identify TBI subgroups based on imaging and blood biomarkers in order to develop precision medicine for TBI.

The TBI Endpoint Development (TED) Initiative[29] began in 2014 with the aim of identifying and validating measures of brain injury and recovery for use in clinical trials to enable the development of precision TBI treatment. TED is supported by DoD; the Food and Drug Administration (FDA); and various public–private partnerships involving academia, industry, philanthropy, and patient advocacy organizations. One impetus for TED was to develop an improved classification system for TBI.

EDUCATION AND AWARENESS-RAISING INITIATIVES

CDC's HEADS UP initiative (see Table A-3) provides information and resources for parents, health care and school professionals, coaches, and athletes aimed at "raising awareness and informing action to improve prevention, recognition, and response to concussion and other serious brain injuries."[30] The program has reportedly "distributed more than 6 million copies of [the] HEADS UP materials and trained over 3 million coaches" (Baldwin et al., 2016).

Since 1986, the nonprofit ThinkFirst National Injury Prevention Foundation has focused on reducing youth and geriatric neurotrauma by developing and providing educational programs on injury prevention education and awareness for children, young adults, parents, and older adults (Youngers et al., 2017).

An effort by DoD's TBICoE (formerly the Defense and Veterans Brain Injury Center [DVBIC]), "A Head for the Future" provides fact sheets on TBI and stories and videos from service members and Veterans.[31]

---

[27] More information about 5P is available at http://www.5pconcussion.com (accessed July 2, 2021) and https://clinicaltrials.gov/ct2/show/NCT01873287 (accessed July 2, 2021).

[28] More information about TRACK-TBI is available at https://tracktbi.ucsf.edu (accessed July 2, 2021).

[29] More information about TED is available at https://tbiendpoints.ucsf.edu (accessed July 2, 2021). See also Manley et al., 2017.

[30] More information about HEADS UP is available at https://www.cdc.gov/headsup/about/index.html (accessed July 2, 2021).

[31] See https://www.health.mil/About-MHS/OASDHA/Defense-Health-Agency/Research-and-Development/Traumatic-Brain-Injury-Center-of-Excellence/A-Head-for-the-Future (accessed August 25, 2021).

TABLE A-3 Selected TBI Educational Efforts

Effort	Key Funders	Year(s)	Target Population(s)	Description
HEADS UP	CDC	2003–present	Youth and elderly	Educational initiative to improve TBI awareness and prevention among youth and elderly
A Head for the Future	DoD	2019	Military personnel	Effort to improve TBI awareness and prevention among service members and Veterans

Note: CDC = Centers for Disease Control and Prevention; DoD = Department of Defense; TBI = traumatic brain injury.

A number of awareness-raising and educational programs are undertaken each March for Brain Injury Awareness Month, led by the Brain Injury Association of America.

In addition, trauma-focused educational efforts may have relevance to TBI. For example, "Stop the Bleed," founded by the American College of Surgeons, is a call-to-action awareness campaign that trains and empowers individuals to respond aptly in a bleeding emergency before professional help arrives. The course is taught by qualified instructors who focus on identification and treatment, as well as the basics of bleeding control through wound packing and pressure dressings.[32]

CARE GUIDELINES

To achieve the best possible outcomes and reduce TBI-related morbidity and mortality, up-to-date, evidence-based guidelines, clinical best practices, and care recommendations are essential (see Table A-4). Much of the current TBI research is focused on addressing the need for such guidelines, and as TBI research advances, guidelines must be continually assessed and revised. Brain Trauma Foundation TBI Guidelines committees[33] have been creating TBI guidelines since 1995. The committees include representatives of various professional societies and academic institutions, including the American Association of Neurological Surgeons (AANS), Congress of Neurological Surgeons (CNS), Army Contracting Command, Aberdeen Proving Ground, Natick Contracting Division, Stanford University, and the Brain Trauma Foundation. The committees create evidence-based guidelines for treating TBI that aim to advance high-quality care and lower TBI-related morbidity and mortality. Since the initial guideline publication in 1995, updated guidelines have been published in 2000, 2007, and 2016.

DoD has established protocols for TBI assessment and return to duty[34] and continues to explore metrics for assessing readiness to return (Scherer et al., 2013). These guidelines are used primarily in military settings to manage mTBI among military personnel.

The International Forum on Consensus in Sport Concussion[35] first established guidelines

---

[32] See https://www.stopthebleed.org (accessed August 25, 2021).

[33] More information about Brain Trauma Foundation TBI Guidelines committees is available at https://www.braintrauma.org/coma/guidelines (accessed July 2, 2021) and https://www.braintrauma.org/uploads/13/06/Guidelines_for_Management_of_Severe_TBI_4th_Edition.pdf (accessed July 2, 2021).

[34] More information about DoD protocols for TBI assessment is available at DoD Clinical Recommendation January 2021, Progressive Return to Activity Following Acute Concussion/Mild Traumatic Brain Injury. https://jts.amedd.army.mil/assets/docs/cpgs/Progressive_Return_to_Activity_Following_Acute_Concussion_mTBI_Clinical_Recommendation_2021.pdf (accessed March 2, 2022).

[35] More information about International Forum on Consensus in Sport Concussion is available at https://waset.org/sports-concussion-prevention-diagnosis-and-treatment-conference-in-august-2021-in-paris (accessed July 2, 2021).

TABLE A-4 Selected TBI Clinical Guidance Development Efforts

Effort	Key Funders	Year(s)	Target Population	Description
Brain Trauma Foundation TBI Guidelines committees	AANS, CNS, Army Contracting Command, Stanford University, Brain Trauma Foundation	1995–present	Specified subpopulations (ex., severe TBI)	Committees formed to support the creation of evidence-based guidelines for TBI care
DoD protocols for TBI assessment and return to duty			Military personnel	Guidelines for military personnel who experience mTBI
International consensus conferences and statements on concussion in sport		2001–present	Sports participants	Forum developed to conduct systematic TBI evidence review every 4 years
Guidelines for disorders of consciousness	ANN, ACRM, NIDILRR	2018	Persons with prolonged disorders of consciousness	Recommendations for patients with prolonged disorders of consciousness
Pediatric mTBI CDC Resources	CDC	2018	Children with mTBI	Guidelines for pediatric mTBI

Note: AANS = American Association of Neurological Surgeons; ACRM = American Congress of Rehabilitation Medicine; ANN = American Academy of Neurology; CDC = Centers for Disease Control and Prevention; CNS = Congress of Neurological Surgeons; DoD = Department of Defense; mTBI = mild traumatic brain injury; NIDILRR = National Institute on Disability, Independent Living, and Rehabilitation Research; TBI = traumatic brain injury.

in 2001, and its sixth conference is scheduled for 2022. Every 4 years, the forum conducts a systematic review of concussion evidence to inform a series of evidence-based statements. The most recent consensus statement was released in 2017 following the fifth international conference (McCrory et al., 2017).

In 2018, the American Academy of Neurology (ANN), American Congress of Rehabilitation Medicine (ACRM), and NIDILRR created new guidelines for disorders of consciousness (Giacino et al., 2018). These guidelines provided updated care recommendations for patients with prolonged disorders of consciousness, such as vegetative states, unresponsive wakefulness syndrome, and minimally conscious states.

CDC's pediatric mTBI guidelines were first published in 2018 (Lumba-Brown et al., 2018).[36] They address diagnosis, prognosis, management, and treatment for pediatric mTBI.

As part of its HEADS UP initiative, a toolkit for healthcare professionals was first developed by CDC in 2003 and rereleased in 2007 (CDC, 2013). The website now includes online training courses for health care providers and youth sports coaches, among other resources.[37]

FEDERAL INVESTMENTS IN TBI RESEARCH

Significant resources have been devoted to TBI over the past decade, including through federal and philanthropic research investments that have supported long-term clinical stud-

---

[36] More information about CDC's pediatric mTBI guidelines is available at https://www.cdc.gov/traumaticbraininjury/PediatricmTBIGuideline.html (accessed July 2, 2021).

[37] See https://www.cdc.gov/headsup/resources/index.html (accessed September 24, 2021).

ies. According to available information, federal agencies invested approximately $330 million in fiscal year 2019 and approximately $2 billion over the 5-year period 2014 to 2019. Information on support for TBI in the *Federal RePORTER* database for 2014 to 2019 shows 5,041 projects with $2,111,385,035 funding involving NIH; the CDMRP; the National Science Foundation; the NIDILRR; the Center for Neuroscience and Regenerative Medicine (based at the Uniformed Services University of the Health Sciences), CDC, the Combat Casualty Care Research Program, the Agency for Healthcare Research and Quality, and the National Institute of Food and Agriculture. TBI projects were also supported at the VA and DVBIC, although this funding was not reported in the available total.[38] NIH estimates of funding for TBI has increased from $87 million in 2014 to $134 million in 2019.[39] Recent annual funding among participating agencies of the NRAP has included funding from DoD ($141 million); VA Office of Research and Development ($41.9 million); NIH ($134 million); NIDILRR ($16 million); and CDC ($3 million), totaling approximately $335.9 million. The most recent request for proposals issued by the CDMRP in Traumatic Brain Injury and Psychological Health, released in August 2021, indicated that $175 million had been allocated to the program.[40]

REFERENCES

Baldwin, G., M. Breiding, and D. Sleet. 2016. Using the public health model to address unintentional injuries and TBI: A perspective from the Centers for Disease Control and Prevention (CDC). *NeuroRehabilitation* 39(3):345-349.

Brain Trauma Blueprint. 2021. *Traumatic brain injury: A new roadmap outlining opportunities, barriers, and recommendations for advancing treatment solutions.* Press release. https://www.braintraumablueprint.org/tbi-new-roadmap-advancing-treatment (accessed July 31, 2021).

CDC (Centers for Disease Control and Prevention). 2013. *HEADS UP in 10 years: The anniversary viewbook of CDC's HEADS UP.* https://www.cdc.gov/headsup/pdfs/HeadsUp_10YrViewBook-a.pdf (accessed September 24, 2021).

Cohen Veterans Bioscience. 2019. Pathways to effective treatments for traumatic brain injuries. *Proceedings of the Second Annual Brain Trauma Blueprint State of the Science Summit.* June 5–6, 2019. https://www.braintrauma blueprint.org/wp-content/uploads/2020/11/braintraumablueprint-tbisummit2019-proceedings.pdf (accessed July 31, 2021).

Dijkers, M., C. Harrison-Felix, and J. Marwitz. 2010. The Traumatic Brain Injury Model Systems history and contributions to clinical service and research. *Journal of Head Trauma Rehabilitation* 25(2):81-91.

DoD (Department of Defense), VA (Department of Veterans Affairs), HHS (Department of Health and Human Services), and ED (Department of Education). 2013. *National research action plan: Responding to the Executive Order Improving Access to Mental Health Services for Veterans, Service Members, and Military Families (August 31, 2012).* https://obamawhitehouse.archives.gov/sites/default/files/uploads/nrap_for_eo_on_mental_health_august_2013.pdf (accessed July 31, 2021).

Giacino, J. T., D. I. Katz, N. D. Schiff, J. Whyte, E. J. Ashman, S. Ashwal, R. Barbano, F. M. Hammond, S. Laureys, G. S. F. Ling, R. Nakase-Richardson, R. T. Seel, S. Yablon, T. S. D. Getchius, G. S. Gronseth, and M. J. Armstrong. 2018. Practice guideline update recommendations summary: Disorders of consciousness: Report of the Guideline Development, Dissemination, and Implementation Subcommittee of the American Academy of Neurology; the American Congress of Rehabilitation Medicine; and the National Institute on Disability, Independent Living, and Rehabilitation Research. *Neurology* 91(10):450-460.

Guskiewicz, K. M., M. McCrea, S. W. Marshall, R. C. Cantu, C. Randolph, W. Barr, J. A. Onate, and J. P. Kelly. 2003. Cumulative effects associated with recurrent concussion in collegiate football players: The NCAA Concussion Study. *Journal of the American Medical Association* 290(19):2549-2555.

---

[38] See https://federalreporter.nih.gov, using a search for "Traumatic Brain Injury" or TBI (accessed May 13, 2021).

[39] Based on NIH Resources—Estimates of Funding for Various Research, Condition, and Disease Categories (RCDC) available at https://report.nih.gov/funding/categorical-spending# (accessed May 13, 2021). Searching "Injury - Traumatic Brain Injury" provided results of 2014 ($87 million); 2015 ($93 million); 2016 ($105 million); 2017 ($116 million); 2018 ($133 million); 2019 ($134 million); 2020 estimated ($143 million); and 2021 estimated ($130 million).

[40] See https://cdmrp.army.mil/funding/tbiphrp (accessed August 25, 2021).

Haarbauer-Krupa, J., M. J. Pugh, E. M. Prager, N. Harmon, J. Wolfe, and K. C. Yaffe. 2021. Epidemiology of chronic effects of traumatic brain injury. *Journal of Neurotrauma* 38(23):3235-3247. https://doi.org/10.1089/neu.2021.0062.

Jaffee, M., and E. M. Martin. 2010. Defense and Veterans Brain Injury Center: Program overview and research initiatives. *Military Medicine* 175(7 Suppl):37-41.

Kochanek, P. M., C. E. Dixon, S. Mondello, K. Wang, A. Lafrenaye, H. M. Bramlett, W. Dietrich, R. L. Hayes, D. A. Shear, J. S. Gilsdorf, M. Catania, S. M. Poloyac, P. E. Empey, T. C. Jackson, and J. T. Povlishock. 2018. Multi-Center pre-clinical consortia to enhance translation of therapies and biomarkers for traumatic brain injury: Operation brain trauma therapy and beyond. *Frontiers in Neurology* 9:640.

Lumba-Brown, A., K. O. Yeates, K. Sarmiento, M. Breiding, T. Haegerich, G. Gioia, M. Turner, et al. 2018. Centers for Disease Control and Prevention guideline on the diagnosis and management of mild traumatic brain injury among children. *JAMA Pediatrics* 172(11):e182853.

Lumba-Brown, A., E. Prager, N. Harmon, M. McCrea, M. Bell, J., Ghajar, S. Pyne, and D. Cifu. 2021. A review of implementation concepts and strategies surrounding traumatic brain injury clinical care guidelines. *Journal of Neurotrauma* 38(23). https://doi.org/10.1089/neu.2021.0067.

Manley, G. T., C. Mac Donald, A. Markowitz, D. Stephenson, A. Robbins, R. Gardner, E. Winkler, Y. Bodien, S. Taylor, J. Yue, L. Kannan, A. Kumar, M. McCrea, K. Wang, and TED Investigators. 2017. The Traumatic Brain Injury Endpoints Development (TED) Initiative: Progress on a public-private regulatory collaboration to accelerate diagnosis and treatment of traumatic brain injury. *Journal of Neurotrauma* 34(19):2721-2730.

McCrory, P., W. Meeuwisse, J. Dvořák, M. Aubry, J. Bailes, S. Broglio, R. Cantu, et al. 2017. Consensus statement on concussion in sport-the 5th international conference on concussion in sport held in Berlin, October 2016. *British Journal of Sports Medicine* 51(11):838-847.

Pugh, M. J., E. Kennedy, E. Prager, J. Humpherys, K. Dams-O'Connor, D. Hack, M. K. McCafferty, J. Wolfe, K. Yaffe, M. McCrea, A. Ferguson, L. Lancashire, J. Ghajar, and A. Lumba-Brown. 2021. Phenotyping the spectrum of traumatic brain injury: A review and pathway to standardization. *Journal of Neurotrauma* 38(23). https://doi.org/10.1089/neu.2021.0059.

Putukian, M., B. D'Alonzo, C. Campbell-McGovern, and D. Wiebe. 2019. The Ivy League-Big Ten Epidemiology of Concussion Study: A report on methods and first findings. *American Journal of Sports Medicine* 47(5):1236-1247.

Scherer, M., M. Weightman, M. Radomski, L. Davidson, and K. McCulloch. 2013. Returning service members to duty following mild traumatic brain injury: exploring the use of dual-task and multitask assessment methods. *Physical Therapy* 93(9):1254-1267

Smith, D., J-P. Dollé, K. E. Ameen-Ali, A. Bretzin, E. Cortes, J. Crary, K. Dams-O'Connor, R. Diaz-Arrastia, B. Edlow, R. Folkerth, L-N. Hazrati, S. Hinds, D. Iacono, V. Johnson, C. D. Keene, J. Kofler, G. Kovacs, E. Lee, G. Manley, D. Meaney, T. Montine, D. Okonkwo, D. Perl, J. Trjanowski, D. Wiebe, K. Yaffe, T. McCabe, and W. Stewart. 2021a. Collaborative Neuropatholoy Network Characterizing ouTcomes of TBI (CONNECT-TBI). *Acta Neuropathologica Communications* 9:32. https://doi.org/10.1186/s40478-021-01122-9.

Smith, D. H., P. Kochanek, S. Rosi, R. Meyer, C. Ferland-Beckham, E. Prager, S. Ahlers, and F. Crawford. 2021b. Roadmap for advancing pre-clinical science in traumatic brain injury. *Journal of Neurotrauma*. https://doi.org/10.1089/neu.2021.0094.

Tso, S., A. Saha, and M. D. Cusimano. 2021. The Traumatic Brain Injury Model Systems National Database: A review of published research. *Neurotrauma Reports* 2(1):149-164.

Ursano, R. J., L. J. Colpe, S. G. Heeringa, R. C. Kessler, M. Schoenbaum, M. B. Stein, and A. S. Collaborators. 2014. The Army study to assess risk and resilience in servicemembers (Army STARRS). *Psychiatry: Interpersonal and Biological Processes* 77(2):107-119.

White House. 2012. *Improving access to mental health services for Veterans, service members, and military families.* Executive Order 13625 of August 31, 2012. https://obamawhitehouse.archives.gov/the-press-office/2012/08/31/executive-order-improving-access-mental-health-services-veterans-service (accessed July 31, 2021).

Youngers, E. H., K. Zundel, D. Gerhardstein, M. Martínez, C. Bertrán, M. Proctor, M. Spatola, and E. Neuwelt. 2017. Comprehensive review of the ThinkFirst injury prevention programs: A 30-year success story for organized neurosurgery. *Neurosurgery* 81(3):416-421.

Zemek, R., M. Osmond, N. Barrowan, and on behalf of the Pediatric Emergency Research Canada (PERC) Concussion Team. 2013. Predicting and Preventing Postconcussive Problems in Paediatrics (5P) study: Protocol for a prospective multientre clinical prediction rule derivation study in children with concussion. *BMJ Open* 3(8):e003550. https://doi.org/10.1136/bmjopen-2013-003550.

Appendix B

Biomarker Development for Diagnosis, Prognosis, and Monitoring of Traumatic Brain Injury

A number of biomarkers are being evaluated for or show promise in providing improved sensitivity for diagnosis, prognosis, and monitoring of traumatic brain injury (TBI). This appendix summarizes developments in this area.

NEUROIMAGING BIOMARKERS

Neuroimaging is an important component in the evaluation of patients with a suspected TBI. Imaging is a critical tool in identifying TBI pathologies that increase a patient's risk of mortality or further neurologic deterioration, and that indicate the need for urgent medical intervention.

Current Options

In clinical settings, computed tomography (CT) remains the standard for imaging of acute TBI because of its ability to identity gross pathologies, such as intracranial hemorrhage, swelling, or presence of foreign objects; its noninvasive nature; and its wide availability across nearly all care settings (e.g., in urban and rural hospitals, trauma centers, and community hospitals). There are established guidelines for diagnosing TBI with CT (Freire-Aragón et al., 2017). In patients with more severe injuries, head CT is preferable in characterizing the type and extent of specific TBI pathologies (e.g., diffuse axonal injury), as well as quantifying the combined contribution of multiple pathologies (e.g., subarachnoid hemorrhage and cortical contusion). However, brain CT scans are limited in detecting and quantifying more subtle neuronal injury.

Magnetic resonance imaging (MRI), the second common neuroimaging method for TBI, can better characterize the nature, locale, and extent of TBI pathology and track the course of pathologies over time relative to CT. Clinicians may use routine MRI when a patient exhibits persistent or worsening symptoms because MRI can provide enhanced anatomic detail compared with CT, giving clinicians greater diagnostic clarity. Currently, MRI is an adjunctive tool in the evaluation of patients whose clinical outcome appears more severe than what would be expected based on brain CT (Currie et al., 2016). Susceptibility artifact-sensitive sequences (e.g., susceptibility-weighted imaging) are also available and provide information on the presence of microhemorrhages within the brain that are less visible on more conventional T2 sequences (Blennow et al., 2016). Given the coexistence of white matter microhemorrhage and diffuse axonal injury, this approach may furnish a better understanding of patients who are symptomatic but have a normal CT. Additional investigation is warranted before changing current clinical practice guidelines, given the lower frequency of these findings in mild TBI and their inconsistent relation to functional outcome (Currie et al., 2016; Pavlovic et al., 2019). However, the subgroup of TBI patients who benefit the most from MRI and optimal time between injury and brain MRI evaluation have not yet been well defined.

In addition to routine CT and MRI imaging, a variety of advanced quantitative techniques demonstrate promise in better characterizing the acute, sub-acute, and chronic phases of TBI; their use in TBI and concussion has been the subject of several recent review papers (Asken et al., 2018b; Irimia et al., 2012; Lindsey et al., 2021; Sharp et al., 2014). Diffusion imaging (including diffusion tensor imaging, diffusion spectrum imaging, and diffusion kurtosis imaging) and volumetric analysis of three-dimensional anatomic imaging may provide insight into gross and microstructural changes following a TBI. These findings may have value in both the short- and longer-term phases of recovery in patients with a broad range of severity of injuries and time since injury. Generally, studies report abnormalities in diffusion imaging metrics across several brain regions, with the most commonly reported findings in the corpus callosum, corona radiata, internal capsule, and cingulum bundle. In adults, there is some evidence of initially increased fractional anisotropy and decreased apparent diffusion coefficient or mean diffusivity in the acute to sub-acute recovery phase, although longitudinal studies do not necessarily suggest a consistent pattern over time (Asken et al., 2018b). Additional longitudinal studies and studies of mild TBI are needed to explore the precise trajectory of change in diffusion metrics over the course of recovery.

Magnetization transfer imaging (MTI) may also add sensitivity to the MRI evaluation of patients with all severities of TBI (Tu et al., 2017; Wilde et al., 2015). MTI examines the presence or absence of macromolecules, which include proteins and phospholipids that coat axonal membranes or myelin sheaths within the white matter. MTI has been used to infer the degree of myelin integrity and Wallerian degeneration, inflammation, and edema in various disease processes, including TBI. More recently, it has been evaluated in experimental models of TBI in relation to histologically verified myelin loss (Lehto et al., 2017). However, reports of utility in patients have been limited relative to other neuroimaging modalities.

Emerging research also suggests that a dysregulation of cerebral blood flow contributes to TBI pathophysiology and acute and chronic symptoms (Ellis et al., 2016). Change in cerebral blood flow following a vasoactive stimulus is defined as cerebrovascular reactivity and can be measured by imaging techniques including CT, MRI, positron emission tomography (PET)/single photon emission computed tomography (SPECT) perfusion techniques, and transcranial Doppler. Cerebrovascular reactivity (CVR) imaging is used for diagnosing and managing many cerebrovascular diseases but has only recently been studied in TBI (Zeiler et al., 2020a). Some work has begun to evaluate CVR as a neuroimaging biomarker of traumatic vascular injury in sports concussion (Churchill et al., 2019, 2020) and moderate to severe TBI (Zeiler et al., 2020b). The aim is to improve TBI management by improving diagnosis and prediction of recovery. Further work is required to determine whether this technique provides accurate, reliable, and reproducible neuroimaging-based measures of CVR and to correlate imaging measures with specific outcomes.

Another method using MRI technology is the use of functional MRI (fMRI). In this method, blood oxygen level dependent (BOLD)-based fMRI sequences are employed, and involve interpretations of neurological activity related to the oxygenation state of blood and hemodynamic response to the activity-related metabolic task. These sequences have been used to identify regions of brain activation that occur under both task-oriented and resting-state conditions that relate to brain injury, and possible symptoms and deficits related to the injury. Additionally, researchers have used fMRI to establish patterns of connectivity between brain regions and to describe how these connections are altered during both normal development and disease. In TBI, task-based fMRI studies have demonstrated alterations in brain activity across a number of cognitive tasks, including working memory, sustained attention, executive function, and language processing (Laatsch and Krisky, 2006; Palacios et al., 2013; Wu et al., 2020). Reduced connectivity has also been shown in brain regions following TBI (Kondziella et al., 2017; Wu et al., 2020).

PET is a neuroimaging technique that allows for detection and localization of radioisotopes associated with biologically active radiopharmaceuticals that aggregate within the brain following administration of the ligand. PET detects high-energy photons that result from positron decay. In TBI, much of the work conducted with PET to date has involved the imaging of glucose metabolism using 18F-fluorodeoxyglucose imaging. These studies have generally demonstrated reductions in glucose metabolism in multiple brain regions of TBI patients, which are reported to relate to the level of consciousness at the time of PET imaging (Shah et al., 2020). Radiopharmaceuticals revealing pathological correlates of long-term neurodegeneration in the setting of TBI have received considerable interest. Specifically, the amyloid imaging agent Pittsburgh Compound-B (11C-PiB) has been used in multiple studies of patients with TBI. Positive findings are demonstrated in some studies (Hong et al., 2014; Kawai et al., 2013), but findings are inconsistent in others (Ayubcha et al., 2021). Perhaps of greater interest are studies evaluating recently available radiopharmaceuticals targeting abnormally phosphorylated paired helical filament tau following TBI. Postmortem examinations of chronic traumatic encephalopathy (CTE) report the pathological finding of abnormal tau aggregation, and there has been significant interest in developing an in vivo biomarker for detecting this condition. To date, several studies have reported tauopathy in individuals with chronic TBI utilizing tau imaging agents (Gorgoraptis et al., 2019; Takahata et al., 2019).

Future Directions and Limits

Additional studies will be needed to determine the possible benefits of various imaging techniques in various TBI patient populations, injury severities, and care settings. Although advanced quantitative techniques have improved understanding of TBI, their role in diagnosis is still developing, and clinical platforms for utilizing these approaches in patient care remain forthcoming. Additional obstacles include difficulties in (1) directly comparing quantitative metrics derived from different scanners or acquisition parameters and (2) the lack of adequate normative data to enable harmonization across centers, the latter of which is being reconciled by the development of a Normative Neuroimaging Library.[1] Finally, while many of these imaging modalities demonstrate statistical relationships with symptom reports, cognitive functioning, and other outcomes, the validation of these biomarkers for diagnostic use in concussion and mild TBI is complicated by the lack of consistent diagnostic criteria and the existence of other indicators of injury. Additionally, anatomic heterogeneity in TBI

---

[1] See https://www.cohenveteransbioscience.org/programs/our-programs/normative-neuroimaging-library (accessed March 2, 2022).

complicates use of common regions of interest in which to focus imaging. It will also be important to determine the need for further development and optimization of informatics platforms to facilitate interpretation of imaging studies, including metrics on the character and degree of TBI pathologies.

BIOFLUID BIOMARKERS

Biomarkers within blood, cerebrospinal fluid (CSF), and saliva show promise in detecting underlying pathologies of TBI and risk for an incomplete recovery.

Current Options

A number of biomarkers are involved in recovery of tissue injury related to a TBI. Specifically, biomarkers include markers of inflammation and blood–brain barrier (BBB) integrity, as well axonal, neuronal, astroglial, and vascular injury. Initially, there is increased flow of immune cells into injured tissue, initiating a debriding process that is essential for tissue recovery. Yet, if this process is too extreme or prolonged, tissue injury can be substantial and can result in more injuries, termed the secondary injury process. Other TBI biomarkers indicate specific brain cell types, including astrocytes and microglia, showing that there is a cascade of biomarker activity that facilitates recovery. When these activities are insufficiently regulated, long-term risks to neurons can result, placing the individual at greater risk for compromise in function and increasing the risk for symptoms and chronic deficits.

The first combination biomarkers to receive Food and Drug Administration (FDA) approval in acute TBI are glial fibrillary acidic protein (GFAP) and ubiquitin carboxyl-terminal hydrolase L1 (UCH-L1) (Bazarian et al., 2018). GFAP is an astroglial intermediate filament structural cytoskeleton protein that is released on injury and cell death; after acute TBI, serum GFAP levels peak 20 hours after injury (Czeiter et al., 2020; Gill et al., 2018; Papa et al., 2019). UCH-L1, a neuron-enriched enzyme involved in ubiquitin turnover, is detectable as early as 1 hour after TBI, peaks at 8 hours, and declines slowly 48 hours after injury (Anderson et al., 2020; Czeiter et al., 2020; Papa et al., 2019). Research has shown high sensitivity and negative predictive value of the brain trauma indicator (BTI) test for predicting traumatic intracranial injuries on head CT scan acutely after TBI, and distinguishing CT-positive, more severely injured from CT-negative, mild TBI patients (Anderson et al., 2020). In more mild cohorts, including sports concussion, elevated GFAP and UCLH1 have been observed days following concussion, indicating that these biomarkers are accurate predictors in even the mildest of brain injuries (McCrea et al., 2020).

S100B, a marker of both astrocyte and oligodendrocyte activity, also shows promise as a biomarker of TBI, with higher levels being associated with greater TBI severity and poorer outcomes (Czeiter et al., 2020; Jones et al., 2020). A phase 1 cohort analysis (N = 1,409) of the ability of point-of-care GFAP and S100B levels to predict intracranial abnormalities at 24 hours after injury across the full TBI spectrum (Glasgow Coma Scale [GSC] 3–15) was conducted by the TRACK-TBI network. Receiver operator characteristic (ROC) curves for the prediction of CT-positive scans after injury had significantly higher area under the curve (AUC) for GFAP and S100B (0.85 and 0.67, respectively) (Okonkwo et al., 2020). The CENTER-TBI project included analyses of six serum biomarkers (S100B, NSE, GFAP, UCH-L1, neurofilament protein-light [NfL], and total tau), and found that GFAP achieved the highest discrimination for predicting CT abnormalities (AUC 0.89), better than any other single candidate protein or combination of biomarkers in the panel (Czeiter et al., 2020). Thus, ongoing studies continue to evaluate these biomarkers with the aim of ultimately determining which biomarkers or combination of biomarkers provide the most diagnostic and prognostic value.

Other proteins may be of value for diagnosis and prediction following a TBI. Specifically, NfL is an intermediate filament that provides cytoskeleton support within neurons (Gaetani et al., 2019). Tau is an axonal protein that is associated with axonal damage, and has been implicated in both short- and long-term outcomes related to TBI (Mckee and Daneshvar, 2015). Serum levels of NfL correlate with CSF levels (Shahim et al., 2020), indicating that NfL has brain-specific activity that can be detected within samples of blood. Recently, it has been shown to be elevated in mild to severe injuries (McCrea et al., 2020; Thelin et al., 2019) and to be elevated years following a TBI, with the highest levels in individuals with more severe chronic symptoms (Guedes et al., 2020b; Shahim et al., 2020). Recent studies of plasma tau in acute sports concussion collected within the first 6–24 hours after injury suggest that higher levels of tau may be prognostic biomarkers of prolonged recovery (Pattinson et al., 2020). Lastly, concentrations of total tau in the blood have been linked to chronic symptoms suggestive of CTE in athletes with high numbers of concussions over their career (Mez et al., 2017).

Researchers are also studying exosomes, which are present in blood and carry biomarkers that may be useful in tracking TBI. Exosomes are lipid-membrane-bound extracellular vesicles whose cargo is rich in microRNA (miRNA) and protein, sequestered from the cytoplasm of the cell of origin. Exosomes are secreted by all cells and are known to have a range of biological functions, including cell-to-cell communication and signaling (Guedes et al., 2020a). Exosomes easily cross the BBB and are abundant in peripheral circulation, and their cell of origin can be identified by the proteins they carry on their membrane. Studies of exosomes show that they coordinate response from TBIs (Manek et al., 2018). Exosomal activity has been shown to remain dysregulated years following the injury and to relate to chronic symptoms (Goetzl et al., 2020; Guedes et al., 2020b). Preclinical studies show that exosomal content can promote improved recovery (Chen et al., 2020; Yang et al., 2019). Therefore, additional studies are needed to better understand the role of exosomes in recovery from TBI and their role in acute and chronic symptoms.

Future Directions and Limits

A challenge for the use of TBI biomarkers relates to both the heterogeneity of TBI pathologies and the broad spectrum of TBI severity (from concussion to coma). No single biomarker reflects all known pathophysiological mechanisms of TBI, particularly given their dynamic trajectories over time. In addition, the "majority of TBI biomarker research has focused on … diagnostic biomarkers of acute TBI within the first 24 hours after injury" (Kenney et al., 2021, p. 66), and few candidates have been identified for the diagnosis of sub-acute (up to 1 week postinjury) or chronic sequelae after TBI (3 months to years). Biomarker profiles between weeks and months will facilitate understanding TBI progression and are discussed further in the section on biomarker monitoring below.

Continued research is needed on the translation of biomarkers to clinical practice, including further validation of candidate biomarkers across diverse patient populations, to determine cutoffs for reliable detection of TBI and the possible impacts of comorbidities (e.g., polytrauma, posttraumatic stress disorder [PTSD], depression) on biomarkers. Further discovery of novel biomarkers that are more sensitive and specific continues to be needed to enable tracking of outcomes. For clinical utility, it will be important to determine the added value of fluid biomarkers over existing TBI clinical and neuroimaging evaluation methods. For widespread implementation within care and community settings, development and validation of accessible, low-resource-burden, cost-effective point-of-care or other quick-delivery modalities for testing options for biomarkers will be critical.

NEUROPHYSIOLOGICAL BIOMARKERS

Although not typically considered "neuroimaging" procedures, a number of prototype technologies intended for clinical evaluation of patients with TBI are in development. These technologies include portable, quantitative electroencephalography (qEEG), eye movement tracking devices, pupilometers, infrared scanners, and others. Some of these technologies have gained clearance from FDA but have minimal penetration in clinical practice, particularly in hospital and trauma care settings.

An electroencephalogram (EEG) records the averaged excitatory and inhibitory postsynaptic potentials of cortical pyramidal neurons, which tend to oscillate at different frequency bands (e.g., delta, theta, alpha, beta, and gamma bands) and involve cortico-cortical and thalamocortical connections. Electrophysiology has the advantage of being inexpensive and easily transportable. This technique also has high temporal resolution and therefore provides information complementary to that derived with such technologies as MRI, which provide high spatial resolution. Several electrophysiological techniques hold promise for detecting mild TBI.

A clinical review of EEG typically involves subjective visual inspection of brain electrical activity, assessment of topography and frequencies, and detection of pathological features. Clinical EEG is generally used to monitor and diagnose epileptic seizures arising in patients with acute TBI. EEG dysfunctions (such as focal slowing) appear to be related to BBB breakdown (Korn et al., 2005; Tomkins et al., 2011). Changes observed in mild TBI clinical EEG have been reported as nonspecific, have low interrater agreement, and may be more useful when used with other approaches, such as qEEG and/or event-related potentials (Gaetz and Bernstein, 2001; Rapp et al., 2015).

qEEG is considered more robust than clinical EEG and given its digital form, involves statistical analyses of the raw signal in order to derive numerical results and relevant information on EEG data. qEEG changes appear to be sensitive to symptoms experienced from mild TBI, particularly balance instability (Thompson et al., 2005). Studies with large sample sizes have also found that qEEG is sensitive for detecting mild TBI (Rapp et al., 2015; Thatcher et al., 2001).

The capacity of EEG determinants—such as coherence, phase, and amplitude difference—to discriminate between mild and severe TBI during the post-acute period is high (sensitivity of 95 percent and specificity of 97 percent) (Thatcher et al., 2001). These results have been cross-validated in a sample of approximately 500 Department of Veterans Affairs (VA) patients (Rapp et al., 2015; Thatcher et al., 2001). Studies using power spectrum analyses have generally shown a decrease in alpha power and an increase in delta, beta, and theta bands. The findings vary in different studies, requiring standardization across sites to improve consistency (Rapp et al., 2015; Thatcher et al., 2001). Additional consideration is required to account appropriately for confounding factors and overlap in populations prone to present with psychiatric disorders (Thornton, 2003). Portable EEG devices have been developed for the assessment of mild TBI in sideline testing (for athletes); in the field (for military personnel); and in more traditional care settings, such as the emergency department. Finally, researchers recently combined transcranial magnetic stimulation (TMS) with EEG to study connectivity changes post-TBI, which may offer a promising avenue for investigating the neural substrates of connectivity dysfunction and reorganization after mild TBI (Coyle et al., 2018).

Event-related potentials (ERPs) allow researchers to understand cognitive processes using time-locked stimuli. P300 is related to attention and working memory. Its amplitude is often related to the amount of attention required by a task, while its latency is related to the time required for stimulus categorization and discrimination (McCarthy and Donchin, 1981). Various studies have investigated ERPs and found altered control of thought processes and emotional processing in individuals with mild TBI and PTSD (Lew et al., 2005; Solbakk et al., 2005). P300 responses were found to be significantly delayed in latency and lower in amplitude in response to angry faces (Lew et al., 2005), suggesting difficulty in recognizing facial affect. Another study showed similar results in response to affective pictures and suggested reduced attentional resources and dysregulation of top-down processing (Lew et al., 2005; Solbakk et al., 2005). Reduced amplitude of P300 (around 40 percent of symptomatic athletes) and increased P300 latencies have also been observed in athletes with a history of concussion (Gaetz and Weinberg, 2000; Lavoie et al., 2004). P300 amplitudes correlate better with the severity of postconcussive symptoms relative to such factors as number of concussions, time since last concussion, severity of injury, or loss of consciousness (Dupuis et al., 2000; Gosselin et al., 2006).

Magnetoencephalography (MEG) records magnetic fields produced by electrical cortical activity and has better temporal resolution than EEG. MEG shows potential for the diagnosis of mild TBI and has revealed abnormal activity in the frontal, parietal, and temporal regions in patients with blast-related mild TBI (Mu et al., 2017). In a recent study, MEG demonstrated sensitivity in detection of changes in individuals with sub-acute/chronic mild TBI (identifying abnormal brain activity in 87 percent of mild TBI patients in delta wave [1–4 Hz]) (Huang et al., 2012). In general, however, MEG has been collected only in small cohorts, is very expensive to acquire, is not transportable, is available in only a few centers in the world, requires specialized expertise for analysis, and is sensitive to cortical but not subcortical changes.

When using electrophysiology as a diagnostic method for individuals with possible exposure to mild TBI, one should keep in mind the impact of common technical difficulties, such as electrical artifacts, electrode placement, skull defects, medication effects, and patient alertness, on interpreting data. For this reason, it may be more appropriate to use approaches such as qEEG and ERPs in conjunction with other techniques, such as neuroimaging and biofluid markers.

Vision and oculomotor assessment using eye tracking devices, saccadometers, and electrooculography has also been used to assess mild TBI and concussion (Cochrane et al., 2019; Ettenhofer et al., 2018, 2020; Hunfalvay et al. 2019; Kelly et al., 2019; Mani et al., 2018; Sussman et al., 2016). This method correlates with concussion symptoms in children and adults and has promising utility as a rapid, objective, and noninvasive aid for diagnosis. Several oculomotor measures, including metrics of fixation, smooth pursuit, saccades (Brooks et al., 2019), and convergence (Santo et al., 2020), have been investigated for use as potential biomarkers of altered brain function after TBI. One study demonstrated that oculomotor assessment may be an indicator of decreased integrity of frontal white matter tracts and of altered attention and working memory functioning (Maruta et al., 2010). Moreover, researchers have developed mobile eye tracking devices, which could benefit future clinical research by capturing eye movements remotely. However, firm consensus is as yet lacking regarding which visuomotor metric is most sensitive to TBI-related change.

Although currently limited, recent data suggest that TMS has prognostic value in detecting neurophysiological changes postconcussion (Major et al., 2015). At 1 to 5 years postconcussion, no differences were observed in the amplitude of motor-evoked potentials (MEP), but an increased motor threshold (i.e., the lowest stimulus intensity to produce a detectable MEP) was found compared with noninjured controls (De Beaumont et al., 2007; Tallus et al., 2012). Another study found a lengthened duration of the cortical silent period (cSP) (i.e., interruption of voluntary muscle contraction after TMS of the contralateral motor cortex) in patients with concussion versus controls (De Beaumont et al., 2007, 2009; Tremblay et al., 2011). Despite finding no intracortical facilitation differences among single-concussion, multiple-concussions, and control groups, studies have found that patients with concussion have longer intracortical inhibition compared with controls (De Beaumont et al., 2009; Tremblay et al., 2011). Two studies found similar long-term neurophysiological changes (more than 5 years postconcussion), such as a lengthened cSP of shorter duration and a longer intracortical inhibition in retired athletes compared with controls (De Beaumont et al., 2009; Pearce et al., 2014). Therefore, long-term changes in intracortical inhibition, as well as increased stimulation threshold and slowed neurological conduction time, may be useful indicators when considering prognosis for mild TBI. Nevertheless, additional studies are needed to confirm the value of TMS as a prognostic tool.

USE OF BIOMARKERS FOR IMPROVED MONITORING AFTER TBI

An additional use of biomarkers is to monitor the changes to a person's condition as it evolves over time. Biomarkers can also be used to monitor and assess treatment effectiveness by narrowly determining target engagement or broadly tracking progressive atrophy and neurodegeneration, reflecting brain cell injury or death. Biomarkers reflecting functional compromise and reversible injury would be powerful tools for monitoring patient status and injury severity in the acute and sub-acute periods, especially after mild TBI, when objective indicators of injury are lacking (e.g., absence of focal lesions); however, this is presently an underdeveloped area of research. Use of biomarker trajectories for monitoring is important for clinical assessment of a patient's status, as well as for readouts of possible toxicity or side effects of an intervention in clinical TBI trials. The concept is to use biomarker profiles to monitor patient status or specific pathophysiological processes. Profiling biomarkers can also be used as predictive or pharmacodynamic indicators of specific progressive TBI mechanisms that are a target of a treatment (e.g., a measure of attenuated inflammation, reduced fiber tract atrophy or neuronal plasticity). Like diagnostic and prognostic biomarkers, monitoring biomarkers can be developed as trajectories of a single biomarker or of a panel of a variety of biomarker types (e.g., imaging, biofluid, physiologic). It is critical to determine biomarker profiles and half-lives in circulation in order to best use temporal profiles to assess severity and status of injury in a TBI patient.

Neuroimaging Biomarkers for Monitoring TBI

TBI can inflict acute irreversible brain damage in the form of neuronal and glial cell death, traumatic axonal injury, and vascular injury. TBI also results in neurological deficits due to metabolic depression, edema, excitotoxicity, and ionic dysregulation (Bergsneider et al., 2001; MacFarlane and Glenn, 2015; Vespa et al., 2005). These pathophysiological injury types occur secondary to the primary traumatic insult and likely compromise function of the neurovascular unit (NVU), which integrates the relationships among capillaries, neuronal networks, and glia (Bartnik-Olson et al., 2014). Knowledge of inflammation, metabolism, and functional homeostasis can provide assessment tools targeting neurological deficits rooted in NVU compromise. Imaging modalities such as MRI, CT, PET, SPECT, and transcranial Doppler (TCD) can show alterations in blood flow or hyperemia (Fatima et al., 2019; Van Horn et al., 2017) and may help identify perilesional or pericontusional "at-risk" tissues. MRI can be used as a tool for identifying regions of the brain that have incurred injury; however, it requires standardization and calibration of instruments to monitor brain health over time, normalization across scanners and recording vocabulary, and deep machine learning algorithms to associate imaging features and clinical phenotypes.

Contrast-enhanced neuroimaging administered in TBI patients may help identify BBB disruption and associated vasogenic edema. Alternatively, diffusion-sensitive techniques, such as diffusion-weighted imaging with calculation of apparent diffusion coefficient maps, may identify restricted diffusion, identifying areas of cytotoxic edema and active necrosis. In the setting of contusion or in brain regions where blood flow is compromised, tissue around the central area of injury may be at risk of deteriorating over time; accordingly, it is called perifocal, pericontusional, or perilesional tissue with blood flow and energy metabolite changes (Vespa et al., 2007; Wu et al., 2013). Metabolic depression not only is present after severe TBI, but it also is a major endophenotype of mild TBI and concussion (Giza et al., 2017). The concept of metabolic vulnerability is broadly accepted as an important mechanism of TBI progression and is a contributor to exacerbated symptoms after repeated mild TBI (Greco et al., 2019). In a small cohort of football players with concussion, arterial spin labeling monitored decreased cerebral blood flow that recovered over various time periods associated with perseverance of psychological symptoms (Meier et al., 2015). Microdialysate measures document low oxygen extraction fraction, decreased oxygen/glucose ratio, and increased lactate/pyruvate ratio (Vespa et al., 2005). Scientists have recently adapted pH-weighted molecular MRI from prior use in brain tumor characterization to monitor metabolic vulnerability due to these secondary injury processes (Ellingson et al., 2019). Chemical exchange saturation transfer imaging monitors cerebral acidosis secondary to TBI and has shown promising correlations with Extended Glasgow Outcome Scale outcomes at 6 months postinjury. This pioneering work is hopeful as it bridges acute pathophysiology of at-risk tissue with accepted outcome measures in the field and provides images of abnormal brain physiology as a consequence of TBI.

Perilesional tissue is a prime target for TBI therapies as it is potentially salvageable; thus, imaging and metabolism-related biomarkers may be very useful as near-term predictive and pharmacodynamic biomarkers. Versions of nuclear spin magnetic resonance spectroscopy (H^1, P^{31}, C^{13}-MRS) are promising imaging modalities for tracking the energy state of the injured brain and metabolic recovery after concussion using such metabolites as N-acetyl aspartate and other compounds (Harris et al., 2015; Stovell et al., 2017; Vagnozzi et al., 2010); however, additional clinical validation and confirmation of selectivity are needed. Metabolic profiling is able to monitor impaired bioenergetic state after mild TBI using gas chromatography mass spectrometry (Wolahan et al., 2015; Yi et al., 2016). Yet, such metabolomic screens need to rigorously assess brain specificity for compounds to be developed into clinically useful monitoring tools. Protein biomarkers of metabolic compromise can be selected more easily for enriched treatment.

Astroglial metabolic biomarkers are prime candidates for tissue compromise, as astrocytes have key functions in the NVU. By wrapping around blood vessels, astrocytes are positioned for direct trauma release of biomarkers into circulation, and astrocyte injury is a known driver of metabolic crisis (Halford et al., 2017). For instance, the brain-specific isoform of the glycolytic enzyme aldolase, ALDOC, is rapidly released from membrane-wounded astrocytes in a human stretch-injury model, as well as in mouse, swine, and rat neurotrauma models in pericontused regions (Halford et al., 2017). Proteomic studies in these trauma models document that release of metabolic enzymes associate with cell wounding early postinjury and are a dominant protein class in CSF proteomes of patients with TBI (Halford et al., 2017; Levine et al., 2016). Profiling metabolic biomarkers could help in assessing the effectiveness of therapies aimed at boosting energy levels in vulnerable brain areas after TBI and are among the most promising approaches currently investigated for clinical translation (Talley Watts et al., 2013).

Neurophysiological Biomarkers to Monitor TBI

Clinicians usually use EEG in the acute stage to monitor seizures in TBI patients but have also used this tool to detect changes in mild TBI over time (months to years) (Nuwer et al., 2005). Claassen and colleagues (2016) found that monitoring of brain activity using EEG can provide insight into the status of minimally conscious patients with TBI. This study showed that EEG measures of behavioral states provide distinctive signatures that complement behavioral assessments of patients with hemorrhage shortly after TBI. More research is needed to link these measures to patient outcomes.

Biofluid Markers to Monitor TBI

To employ biofluid markers successfully as TBI monitoring tools, it will be critical to gain more comprehensive insight on their trajectory, including release; presence in CSF; and, for noninvasive tracking, their appearance in blood, degradation, and clearance after injury. The temporal profiles of GFAP, UCH-L1, and S100B have been partially described, yet correlations with underlying pathophysiological processes leading to their temporal profiles are still largely elusive (Ercole et al., 2016; Papa et al., 2019; Thelin et al., 2017). A recent pilot study showed that percent change in serum UCH-L1 and S100B improved discrimination between athletes with and without concussion, versus analysis of these markers' serum levels at any separate time points (Meier et al., 2017). Monitoring of percent change, accomplished by comparing individuals' change to preinjury or preseason levels, reduces noise from large interindividual heterogeneity. Yet most emergency care providers do not know individual baseline biomarker levels of patients with mild TBI, and most rely on generalized reference values. In this case, carefully monitoring repeated measurements can provide a patient's rate of change, allowing for individualized profiling during acute care.

Measuring S100B levels in serum (and more recently in saliva) has been shown to be a useful marker in assessing brain tissue after TBI (Asken et al., 2018a). This biomarker is already assisting clinicians and researchers, primarily in Europe (Calcagnile et al., 2012). However, its lack of specificity due to its presence following orthopedic trauma outside the brain has limited its use in polytrauma (Papa et al., 2014); thus, this biomarker has not been widely used in North America. However, clinicians have successfully implemented S100B monitoring to evaluate the need for head CT in patients with mild TBI and to detect secondary injury progression (Thelin et al., 2017). Persistently elevated total tau levels in preliminary studies of athletes were associated with persistent postconcussive symptoms compared with athletes with normal or only mildly elevated plasma tau measures whose symptoms resolved and who returned to full competition (Gill et al., 2017). Thus, tau may be a potential biomarker for monitoring recovery in athletes with TBI and could be used as a guide to determine when it is safe to return to play. Despite limited knowledge of biomarker kinetics, these are promising findings that provide approaches for the use of biomarkers to diagnose and monitor the progression of TBI sequelae, personalize individual patient care, and help predict outcomes.

REFERENCES

Anderson, T. N., J. Hwang, M. Munar, L. Papa, H. E. Hinson, A. Vaughan, and S. E. Rowell. 2020. Blood-based biomarkers for prediction of intracranial hemorrhage and outcome in patients with moderate or severe traumatic brain injury. *Journal of Trauma and Acute Care Surgery* 89(1):80-86.

Asken, B. M., R. Bauer, S. DeKosky, A. Svingos, G. Hromas, J. Boone, D. DuBose, R. Hayes, and J. Clugston. 2018a. Concussion BASICS III: Serum biomarker changes following sport-related concussion. *Neurology* 91(23):e2133-e2143.

Asken, B. M., S. T. DeKosky, J. R. Clugston, M. S. Jaffee, and R. M. Bauer. 2018b. Diffusion tensor imaging (DTI) findings in adult civilian, military, and sport-related mild traumatic brain injury (mTBI): A systematic critical review. *Brain Imaging and Behavior* 12(2):585-612.

Ayubcha, C., M. E. Revheim, A. Newberg, M. Moghbel, C. Rojulpote, T. J. Werner, and A. Alavi. 2021. A critical review of radiotracers in the positron emission tomography imaging of traumatic brain injury: FDG, tau, and amyloid imaging in mild traumatic brain injury and chronic traumatic encephalopathy. *European Journal of Nuclear Medicine and Molecular Imaging* 48(2):623-641.

Bartnik-Olson, B. L., B. Holshouser, H. Wang, M. Grube, K. Tong, V. Wong, and S. H. Ashwal. 2014. Impaired neurovascular unit function contributes to persistent symptoms after concussion: A pilot study. *Journal of Neurotrauma* 31(17):1497-1506.

Bazarian, J. J., P. Biberthaler, R. D. Welch, L. M. Lewis, P. Barzo, V. Bogner-Flatz, P. G. Brolinson, A. Büki, J. Y. Chen, R. H. Christenson, D. Hack, J. S. Huff, S. Johar, J. D. Jordan, B. A. Leidel, T. Lindner, E. Ludington, D. O. Okonkwo, J. Ornato, W. F. Peacock, K. Schmidt, J. A. Tyndall, A. Vossough, and A. S. Jagoda. 2018. Serum GFAP and UCH-L1 for prediction of absence of intracranial injuries on head CT (ALERT-TBI): A multicentre observational study. *Lancet Neurology* 17(9):782-789.

Bergsneider, M., D. Hovda, D. McArthurs, M. Etchepare, S. Huang, N. Sehati, P. Satz, M. Phelps, and D. Becker. 2001. Metabolic recovery following human traumatic brain injury based on FDG-PET: time course and relationship to neurological disability. *Journal of Head Trauma Rehabilitation* 16(2):135-148.

Blennow, K., D. L. Brody, P. M. Kochanek, H. Levin, A. McKee, G. M. Ribbers, K. Yaffe, and H. Zetterberg. 2016. Traumatic brain injuries. *Nature Reviews: Disease Primers* 2:16084.

Brooks, J. S., W. Smith, B. Webb, M. Heath, and J. Dickey. 2019. Development and validation of a high-speed video system for measuring saccadic eye movement. *Behavior Research Methods* 51(5):2302-2309.

Calcagnile, O., L. Undén, and J. Undén. 2012. Clinical validation of S100B use in management of mild head injury. *BMC Emergency Medicine* 12:13.

Chen, Y., J. Li, B. Ma, N. Li, S. Wang, Z. Sun, C. Xue, Q. Han, J. Wei, and R. C. Zhao. 2020. MSC-derived exosomes promote recovery from traumatic brain injury via microglia/macrophages in rat. *Aging* 12(18):18274-18296.

Churchill, N. W., M. G. Hutchison, S. J. Graham, and T. A. Schweizer. 2019. Evaluating cerebrovascular reactivity during the early symptomatic phase of sport concussion. *Journal of Neurotrauma* 36(10):1518-1525.

Churchill, N. W., M. G. Hutchison, S. J. Graham, and T. A. Schweizer. 2020. Cerebrovascular reactivity after sport concussion: From acute injury to 1 year after medical clearance. *Frontiers in Neurology* 11:558.

Claassen, J., A. Velazquez, E. Meyers, J. Witsch, M. Falo, S. Park, S. Agarwal, J. M. Schmidt, N. Schiff, J. Sitt, L. Naccache, E. Connolly, and H. P. Frey. 2016. Bedside quantitative electroencephalography improves assessment of consciousness in comatose subarachnoid hemorrhage patients. *Annals of Neurology* 80(4):541-553.

Cochrane, G. D., J. Christy, A. Almutairi, C. Busettini, M. Swanson, and K. Weise. 2019. Visuo-oculomotor function and reaction times in athletes with and without concussion. *Optometry and Vision Science* 96(4):256-265.

Coyle, H. L., J. Ponsford, and K. Hoy. 2018. Understanding individual variability in symptoms and recovery following mTBI: A role for TMS-EEG? *Neuroscience & Biobehavioral Reviews* 92:140-149.

Currie, S., N. Saleem, J. A. Straiton, J. Macmullen-Price, D. J. Warren, and I. J. Craven. 2016. Imaging assessment of traumatic brain injury. *Postgraduate Medical Journal* 92(1083):41-50.

Czeiter, E., K. Amrein, B. Y. Gravesteijn, F. Lecky, D. K. Menon, S. Mondello, V. Newcombe, S. Richter, E. W. Steyerberg, T. V. Vyvere, J. Verheyden, H. Xu, Z. Yang, A. Maas, K. Wang, A. Büki, and CENTER-TBI Participants and Investigators. 2020. Blood biomarkers on admission in acute traumatic brain injury: Relations to severity, CT findings and care path in the CENTER-TBI study. *EBioMedicine* 56:102785.

De Beaumont, L., M. Lassonde, S. Leclerc, and H. Théoret. 2007. Long-term and cumulative effects of sports concussion on motor cortex inhibition. *Neurosurgery* 61(2):329-336; discussion 336-337.

De Beaumont, L., H. Théoret, D. Mongeon, J. Messier, S. Leclerc, S. Tremblay, D. Ellemberg, and M. Lassonde. 2009. Brain function decline in healthy retired athletes who sustained their last sports concussion in early adulthood. *Brain* 132(Pt 3):695-708.

Dupuis, F., K. M. Johnston, M. Lavoie, F. Lepore, and M. Lassonde. 2000. Concussions in athletes produce brain dysfunction as revealed by event-related potentials. *NeuroReport* 11(18):4087-4092.

Ellingson, B. M., J. Yao, C. Raymond, A. Chakhoyan, K. Khatibi, N. Salamon, J. P. Villablanca, I. Wanner, C. R. Real, A. Laiwalla, D. L. McArthur, M. M. Monti, D. A. Hovda, and P. M. Vespa. 2019. pH-weighted molecular MRI in human traumatic brain injury (TBI) using amine proton chemical exchange saturation transfer echoplanar imaging (CEST EPI). *NeuroImage: Clinical* 22:101736.

Ellis, M. J., L. N. Ryner, O. Sobczyk, J. Fierstra, D. J. Mikulis, J. A. Fisher, J. Duffin, and W. A. Mutch. 2016. Neuroimaging assessment of cerebrovascular reactivity in concussion: Current concepts, methodological considerations, and review of the literature. *Frontiers in Neurology* 7:61.

Ercole, A., E. P. Thelin, A. Holst, B. M. Bellander, and D. W. Nelson. 2016. Kinetic modelling of serum S100b after traumatic brain injury. *BMC Neurology* 16:93.

Ettenhofer, M. L., J. N. Hershaw, J. R. Engle, and L. D. Hungerford. 2018. Saccadic impairment in chronic traumatic brain injury: Examining the influence of cognitive load and injury severity. *Brain Injury* 32(13-14):1740-1748.

Ettenhofer, M. L., S. I. Gimbel, and E. Cordero. 2020. Clinical validation of an optimized multimodal neurocognitive assessment of chronic mild TBI. *Annals of Clinical and Translational Neurology* 7(4):507-516.

Fatima, N., A. Shuaib, T. S. Chughtai, A. Ayyad, and M. Saqqur. 2019. The role of transcranial doppler in traumatic brain injury: A systemic review and meta-analysis. *Asian Journal of Neurosurgery* 14(3):626-633.

Freire-Aragón, M. D., A. Rodríguez-Rodríguez, and J. J. Egea-Guerrero. 2017. Update in mild traumatic brain injury. Actualización en el traumatismo craneoencefálico leve. *Medicina Clínica* 149(3):122-127.

Gaetani, L., K. Blennow, P. Calabresi, M. Di Filippo, L. Parnetti, and H. Zetterberg. 2019. Neurofilament light chain as a biomarker in neurological disorders. *Journal of Neurology, Neurosurgery, and Psychiatry* 90(8):870-881.

Gaetz, M., and D. Bernstein. 2001. The current status of electrophysiologic procedures for the assessment of mild traumatic brain injury. *Journal of Head Trauma Rehabilitation* 16(4):386-405.

Gaetz, M., and H. Weinberg. 2000. Electrophysiological indices of persistent post-concussion symptoms. *Brain Injury* 14(9):815-832.

Gill, J., K. Merchant-Borna, A. Jeromin, W. Livingston, and J. Bazarian. 2017. Acute plasma tau relates to prolonged return to play after concussion. *Neurology* 88(6):595-602.

Gill, J., L. Latour, R. Diaz-Arrastia, V. Motamedi, C. Turtzo, P. Shahim, S. Mondello, C. DeVoto, E. Veras, D. Hanlon, L. Song, and A. Jeromin. 2018. Glial fibrillary acidic protein elevations relate to neuroimaging abnormalities after mild TBI. *Neurology* 91(15):e1385-e1389.

Giza, C. C., M. L. Prins, and D. A. Hovda. 2017. It's not all fun and games: Sports, concussions, and neuroscience. *Neuron* 94(6):1051-1055.

Goetzl, E. J., C. B. Peltz, M. Mustapic, D. Kapogiannis, and K. Yaffe. 2020. Neuron-derived plasma exosome proteins after remote traumatic brain injury. *Journal of Neurotrauma* 37(2):382-388.

Gorgoraptis, N., L. M. Li, A. Whittington, K. A. Zimmerman, L. M. Maclean, C. McLeod, E. Ross, A. Heslegrave, H. Zetterberg, J. Passchier, P. M. Matthews, R. N. Gunn, T. M. McMillan, and D. J. Sharp. 2019. In vivo detection of cerebral tau pathology in long-term survivors of traumatic brain injury. *Science Translational Medicine* 11(508):eaaw1993.

Gosselin, N., M. Thériault, S. Leclerc, J. Montplaisir, and M. Lassonde. 2006. Neurophysiological anomalies in symptomatic and asymptomatic concussed athletes. *Neurosurgery* 58(6):1151-1161.

Greco, T., L. Ferguson, C. Giza, and M. L. Prins. 2019. Mechanisms underlying vulnerabilities after repeat mild traumatic brain injuries. *Experimental Neurology* 317:206-213.

Guedes, V. A., C. Devoto, J. Leete, D. Sass, J. D. Acott, S. Mithani, and J. M. Gill. 2020a. Extracellular vesicle proteins and microRNAs as biomarkers for traumatic brain injury. *Frontiers in Neurology* 11:663.

Guedes, V. A., K. Kenney, P. Shahim, B. X. Qu, C. Lai, C. Devoto, W. C. Walker, T. Nolen, R. Diaz-Arrastia, J. M. Gill, and CENC Multisite Observational Study Investigators. 2020b. Exosomal neurofilament light: A prognostic biomarker for remote symptoms after mild traumatic brain injury? *Neurology* 94(23):e2412-e2423.

Halford, J., S. Shen, K. Itamura, J. Levine, A. C. Chong, G. Czerwieniec, T. C. Glenn, D. A. Hovda, P. Vespa, R. Bullock, W. D. Dietrich, S. Mondello, J. A. Loo, and I. B. Wanner. New astroglial injury-defined biomarkers for neurotrauma assessment. *Journal of Cerebral Blood Flow and Metabolism* 37(10):3278-3299.

Harris, J. L., I. Y. Choi, and W. M. Brooks. 2015. Probing astrocyte metabolism in vivo: Proton magnetic resonance spectroscopy in the injured and aging brain. *Frontiers in Aging Neuroscience* 7:202.

Hong, Y. T., T. Veenith, D. Dewar, J. G. Outtrim, V. Mani, C. Williams, S. Pimlott, P. J. Hutchinson, A. Tavares, R. Canales, C. A. Mathis, W. E. Klunk, F. I. Aigbirhio, J. P. Coles, J. C. Baron, J. D. Pickard, T. D. Fryer, W. Stewart, and D. K. Menon. 2014. Amyloid imaging with carbon 11-labeled Pittsburgh compound B for traumatic brain injury. *JAMA Neurology* 71(1):23-31.

Huang, M. X., S. Nichols, A. Robb, A. Angeles, A. Drake, M. Holland, S. Asmussen, J. D'Andrea, W. Chun, M. Levy, L. Cui, T. Song, D. G. Baker, P. Hammer, R. McLay, R. J. Theilmann, R. Coimbra, M. Diwakar, C. Boyd, J. Neff, T. T. Liu, J. Webb-Murphy, R. Farinpour, C. Cheung, D. L. Harrington, D. Heister, and R. R. Lee. 2012. An automatic MEG low-frequency source imaging approach for detecting injuries in mild and moderate TBI patients with blast and non-blast causes. *Neuroimage* 61(4):1067-1082.

Hunfalvay, M., C. M. Roberts, N. Murray, A. Tyagi, H. Kelly, and T. Bolte. 2019. Horizontal and vertical self-paced saccades as a diagnostic marker of traumatic brain injury. *Concussion* 4(1):CNC60.

Irimia, A., B. Wang, S. R. Aylward, M. W. Prastawa, D. F. Pace, G. Gerig, D. A. Hovda, R. Kikinis, P. M. Vespa, and J. D. Van Horn. 2012. Neuroimaging of structural pathology and connectomics in traumatic brain injury: Toward personalized outcome prediction. *NeuroImage: Clinical* 1(1):1-17.

Jones, C., C. Harmon, M. McCann, H. Gunyan, and J. J. Bazarian. 2020. S100B outperforms clinical decision rules for the identification of intracranial injury on head CT scan after mild traumatic brain injury. *Brain Injury* 34(3):407-414.

Kawai, N., M. Kawanishi, N. Kudomi, Y. Maeda, Y. Yamamoto, Y. Nishiyama, and T. Tamiya. 2013. Detection of brain amyloid ß deposition in patients with neuropsychological impairment after traumatic brain injury: PET evaluation using Pittsburgh Compound-B. *Brain Injury* 27(9):1026-1031.

Kelly, K. M., A. Kiderman, S. Akhavan, M. Quigley, E. Snell, E. Happy, A. Synowiec, E. Miller, M. Bauer, L. Oakes, Y. Eydelman, C. Gallagher, T. Dinehart, J. Schroeder, and R. Ashmore. 2019. Oculomotor, vestibular, and reaction time effects of sports-related concussion: video-oculography in assessing sports-related concussion. *Journal of Head Trauma Rehabilitation* 34(3):176-188.

Kenney, K., J. K. Werner, and J. M. Gill. 2021. 7-Proteomic, genetic, and epigenetic biomarkers in traumatic brain injury. In *Brain Injury Medicine: Board Review, First Edition* (pp. 66-70). Editors: B. C. Eapen and D. X. Cifu. Philadelphia, PA: Elsevier.

Kondziella, D., P. M. Fisher, V. A. Larsen, J. Hauerberg, M. Fabricius, K. Møller, and G. M. Knudsen. 2017. Functional MRI for Assessment of the Default Mode Network in Acute Brain Injury. *Neurocritical Care* 27(3):401-406.

Korn, A., H. Golan, I. Melamed, R. Pascual-Marqui, and A. Friedman. 2005. Focal cortical dysfunction and blood-brain barrier disruption in patients with postconcussion syndrome. *Journal of Clinical Neurophysiology* 22(1):1-9.

Laatsch, L., and C. Krisky. 2006. Changes in fMRI activation following rehabilitation of reading and visual processing deficits in subjects with traumatic brain injury. *Brain Injury* 20(13-14):1367-1375.

Lavoie, M. E., F. Dupuis, K. M. Johnston, S. Leclerc, and M. Lassonde. 2004. Visual p300 effects beyond symptoms in concussed college athletes. *Journal of Clinical and Experimental Neuropsychology* 26(1):55-73.

Lehto, L. J., A. Sierra, and O. Gröhn. 2017. Magnetization transfer SWIFT MRI consistently detects histologically verified myelin loss in the thalamocortical pathway after a traumatic brain injury in rat. *NMR in Biomedicine* 30(2):10.1002/nbm.3678.

Levine, J., E. Kwon, P. Paez, W. Yan, G. Czerwieniec, J. A. Loo, M. V. Sofroniew, and I. B. Wanner. 2016. Traumatically injured astrocytes release a proteomic signature modulated by STAT3-dependent cell survival. *Glia* 64(5):668-694.

Lew, H. L., J. H. Poole, J. Y. Chiang, E. H. Lee, E. S. Date, and D. Warden. 2005. Event-related potential in facial affect recognition: potential clinical utility in patients with traumatic brain injury. *Journal of Rehabilitation Research and Development* 42(1):29-34.

Lindsey, H. M., C. B. Hodges, K. M. Greer, E. A. Wilde, and T. L. Merkley. 2021. Diffusion-weighted imaging in mild traumatic brain injury: A systematic review of the literature. *Neuropsychology Review.* https://doi.org/10.1007/s11065-021-09485-5.

MacFarlane, M. P., and L. Glenn. 2015. Neurochemical cascade of concussion. *Brain Injury* 29(2):139-153.

Major, B. P., M. A. Rogers, and A. J. Pearce. 2015. Using transcranial magnetic stimulation to quantify electrophysiological changes following concussive brain injury: a systematic review. *Clinical and Experimental Pharmacology & Physiology* 42(4):394-405.

Manek, R., A. Moghieb, Z. Yang, D. Kumar, F. Kobessiy, G. A. Sarkis, V. Raghavan, and K. Wang. 2018. Protein biomarkers and neuroproteomics characterization of microvesicles/exosomes from human cerebrospinal fluid following traumatic brain injury. *Molecular Neurobiology* 55(7):6112-6128.

Mani, R., L. Asper, and S. K. Khuu. 2018. Deficits in saccades and smooth-pursuit eye movements in adults with traumatic brain injury: a systematic review and meta-analysis. *Brain Injury* 32(11):1315-1336.

Maruta, J., M. Suh, S. N. Niogi, P. Mukherjee, and J. Ghajar. 2010. Visual tracking synchronization as a metric for concussion screening. *Journal of Head Trauma Rehabilitation* 25(4):293-305.

McCarthy, G. and E. Donchin. 1981. A metric for thought: a comparison of P300 latency and reaction time. *Science* 211(4477):77-80.

McCrea, M., S. P. Broglio, T. W. McAllister, J. Gill, C. C. Giza, D. L. Huber, J. Harezlak, K. L. Cameron, M. N. Houston, G. McGinty, J. C. Jackson, K. Guskiewicz, J. Mihalik, M. A. Brooks, S. Duma, S. Rowson, L. D. Nelson, P. Pasquina, T. B. Meier, CARE Consortium Investigators, T. Foroud, B. P. Katz, A. J. Saykin, D. E. Campbell, S. J. Svoboda, J. Goldman, and J. DiFiori. 2020. Association of blood biomarkers with acute sport-related concussion in collegiate athletes: Findings from the NCAA and Department of Defense CARE Consortium. *JAMA Network Open* 3(1):e1919771.

Mckee, A. C., and D. H. Daneshvar. 2015. The neuropathology of traumatic brain injury. *Handbook of Clinical Neurology* 127:45-66.

Meier, T. B., P. S. Bellgowan, R. Singh, R. Kuplicki, D. W. Polanski, and A. R. Mayer. 2015. Recovery of cerebral blood flow following sports-related concussion. *JAMA Neurology* 72(5):530-538.

Meier, T. B., L. D. Nelson, D. L. Huber, J. J. Bazarian, R. L. Hayes, and M. A. McCrea. 2017. Prospective assessment of acute blood markers of brain injury in sport-related concussion. *Journal of Neurotrauma* 34(22):3134-3142.

Mez, J., D. H. Daneshvar, P. T. Kiernan, B. Abdolmohammadi, V. E. Alvarez, B. R. Huber, M. L. Alosco, T. M. Solomon, C. J. Nowinski, L. McHale, K. A. Cormier, C. A. Kubilus, B. M. Martin, L. Murphy, C. M. Baugh, P. H. Montenigro, C. E. Chaisson, Y. Tripodis, N. W. Kowall, J. Weuve, M. D. McClean, R. C. Cantu, L. E. Goldstein, D. I. Katz, R. A Stern, T. D. Stein, and A. C. McKee. 2017. Clinicopathological evaluation of chronic traumatic encephalopathy in players of American football. *Journal of the American Medical Association* 318(4):360-370.

Mu, W., E. Catenaccio, and M. L. Lipton. 2017. Neuroimaging in blast-related mild traumatic brain injury. *Journal of Head Trauma Rehabilitation* 32(1):55-69.

Nuwer, M. R., D. A. Hovda, L. M. Schrader, and P. M. Vespa. 2005. Routine and quantitative EEG in mild traumatic brain injury. *Clinical Neurophysiology* 116(9):2001-2025.

Okonkwo, D. O.,R. C. Puffer, A. M. Puccio, E. L. Yuh, J. K. Yue, R. Diaz-Arrastia, F. K. Korley, K. Wang, X. Sun, S. R. Taylor, P. Mukherjee, A. J. Markowitz, S. Jain, G. T. Manley, and Transforming Research and Clinical Knowledge in Traumatic Brain Injury (TRACK-TBI) Investigators. 2020. Point-of-care platform blood biomarker testing of glial fibrillary acidic protein versus S100 calcium-binding protein B for prediction of traumatic brain injuries: A Transforming Research and Clinical Knowledge in Traumatic Brain Injury Study. *Journal of Neurotrauma* 37(23):2460-2467.

Palacios, E. M., SR. Sala-Llonch, C. Junque, D. Fernandez-Espejo, T. Roig, J. M. Tormos, N. Bargallo, and P. Vendrell. 2013. Long-term declarative memory deficits in diffuse TBI: Correlations with cortical thickness, white matter integrity and hippocampal volume. *Cortex* 49(3):646-657.

Papa, L., S. Silvestri, G. M. Brophy, P. Giordano, J. L. Falk, C. F. Braga, C. N. Tan, N. J. Ameli, J. A. Demery, N. K. Dixit, N. M. E. Mendes, R. L. Hayes, K. K. Wang, and C. S. Robertson. 2014. GFAP out-performs S100beta in detecting traumatic intracranial lesions on computed tomography in trauma patients with mild traumatic brain injury and those with extracranial lesions. *Journal of Neurotrauma* 31(22):1815-1822.

Papa, L., M. R. Zonfrillo, R. D. Welch, L. M. Lewis, C. F. Braga, C. N. Tan, N. J. Ameli, M. A. Lopez, C. A. Haeussler, D. Mendez Giordano, P. A. Giordano, J. Ramirez, and M. K. Mittal. 2019. Evaluating glial and neuronal blood biomarkers GFAP and UCH-L1 as gradients of brain injury in concussive, subconcussive and non-concussive trauma: a prospective cohort study. *BMJ Paediatrics Open* 3(1):e000473.

Pattinson, C. L., T. B. Meier, V. A. Guedes, C. Lai, C. Devoto, T. Haight, S. P. Broglio, T. McAllister, C. Giza, D. Huber, J. Harezlak, K. Cameron, G. McGinty, J. Jackson, K. Guskiewicz, J. Mihalik, A. Brooks, S. Duma, S. Rowson, L. D. Nelson, P. Pasquina, M. McCrea, J. M. Gill, and CARE Consortium Investigators. 2020. Plasma Biomarker concentrations associated with return to sport following sport-related concussion in collegiate athletes—A Concussion Assessment, Research, and Education (CARE) Consortium Study. *JAMA Network Open* 3(8):e2013191.

Pavlovic, D., S. Pekic, M. Stojanovic, and V. Popovic. 2019. Traumatic brain injury: Neuropathological, neurocognitive and neurobehavioral sequelae. *Pituitary* 22(3):270-282.

Pearce, A. J., K. Hoy, M. A. Rogers, D. T. Corp, J. J. Maller, H. G. Drury, and P. B. Fitzgerald. 2014. The long-term effects of sports concussion on retired Australian football players: A study using transcranial magnetic stimulation. *Journal of Neurotrauma* 31(13):1139-1145.

Rapp, P. E., D. O. Keyser, A. Albano, R. Hernandez, D. B. Gibson, R. A. Zambon, W. D. Hairston, J. D. Hughes, A. Krystal, and A. S. Nichols. 2015. Traumatic brain injury detection using electrophysiological methods. *Frontiers in Human Neuroscience* 9:11.

Santo, A. L., M. L. Race, and E. F. Teel. 2020. Near point of convergence deficits and treatment following concussion: A systematic review. *Journal of Sport Rehabilitation* 29(8):1179-1193.

Shah, S. A., R. J. Lowder, and A. Kuceyeski. 2020. Quantitative multimodal imaging in traumatic brain injuries producing impaired cognition. *Current Opinion in Neurology* 33(6):691-698.

Shahim, P., A. Politis, A. van der Merwe, B. Moore, V. Ekanayake, S. M. Lippa, Y. Y. Chou, D. L. Pham, J. A. Butman, R. Diaz-Arrastia, H. Zetterberg, K. Blennow, J. M. Gill, D. L. Brody, and L. Chan. 2020. Time course and diagnostic utility of NfL, tau, GFAP, and UCH-L1 in subacute and chronic TBI. *Neurology* 95(6):e623-e636.

Sharp, D. J., G. Scott, and R. Leech. 2014. Network dysfunction after traumatic brain injury. *Nature Reviews: Neurology* 10(3):156-166.

Solbakk, A. K., I. Reinvang, S. Svebak, C. S. Nielsen, and K. Sundet. 2005. Attention to affective pictures in closed head injury: Event-related brain potentials and cardiac responses. *Journal of Clinical and Experimental Neuropsychology* 27(2):205-223.

Stovell, M. G., J. L. Yan, A. Sleigh, M. O. Mada, T. A. Carpenter, P. Hutchinson, and K. Carpenter. 2017. Assessing metabolism and injury in acute human traumatic brain injury with magnetic resonance spectroscopy: Current and future applications. *Frontiers in Neurology* 8:426.

Sussman, E. S., A. L. Ho, A. V. Pendharkar, and J. Ghajar. 2016. Clinical evaluation of concussion: The evolving role of oculomotor assessments. *Neurosurgical Focus* 40(4):E7.

Takahata, K., Y. Kimura, N. Sahara, S. Koga, H. Shimada, M. Ichise, F. Saito, S. Moriguchi, S. Kitamura, M. Kubota, S. Umeda, F. Niwa, J. Mizushima, Y. Morimoto, M. Funayama, H. Tabuchi, K. F. Bieniek, K. Kawamura, M-R. Zhang, D. W. Dickson, M. Mimura, M. Kato, T. Suhara, and M. Higuchi. 2019. PET-detectable tau pathology correlates with long-term neuropsychiatric outcomes in patients with traumatic brain injury. *Brain* 142(10):3265-3279.

Talley Watts, L., S. Sprague, W. Zheng, R. J. Garling, D. Jimenez, M. Digicaylioglu, and J. Lechleiter. 2013. Purinergic 2Y1 receptor stimulation decreases cerebral edema and reactive gliosis in a traumatic brain injury model. *Journal of Neurotrauma* 30(1):55-66.

Tallus, J., P. Lioumis, H. Hämäläinen, S. Kähkönen, and O. Tenovuo. 2012. Long-lasting TMS motor threshold elevation in mild traumatic brain injury. *Acta Neurologica Scandinavica* 126(3):178-182.

Thatcher, R. W., D. M. North, R. T. Curtin, R. A. Walker, C. J. Biver, J. F. Gomez, and A. M. Salazar. 2001. An EEG severity index of traumatic brain injury. *Journal of Neuropsychiatry and Clinical Neurosciences* 13(1):77-87.

Thelin, E. P., D. W. Nelson, and B. M. Bellander. 2017. A review of the clinical utility of serum S100B protein levels in the assessment of traumatic brain injury. *Acta Neurochirurgica1* 59(2):209-225.

Thelin, E., F. Al Nimer, A. Frostell, H. Zetterberg, K. Blennow, H. Nyström, M. Svensson, B. M. Bellander, F. Piehl, and D. W. Nelson. 2019. A serum protein biomarker panel improves outcome prediction in human traumatic brain injury. *Journal of Neurotrauma* 36(20):2850-2862.

Thompson, J., W. Sebastianelli, and S. Slobounov. 2005. EEG and postural correlates of mild traumatic brain injury in athletes. *Neuroscience Letters* 377(3):158-163.

Thornton, K. 2003. The electrophysiological effects of a brain injury on auditory memory functioning. The qEEG correlates of impaired memory. *Archives of Clinical Neuropsychology* 18(4):363-378.

Tomkins, O., A. Feintuch, M. Benifla, A. Cohen, A. Friedman, and I. Shelef. 2011. Blood-brain barrier breakdown following traumatic brain injury: A possible role in posttraumatic epilepsy. *Cardiovascular Psychiatry and Neurology* 2011:765923. https://doi.org/10.1155/2011/765923.

Tremblay, S., L. de Beaumont, M. Lassonde, and H. Théoret. 2011. Evidence for the specificity of intracortical inhibitory dysfunction in asymptomatic concussed athletes. *Journal of Neurotrauma* 28(4):493-502.

Tu, T. W., J. D. Lescher, R. A. Williams, N. Jikaria, L. C. Turtzo, and J. A. Frank. 2017. Abnormal injury response in spontaneous mild ventriculomegaly wistar rat brains: A pathological correlation study of diffusion tensor and magnetization transfer imaging in mild traumatic brain injury. *Journal of Neurotrauma* 34(1):248-256.

Vagnozzi, R., S. Signoretti, L. Cristofori, F. Alessandrini, R. Floris, E. Isgrò, A. Ria, S. Marziali, G. Zoccatelli, B. Tavazzi, F. Del Bolgia, R. Sorge, S. P. Broglio, T. K. McIntosh, and G. Lazzarino. 2010. Assessment of metabolic brain damage and recovery following mild traumatic brain injury: A multicentre, proton magnetic resonance spectroscopic study in concussed patients. *Brain* 133(11):3232-3242.

Van Horn, J. D., A. Bhattrai, and A. Irimia. 2017. Multimodal imaging of neurometabolic pathology due to traumatic brain injury. *Trends in Neurosciences* 40(1):39-59.

Vespa, P., M. Bergsneider, N. Hattori, H. M. Wu, S. C. Huang, N. A. Martin, T. C. Glenn, D. L. McArthur, and D. A. Hovda. 2005. Metabolic crisis without brain ischemia is common after traumatic brain injury: A combined microdialysis and positron emission tomography study. *Journal of Cerebral Blood Flow and Metabolism* 25(6):763-774.

Vespa, P. M., K. O'Phelan, D. McArthur, C. Miller, M. Eliseo, D. Hirt, T. Glenn, and D. A. Hovda. 2007. Pericontusional brain tissue exhibits persistent elevation of lactate/pyruvate ratio independent of cerebral perfusion pressure. *Critical Care Medicine* 35(4):1153-1160.

Wilde, E. A., S. Bouix, D. F. Tate, A. P. Lin, M. R. Newsome, B. A. Taylor, J. R. Stone, J. Montier, S. E. Gandy, B. Biekman, M. E. Shenton, and G. York. 2015. Advanced neuroimaging applied to veterans and service personnel with traumatic brain injury: state of the art and potential benefits. *Brain Imaging and Behavior* 9(3):367-402.

Wolahan, S. M., D. Hirt, and T. C. Glenn. 2015. Translational metabolomics of head injury: Exploring dysfunctional cerebral metabolism with ex vivo NMR spectroscopy-based metabolite quantification. *Brain Neurotrauma: Molecular, Neuropsychological, and Rehabilitation Aspects*. Boca Raton, FL: F. H. Kobeissy.

Wu, H. M., S. C. Huang, P. Vespa, D. A. Hovda, and M. Bergsneider. 2013. Redefining the pericontusional penumbra following traumatic brain injury: Evidence of deteriorating metabolic derangements based on positron emission tomography. *Journal of Neurotrauma* 30(5):352-360.

Wu, S. J., L. M. Jenkins, A. C. Apple, J. Petersen, F. Xiao, L. Wang, and F. G. Yang. 2020. Longitudinal fMRI task reveals neural plasticity in default mode network with disrupted executive-default coupling and selective attention after traumatic brain injury. *Brain Imaging and Behavior* 14(5):1638-1650.

Yang, Y., Y. Ye, C. Kong, X. Su, X. Zhang, W. Bai, and X. He. 2019. MiR-124 enriched exosomes promoted the M2 polarization of microglia and enhanced hippocampus neurogenesis after traumatic brain injury by inhibiting TLR4 pathway. *Neurochemical Research* 44(4):811-828.

Yi, L., S. Shi, Y. Wang, W. Huang, Z. A. Xia, Z. Xing, W. Peng, and Z. Wang. 2016. Serum metabolic profiling reveals altered metabolic pathways in patients with post-traumatic cognitive impairments. *Scientific Reports* 6:21320.

Zeiler, F. A., M. Aries, M. Cabeleira, T. A. van Essen, N. Stocchetti, D. K. Menon, I. Timofeev, M. Czosnyka, P. Smielewski, P. Hutchinson, A. Ercole, and CENTER-TBI High Resolution ICU (HR ICU) Sub-Study Participants and Investigators. 2020a. Statistical cerebrovascular reactivity signal properties after secondary decompressive craniectomy in traumatic brain injury: A CENTER-TBI pilot analysis. *Journal of Neurotrauma* 37(11):1306-1314.

Zeiler, F. A., A. Ercole, M. Czosnyka, P. Smielewski, G. Hawryluk, P. Hutchinson, D. K. Menon, and M. Aries. 2020b. Continuous cerebrovascular reactivity monitoring in moderate/severe traumatic brain injury: A narrative review of advances in neurocritical care. *British Journal of Anaesthesia* S0007-0912(19):30966-3.

Appendix C

Information Sources and Methods

The committee was tasked with examining the landscape of traumatic brain injury (TBI) research and care, from acute care through rehabilitation and recovery. The committee was asked to produce a report identifying major barriers and knowledge gaps that are impeding progress in the field, highlighting opportunities for collaborative action that could accelerate progress in TBI research and care, and providing a roadmap for advancing research and clinical care to help guide the field over the next decade.

COMMITTEE COMPOSITION

The National Academies of Sciences, Engineering, and Medicine appointed a committee of 18 experts to carry out the statement of task for this study. The committee members brought expertise in basic, translational, and clinical research on TBI; epidemiology; neurotrauma; systems of care for TBI, from acute emergency medicine and trauma care through rehabilitation and community reintegration; neuropsychology and mental health; and health sciences and health care policy. Appendix B provides biographical information for each committee member.

MEETINGS AND INFORMATION-GATHERING ACTIVITIES

The committee deliberated from approximately December 2020 to January 2022 to conduct its assessment and prepare its final report. To address its task, the committee analyzed information obtained from a review of the available literature and other publicly available resources and undertook information-gathering activities that included inviting stakeholders to share perspectives during virtual public workshop sessions, holding webinars, and soliciting public input online.

Literature Review

Several strategies were used to identify literature relevant to the committee's charge. A search of bibliographic databases, including PubMed, Scopus, ProQuest Research Library, Medline, and LexisNexis, was conducted to obtain articles from peer-reviewed journals that addressed clinical care and research associated with TBI. Staff reviewed recent news and literature to identify articles relevant to the committee's charge and created a database of references. In addition, committee members, speakers, sponsors, and other interested parties submitted articles, reports, and statements on these topics. The committee's database included several hundred relevant articles and reports, and was updated throughout the study process.

Public Meetings and Webinars

Sessions at meetings and webinars held over the course of the study enabled the committee to obtain input from a range of stakeholders and members of the public. The committee's first meeting, held virtually in December 2020, provided an opportunity for the committee to discuss its statement of task with the sponsoring organization.

The committee held a series of virtual public workshop sessions over 4 days—March 16, March 18, March 30, and April 1, 2021. Day 1 explored patient and family experiences with TBI care and needs for improvement. Day 2 examined provider and researcher perspectives on TBI acute and post-acute care, along with research needed to address current gaps. Day 3 explored systems issues for TBI care and research, and highlighted opportunities to learn from systems of care in other diseases, such as stroke and Alzheimer's disease. Finally, Day 4 identified actions with the potential to help bring an improved vision of TBI care and research to fruition.

In May and June 2021, the committee held additional public webinars on the state of care and research in the areas of disorders of consciousness and TBI rehabilitation care and research. Speakers who provided input to the committee in its meeting and webinar sessions are listed below.

Recordings from these workshop and webinar sessions are available from the study website. Direct links are:

- Workshop March 16: https://www.nationalacademies.org/event/03-16-2021/accelerating-progress-in-traumatic-brain-injury-research-and-care-virtual-workshop-day-1
- Workshop March 18: https://www.nationalacademies.org/event/03-18-2021/accelerating-progress-in-traumatic-brain-injury-research-and-care-virtual-workshop-day-2
- Workshop March 30: https://www.nationalacademies.org/event/03-30-2021/accelerating-progress-in-traumatic-brain-injury-research-and-care-virtual-workshop-day-3
- Workshop April 1: https://www.nationalacademies.org/event/04-01-2021/accelerating-progress-in-traumatic-brain-injury-research-and-care-virtual-workshop-day-4
- Webinar on Disorders of Consciousness: https://www.nationalacademies.org/event/05-24-2021/accelerating-progress-in-traumatic-brain-injury-research-and-care-webinar-on-disorders-of-consciousness

- Webinar on Rehabilitation Care and Research: https://www.nationalacademies.org/event/06-15-2021/accelerating-progress-in-traumatic-brain-injury-research-and-care-webinar-on-rehabilitation-care-and-research

Public Comments

The committee's information-gathering sessions provided opportunities to interact with a variety of stakeholders. The virtual public workshop session on March 16 also included a public comment period, in which the committee invited input from any interested party.

The committee worked to make its activities as transparent and accessible as possible. The study website, hosted by the National Academies, was updated regularly to reflect recent and planned committee activities. Study outreach included a study-specific email address for comments and questions. A subscription to email updates was available for sharing further information and providing additional comments and input to the committee.

Live video streams with closed captioning were provided during the information-gathering sessions. Information provided to the committee from outside sources or through online comments is available by request through the National Academies' Public Access Records Office.

Consulted Experts

The following individuals were invited speakers at the committee's information-gathering sessions.

Gregory Albers
Professor, Neurology & Neurological Sciences and Director, Stanford Stroke Center
Stanford University

Jandel Allen-Davis
President and Chief Executive Officer
Craig Hospital

Rinad Beidas
Associate Professor, Psychiatry, Medical Ethics and Health Policy, and Medicine, Perelman School of Medicine, and Director, Penn Implementation Science Center
University of Pennsylvania

Patrick Bellgowan
Deputy Associate Director, National Institute of Neurological Disorders and Stroke
National Institutes of Health

Lisa Brandt
Individual Testimony

David Brody
Director of Center for Neuroscience and Regenerative Medicine
Uniformed Services University of the Health Sciences

David Cifu
Senior TBI Specialist, Veterans Health Administration, and Associate Dean of Innovation and Systems Integration and Chair, Department of Physical Medicine and Rehabilitation
Virginia Commonwealth University

Susan Connors
President and Chief Executive Officer
Brain Injury Association of America

John Corrigan
Emeritus Professor, Department of Physical Medicine and Rehabilitation, and Director, Ohio Valley Center for Brain Injury Prevention and Rehabilitation
The Ohio State University

Ramon Diaz-Arrastia
Director, Traumatic Brain Injury Clinical
Research Center, and Associate Director for
Clinical Research, Center for
Neurodegeneration and Repair
University of Pennsylvania

Alberto Esquenazi
Chief Medical Officer and Chairman,
Department of Physical Medicine and
Rehabilitation
MossRehab, Einstein Healthcare Network

Kimberly Frey
Director of Speech-Language Pathology
Craig Hospital

Kelli Williams Gary
Assistant Professor and Dissemination
Coordinator for VCU TBI Model Systems,
Department of Physical Medicine &
Rehabilitation
Virginia Commonwealth University

Joseph Giacino
Director of Rehabilitation
Neuropsychology, Department of Physical
Medicine and Rehabilitation, Spaulding
Rehabilitation Hospital
Neuropsychologist, Department of
Psychiatry, Massachusetts General Hospital

Yael Goverover
Post-Professional Program Director and
Professor of Occupational Therapy, Stein-
hardt School of Culture, Education, and
Human Development
New York University

Magali Haas
Chief Executive Officer and President
Cohen Veterans Bioscience

Scott Hamilton
Individual Testimony

Flora Hammond
Chair, Department of Physical Medicine &
Rehabilitation
Indiana University School of Medicine

Ramona Hicks
Director of Science and Technology
One Mind

Julia Iyasere
Executive Director, Dalio Center for Health
Justice
NewYork-Presbyterian Hospital

Katherine Lee
Office of the Assistant Secretary of Defense
for Health Affairs
Department of Defense

Roger Lewis
Professor and Chair, Department of
Emergency Medicine
Harbor-UCLA Medical Center

Monica Lichi
Director, Ohio Brain Injury Program, and
Director, Ohio Valley Center for Brain
Injury Prevention & Rehabilitation
The Ohio State University

Kedar Mate
President and Chief Executive Officer
Institute for Healthcare Improvement

Thomas Mayer
Medical Director
NFL Players Association

Joe McCannon
Co-Founder and Coach
Billions Institute

Karen McCulloch
Professor and Director, Neurologic Physical
Therapy Residency
University of North Carolina School of
Medicine

Karen McQuillan
Clinical Nurse Specialist
University of Maryland

Bruce Miller
Director, Memory and Aging Center, and
Co-Director, Global Brain Health Institute
University of California, San Francisco

Megan Moore
Sidney Miller Endowed Associate Professor
in Direct Practice
University of Washington

Risa Nakase-Richardson
Clinical Neuropsychologist, James A. Haley
Veterans' Hospital and Associate Professor.
Department of Medicine, Pulmonary and
Sleep Medicine Section, University of South
Florida
Department of Veterans Affairs

David Okonkwo
Professor and Director, Neurotrauma
Clinical Trials Center
University of Pittsburgh

Paul Perrin
Associate Professor and Director, Health
Psychology Doctoral Program
Virginia Commonwealth University

Terri Pogoda
Center for Healthcare Organization &
Implementation Research, VA Boston
Healthcare System and Research
Associate Professor, Boston University
School of Public Health
Department of Veterans Affairs

Travis Polk
Director, Combat Casualty Care Research
Program
Department of Defense

Dorothy R. Porcello
Supervisor, Outpatient Traumatic Brain
Injury (TBI) and Department of
Neuro Occupational Therapy
Walter Reed National Military Medical
Center

Keith Primeau
Individual Testimony

Aemon Purser
Individual Testimony

James Robinson
Senior Director of Resident Risk
Management, Safety, and Preparedness
Spectrum Retirement Communities

Elizabeth Rotenberry
Fellows Program Manager and Dole
Caregiver Fellow Alumna
Elizabeth Dole Foundation

Angelle Sander
Director, Division of Clinical
Neuropsychology and Rehabilitation
Psychology
Baylor College of Medicine

Joel Scholten
Associate Chief of Staff for Rehabilitation
Services for the Veterans Affairs Medical
Center
Veterans Health Administration

Richard Sidwell
Trauma Surgery and Surgical Critical Care
The Iowa Clinic

Deborah Stein
Professor and Chief of Surgery, Zuckerberg
San Francisco General and Vice Chair of
Trauma and Critical Care Surgery
University of California, San Francisco

Pimjai Sudsawad
Knowledge Translation Program Coordinator
National Institute on Disability,
Independent Living, and Rehabilitation
Research

Kristine Swift
Individual Testimony

Hilaire Thompson
Joanne Montgomery Endowed Professor
and Assistant Vice Provost for Academic
Personnel
University of Washington School of Nursing

Jeffrey Upperman
Professor and Chair, Department of
Pediatric Surgery
Vanderbilt University Medical Center

Mary Voegeli
Nurse Practitioner, Physical Medicine and
Rehabilitation
Medical College of Wisconsin and Froedert
Hospital

John Whyte
Former Director, Moss Rehabilitation
Research Institute and Founding Director,
TBI Rehabilitation Research Laboratory
Moss Rehabilitation Research Institute

David Wright
Professor and Chair, Department of
Emergency Medicine
Emory University

Kristine Yaffe
Professor of Psychiatry, Neurology and
Epidemiology, Roy and Marie Scola
Endowed Chair, and Vice Chair of Research
in Psychiatry
University of California, San Francisco

Appendix D

Committee Member and Staff Biographies

COMMITTEE MEMBERS

Donald Berwick, M.D., M.P.P., FRCP (London) (*Chair*), is the president emeritus and a senior fellow at the Institute for Healthcare Improvement and a former administrator of the Centers for Medicare & Medicaid Services. A pediatrician by background, Dr. Berwick has served on the faculty of the Harvard Medical School and the Harvard T.H. Chan School of Public Health, and on the staff of Boston's Children's Hospital Medical Center, Massachusetts General Hospital, and Brigham and Women's Hospital. He has also served as the vice chair of the United States Preventive Services Task Force, the first "independent member" of the American Hospital Association Board of Trustees, and the chair of the National Advisory Council of the Agency for Healthcare Research and Quality. He served two terms on the Institute of Medicine's (IOM's) Governing Council, was a member of the IOM's Global Health Board, and served on President Clinton's Advisory Commission on Consumer Protection and Quality in the Healthcare Industry. Recognized as a leading authority on health care quality and improvement, Dr. Berwick has received numerous awards for his contributions. In 2005, he was appointed Honorary Knight Commander of the British Empire by Her Majesty Queen Elizabeth II in recognition of his work with the British National Health Service. Dr. Berwick is the author or co-author of more than 200 scientific articles and 6 books.

Jennifer Bogner, Ph.D., ABPP-Rp, FACRM, is a professor and the Bert C. Wiley, MD Endowed Chair in Physical Medicine and Rehabilitation at The Ohio State University. Dr. Bogner is the project director for the Ohio Regional Traumatic Brain Injury (TBI) Model Systems, 1 site of 16 distributed nationally and funded by the National Institute on Disability, Independent Living, and Rehabilitation Research. The TBI Model Systems have been conducting national longitudinal and interventional studies on TBI for the past 35 years, and the Ohio Regional TBI Model System has been a site since 1997. The overarching goal of Dr. Bogner's research has been to improve long-term outcomes after TBI. Specific areas of research include using causal inference methods to evaluate the comparative effectiveness of rehabilitation interventions; prevention and treatment of substance misuse following TBI; evaluating the impact of lifetime exposure to TBI on quality of life; and the development and validation of measurement tools to support rehabilitation research and clinical practice. Dr. Bogner previously chaired the Brain Injury Interdisciplinary Special Interest Group of the American Congress of Rehabilitation Medicine. She received the Roger G. Barker Distinguished Research Contribution Award from the American Psychological Association Division of Rehabilitation Psychology and the William Fields Caveness Award from the Brain Injury Association of America.

Matthew E. Fink, M.D., is the Louis and Gertrude Feil Professor and the chair of the Department of Neurology at Weill Cornell Medical College and the neurologist-in-chief, the chief of the Division of Stroke and Critical Care Neurology, and the vice chair of the Medical Board at NewYork-Presbyterian Hospital/Weill Cornell Medical Center. Dr. Fink was a founding member and the chair of the Critical Care Section of the American Academy of Neurology and the Research Section for Neurocritical Care of the World Federation of Neurology. He is board certified in internal medicine, neurology, critical care medicine, vascular neurology, and neurocritical care. He has been elected as a fellow of the American Neurological Association, the American Academy of Neurology, and the Stroke Council of the American Heart Association. Throughout his career, Dr. Fink has been involved in the education and training of students, residents, and fellows in the field of stroke and critical care neurology, as well as an active participant in clinical research within this field. He is a leader in this new specialty, having lectured widely and published numerous research and clinical articles in the field of stroke and critical care. In addition, he currently serves as the editor of the monthly publication *Neurology Alert* and is the past president of the New York State Neurological Society.

Jessica Gill, Ph.D., R.N., is a Bloomberg Distinguished Professor in the Schools of Nursing and Medicine at Johns Hopkins University. She previously served as a senior investigator with the National Institute of Nursing Research (NINR) at the National Institutes of Health (NIH) and as the deputy director of NINR. Dr. Gill's current research focuses on revealing the mechanisms underlying differential responses to combat trauma and traumatic brain injury (TBI). Dr. Gill is a leader in research focused on identifying blood-based biomarkers that predict poor recovery from traumatic brain injuries, concussions, and blast. She leads biomarker methods and clinical trial design within national and international funded consortiums, and analyzes these samples in her laboratory at NIH. Specifically, Dr. Gill's laboratory has developed novel methods to understand central processes using peripheral blood, to allow for a better understanding of the mechanisms of neuronal recovery from brain injuries. Her research combines biological methods—including proteomics and epigenetics—with neuronal imaging to follow patients during their immediate recoveries and for years afterward to better understand risk and resiliency factors related to clinical outcomes. She will be appointed as a member the National Academy of Medicine in 2022.

Odette Harris, M.D., M.P.H., is a professor of neurosurgery and the vice chair and the director of the Brain Injury Program at Stanford University. She is a fellow of the American Association of Neurological Surgeons, a member of the Congress of Neurological Surgeons, and a fellow of the Aspen Global Leadership Network. Dr. Harris manages and coordinates the medical and surgical care of patients suffering from traumatic brain injury (TBI) who are admitted to the Stanford System. She focuses on implementing and streamlining current treatment algorithms aimed at improving the outcomes of this growing population. Dr. Harris is also the deputy chief of staff of rehabilitation and the site director and the principal investigator of the Traumatic Brain Injury Center of Excellence (TBICoE) at the VA Palo Alto Health Care System. The primary focus of TBICoE is TBI-specific evaluation, treatment, and follow-up care for all military personnel, Veterans, and their dependents.

Sidney Hinds II, M.D., Colonel (U.S. Army [Retired]), is the vice president for brain health strategy and research at the Wounded Warrior Project; the co-principal investigator and the lead for external collaborations for the Long-Term Impact of Military-Relevant Brain Injury Consortium; and a consultant with SCS Consulting, LLC. Dr. Hinds is a neurologist and a nuclear medicine physician with more than 30 years of military medical experience. He most recently served as the brain health research coordinator for the Department of Defense (DoD) Blast Injury Research Coordinating Office and as the medical advisor to the principal assistant for research and technology of the Medical Research and Materiel Command in Fort Detrick, Maryland. He was the national director of the Defense and Veterans Brain Injury Center from July 1, 2013, to March 16, 2016, collaborating, advising, and promoting military-relevant neurological and psychological medical and nonmedical research efforts within DoD and with external partners. Prior to that, he served as the deputy director of the Armed Forces Radiobiology Research Institute for Military Medical Operations, the in-theater neurology consultant in Afghanistan (Operation Enduring Freedom), and the chief of nuclear medicine services at Walter Reed National Military Medical Center.

Frederick Korley, M.D., Ph.D., is an associate professor of emergency medicine at the University of Michigan. His research is focused on the development of diagnostics and therapeutics for traumatic brain injury (TBI). Dr. Korley holds two patents for biofluid-based biomarkers for diagnosing TBI and prognosticating TBI outcome. He is the co-investigator of the largest observational study of TBI in the United States (Transforming Research and Clinical Knowledge in TBI). In collaboration with colleagues in engineering, Dr. Korley is developing a credit card–sized microfluidic device for point-of-care measurement of TBI biofluid-based biomarkers. He is also the principal investigator of two federally funded, multicenter studies run by the Strategies to Innovate Emergency Clinical Care Trials Network, investigating the use of biofluid-based biomarkers for subject selection in clinical trials and for monitoring individual patient response to promising neuroprotective agents. In addition, he is the principal investigator of a Phase II adaptive design, multicenter clinical trial funded by the National Institute of Neurological Disorders and Stroke, investigating the optimal treatment parameters of hyperbaric oxygen for treating severe TBI.

Ellen J. MacKenzie, Ph.D., M.Sc., is the dean of the Johns Hopkins Bloomberg School of Public Health. A leading expert in injury prevention and health services and outcomes research, Dr. MacKenzie was named a Bloomberg Distinguished Professor in 2017, recognizing her interdisciplinary work in trauma care and rehabilitation. She founded the Major Extremity Trauma Research Consortium, a national network of more than 50 civilian and military trauma centers. In 2018, she was elected to the National Academy of Medicine. Before becoming dean, Dr. MacKenzie held key leadership positions at the Bloomberg School, including the chair of the Department of Health Policy and Management, the director of the Center for Injury Research and Policy, and the senior associate dean for academic affairs. She has joint appointments in the Department of Biostatistics and the School of Medicine's departments of orthopaedics, physical medicine and rehabilitation, and emergency medicine. The Centers for Disease Control and Prevention named Dr. MacKenzie one of 20 leaders and visionaries who have had a transformative effect on the field of violence and injury prevention in the past 20 years.

Geoffrey Manley, M.D., Ph.D., is the chief of neurosurgery at Zuckerberg San Francisco General Hospital (ZSFG), where he co-directs the Brain and Spinal Injury Center, and is a professor and the vice chair of neurosurgery at the University of California, San Francisco. Dr. Manley is an internationally recognized expert in neurotrauma. In addition to a robust clinical practice at ZSFG, which is San Francisco and the Greater Bay Area's Level 1 trauma center, he coordinates and leads national and international clinical research efforts in the study of the short- and long-term effects of traumatic brain injury (TBI). Dr. Manley is the contact principal investigator and the co-founder of the Transforming Research and Clinical Knowledge in TBI (TRACK-TBI) NETWORK, an innovative, precision medicine–driven consortium that will test Phase II TBI drugs. The TRACK-TBI studies have created a modern precision medicine information commons for TBI that integrate clinical, imaging, proteomic, genomic, and outcome biomarkers to drive the development of a new TBI disease classification system, which could revolutionize diagnosis, direct patient-specific treatment, and improve outcomes. Dr. Manley's nearly 300 published manuscripts reflect a wide range of research interests from molecular aspects of brain injury to the clinical care of TBI. He sits on the National Academies of Sciences, Engineering, and Medicine's Committee on VA Examinations for Traumatic Brain Injury; has served as a consultant for the World Health Organization's Prehospital Guidelines Committee; and serves on numerous clinical research committees for the National Institutes of Health, the Centers for Disease Control and Prevention, and the Department of Defense.

Susan Margulies, Ph.D., is an assistant director of the National Science Foundation, leading the Directorate for Engineering, and a professor in the Wallace H. Coulter Department of Biomedical Engineering, jointly housed in the College of Engineering at the Georgia Institute of Technology and the School of Medicine at Emory University. She is the Georgia Research Alliance Eminent Scholar in Injury Biomechanics and previously served as the chair of the department. Using an integrated biomechanics approach consisting of relevant animal models, cell and tissue experiments, and complementary computational models and human studies, Dr. Margulies's research has generated new knowledge about the structural and functional responses of the brain and lung to their mechanical environment. Her lab has pioneered new methods for measuring functional effects of large or repeated tissue distortions; identified injury tolerances, response cascades, and causal signaling pathways; and translated these discoveries to preclinical therapeutic trials to mitigate and prevent brain and lung injuries in children and adults. Dr. Margulies is a fellow of the American Society of Mechanical Engineers, the Biomedical Engineering Society, and the American Institute for Medical and Biological Engineering. She is a member of the National Academy of Engineering and the National Academy of Medicine. Any opinions, findings, and conclusions or recommendations expressed in this report are those of Dr. Margulies and do not necessarily reflect the views of the National Science Foundation.

Christina L. Master, M.D., is a professor of clinical pediatrics at the University of Pennsylvania Perelman School of Medicine, and a pediatric and adolescent primary care sports medicine specialist, as well as an academic general pediatrician, at the Children's Hospital of Philadelphia (CHOP). She is board certified in pediatrics, sports medicine, and brain injury medicine, and is also an elected fellow of the American College of Sports Medicine, the American Medical Society for Sports Medicine, and the American Academy of Pediatrics. Dr. Master treats more than 800 children, youth, and young adults with concussions annually in her clinical sports medicine practice, while also continuing in her 29th year of general academic pediatric practice. She is the co-founding director of the Minds Matter

Concussion Program, a CHOP Frontier Program that provides comprehensive, cutting-edge, multidisciplinary clinical care and rehabilitation for concussion, as well as community advocacy and outreach, while advancing the field of concussion and mild traumatic brain injury in children, youth, and young adults through translational clinical research. Dr. Master's particular research emphasis focuses on furthering understanding of visual deficits following concussion, their role in those with persistent postconcussive symptoms, and visual deficits as a target for active intervention and treatment, as well as developing objective physiological measures as quantitative biomarkers of injury and recovery.

Michael McCrea, Ph.D., is a tenured professor, an eminent scholar, and the vice chair of research in the Department of Neurosurgery at the Medical College of Wisconsin (MCW), where he also serves as the co-director for the MCW Center for Neurotrauma Research. Dr. McCrea is the past president of both the American Academy of Clinical Neuropsychology and the American Psychological Association's Society for Clinical Neuropsychology. He has been an active researcher in the neurosciences, with hundreds of scientific publications, book chapters, and national and international lectures on the topic of traumatic brain injury (TBI). Dr. McCrea has led several large, multicenter studies on the effects of TBI and concussion. He currently is the co-principal investigator on the Concussion Assessment, Research and Education Consortium, established by the National Collegiate Athletic Association and the Department of Defense, as well as several other large-scale studies investigating the acute and chronic effects of TBI in various populations at risk. He is also a key investigator on the Transforming Research and Clinical Knowledge in TBI and TBI Endpoint Development studies. Dr. McCrea has served on several national and international expert panels related to research and clinical care for TBI over the past two decades.

Helene Moriarty, Ph.D., R.N., FAAN, is a professor and the Diane and Robert Moritz, Jr. Endowed Chair in Nursing Research at the Villanova University M. Louise Fitzpatrick College of Nursing and a nurse scientist at the Corporal Michael J. Crescenz VA Medical Center. She is also a member of the NewCourtland Center for Transitions and Health, a research center at the University of Pennsylvania School of Nursing. Dr. Moriarty's research has led to novel insights and health care approaches for Veterans with traumatic brain injury (TBI) and their families. This research is one of the first scientific efforts to engage family members as integral partners in the care of Veterans with TBI and to address the health of family caregivers. Her completed National Institutes of Health (NIH)-funded randomized controlled trial evaluated the impact of an innovative rehabilitation intervention, the Veterans' In-home Program (VIP), for Veterans with TBI and their families. Building on the VIP, Dr. Moriarty's current NIH-funded research tests a rehabilitation approach that addresses critical gaps in services and research for civilians and Veterans with chronic TBI symptoms and their families. She has held leadership roles within the VA health system and serves as a member of the American Academy of Nursing's Expert Panel on Military and Veterans Health; in 2019, she was appointed to the VA Nursing Research Field Advisory Committee charged with developing and implementing the strategic plan for nursing research for the VA health system.

Corinne Peek-Asa, Ph.D., is the vice chancellor for research at the University of California, San Diego (UCSD). She was formerly the Lowell Battershell University Distinguished Professor and the associate dean for research for the University of Iowa College of Public Health. She served on the faculty of the University of California, Los Angeles, until 2001, served on the University of Iowa faculty until 2021, and joined UCSD in 2022. Dr. Peek-Asa's area of expertise is injury and violence prevention, including global road traffic safety, interpersonal violence, workplace violence, and acute care. Her work has addressed the full spectrum of mild to severe traumatic brain injuries (TBIs), from prevention to outcomes. She has conducted research on the impact of gender on TBI outcomes and the impact of trauma systems on TBI patients reaching definitive care. She served on the Big Ten-Ivy League Concussion Taskforce, including the data committee. Dr. Peek-Asa has conducted international TBI research, including a role as the principal investigator on a project with the National Institutes of Health and the National Institute of Neurological Disorders and Stroke that established prospective TBI registries in four countries. She was elected to the National Academy of Medicine in 2020.

Thomas M. Scalea, M.D., is the physician-in-chief at the R Adams Cowley Shock Trauma Center at the University of Maryland. As the director, he serves at the level of chair within the school and hospital. As the physician-in-chief, he is responsible for clinical care in all medical administrative functions of the Shock Trauma Center. Under Dr. Scalea's leadership, the Center's faculty is responsible for the bulk of emergency general surgery patients at the University of Maryland Medical Center. His group has built a region-wide critical care program and is now responsible for 9 intensive care units and more than 100 beds. Additionally, Dr. Scalea has reorganized both research and education in the Program in Trauma. He established the G.O. Team, a rapid response team consisting of an anesthesiologist, surgeon, critical care medicine specialist, and certified registered nurse anesthetist. The G.O. team serves as a specialized component of Maryland's statewide emergency medical system to expedite critical care interventions. In 2008 and 2011, Dr. Scalea traveled to Iraq and Afghanistan to observe the Wounded Warrior Care System and provide recommendations on how to improve the system, as well as to determine how to continually refine trauma training. He also served as the senior visiting surgeon at the Landstuhl Regional Medical Center, providing care for injured soldiers as they were evacuated from Iraq.

Eric B. Schoomaker, M.D., Ph.D., FACP, Lieutenant General (U.S. Army [Retired]), was the 42nd U.S. Army surgeon general/commanding general of the U.S. Army Medical Command prior to his retirement in 2012. He then served as a professor and the vice chair for leadership, centers, and programs in the Department of Military and Emergency Medicine at the Uniformed Services University of the Health Sciences; he is currently an emeritus professor, having retired in 2019. Dr. Schoomaker promotes complementary and integrative health and medicine in the shift from a disease management–focused health care system to a system focused on the improvement of health and well-being, as well as leadership education. His assignments included command of the Walter Reed Army Medical Center and the Eisenhower Army Medical Center; two Army regional medical commands; and the Army's Medical Research and Materiel Command at Fort Detrick, Maryland. Dr. Schoomaker has received numerous military awards, including those from France and Germany; the 2012 Dr. Nathan Davis Award from the American Medical Association for outstanding government service; an honorary doctorate of science from Wake Forest University; a doctorate of letters in medicine from the Baylor College of Medicine; and the Philipp M. Lippe Award from the American Academy of Pain Medicine for outstanding contributions to the social and political aspect of pain medicine. He currently works part-time as a senior physician advisor to the Veterans Health Administration.

Martin Schreiber, M.D., is a professor of surgery; the chief of the Division of Trauma, Critical Care, and Acute Care Surgery; and the director of the Donald D. Trunkey Center for Civilian and Combat Casualty Care at Oregon Health & Science University. He is an adjunct professor of surgery at the Uniformed Services University of the Health Sciences. He is also a colonel in the U.S. Army Reserve. Dr. Schreiber's training includes significant military instruction and practice, including direct clinical experience as a military surgeon in Afghanistan. Dr. Schreiber has served as the director of the Joint Theater Trauma System for Iraq and Afghanistan. He also serves as a subject-matter expert on several Department of Defense committees, including the Committee on Surgical Combat Casualty Care (since 2016); the Tactical Combat Casualty Care Subject Matter Expert Panel (since 2018); and, as chair, the Committee on Surgical Combat Casualty Care (since 2019). Dr. Schreiber is the head of the Trauma Research Laboratory. He has been awarded the lifetime achievement award in trauma resuscitation science by the American Heart Association and the Asmund S. Laerdal Memorial Award for extensive involvement in resuscitation research and publishing from the Society of Critical Care Medicine.

Monica S. Vavilala, M.D., directs the Harborview Injury Prevention and Research Center (HIPRC), one of nine injury control centers funded by the Centers for Disease Control and Prevention; she is the only anesthesiologist in the country to hold this position. She is also a professor with tenure of anesthesiology and pain medicine and pediatrics and an adjunct professor of neurological surgery, radiology, and health services at the University of Washington. Dr. Vavilala has clinical expertise in neuroanesthesiology, pediatric trauma, and acute care of patients with traumatic brain injury (TBI). She is a translational TBI researcher and works from bench to bedside to improve care and outcomes after TBI. Dr. Vavilala cofounded the injury and health equity initiative at HIPRC and aims to improve outcomes for groups at greatest risk of injury, including children, the elderly, the poor, underrepresented minorities, and residents of rural areas. She serves on the adult and pediatric Brain Trauma Foundation Guidelines Committees. Dr. Vavilala has received funding from the National Institutes of Health for more than 20 years and has published more than 350 peer-reviewed papers.

NATIONAL ACADEMY OF MEDICINE FELLOW IN OSTEOPATHIC MEDICINE

Julieanne P. Sees, DO, FAAOS, FAOA, FAOAO, is a pediatric neuro-orthopaedic surgeon with dual fellowship training in pediatric orthopaedics and neuro-orthopaedic surgery who has focused care for children and young adults with neuromuscular conditions and chronic brain disease. An active member of the osteopathic medical profession, Dr. Sees serves on the American Osteopathic Association Board of Trustees, the American Osteopathic Foundation Board of Directors, and the American Osteopathic Academy of Orthopedics. She also serves as the president of the Delaware State Osteopathic Medical Society and the webmaster for the American Academy for Cerebral Palsy and Developmental Medicine. She teaches all levels of both osteopathic and allopathic medicine with academic affiliate professorships at the Campbell University Jerry M. Wallace School of Osteopathic Medicine, the Rowan University College of Osteopathic Medicine, and the Midwestern University Chicago College of Osteopathic Medicine. Dr. Sees has authored more than 65 peer-reviewed publications and book chapters and made more than 180 national and international conference presentations and instructional courses. Her scientific and health care advocacy research includes best practices within neuro-orthopaedics and developmental disorders, complex motor conditions and gait abnormalities, physician professional development, clinician well-being, and emerging leadership in health and medicine. Dr. Sees was named an emerging leader of both the American Osteopathic Foundation and the Chicago College of Osteopathic Medicine Alumni Association and a fellow of both the American Orthopedic Association and the American Osteopathic Academy of Orthopedics. She obtained her B.A. in chemistry/religious studies as a Division I scholarly athlete from the College of the Holy Cross, earned her M.D. from the Midwestern University Chicago College of Osteopathic Medicine, and completed an orthopaedic residency at the former University of Medicine and Dentistry of New Jersey School of Osteopathic Medicine.

STAFF

Katherine Bowman, Ph.D. (*Study Director*), is a senior program officer with the Board on Health Sciences Policy. Her activities focus on the implications of developments in science and technology. Dr. Bowman served as the co-director of the report *Heritable Human Genome Editing* (2020), with colleagues at The Royal Society, and as the director of the 2017 report *Human Genome Editing: Science, Ethics, and Governance*. Other recent studies in which she was involved include *Biodefense in the Age of Synthetic Biology* (2018) and *Microbiomes of the Built Environment: A Research Agenda for Indoor Microbiology, Human Health, and Buildings* (2017). Dr. Bowman also takes part in international activities that explore advances in science and their potential impacts for biological and chemical security. She received her Ph.D. in biomedical engineering from Johns Hopkins University.

Clare Stroud, Ph.D., is a senior program officer with the National Academies of Sciences, Engineering, and Medicine. In this capacity, she serves as the director of the Forum on Neuroscience and Nervous System Disorders, which brings together leaders from government, academia, industry, and nonprofit organizations to discuss key challenges and emerging issues in neuroscience research, development of therapies for nervous system disorders, and related ethical and societal issues. She recently served as the director of reports titled *Meeting the Challenge of Caring for Persons Living with Dementia and Their Care Partners and Caregivers: A Way Forward* and *Preventing Cognitive Decline and Dementia: A Way Forward* and as the senior program officer for the report *Medications for Opioid Use Disorder Save Lives*. Dr. Stroud first joined the National Academies as a science and technology policy graduate fellow. She has also been an associate at AmericaSpeaks, a nonprofit organization that engaged citizens in decision making on important public policy issues. Dr. Stroud received her Ph.D. from the University of Maryland, College Park, with research focused on the cognitive neuroscience of language. She received her bachelor's degree from Queen's University in Canada and spent 1 year at the University of Salamanca in Spain.

Chanel Matney, Ph.D., is a program officer with the Forum on Neuroscience and Nervous System Disorders. She also serves as the mentorship and professional development coordinator with the National Science Policy Network, a virtual community of early-career scientists and engineers that provides its members with access to resources, funding, opportunities, and programmatic support on issues related to science policy and advocacy. Dr. Matney has served as an intern, an analyst, and a fellow with various science and technology policy nonprofits. She has served as a California Council of Science and Technology science fellow, working on education policy, and as a committee staffer in the California state legislature, working on transportation issues. Her thesis work mapped the organization of cortical circuits using anatomical tracing and electrophysiology. As a graduate student, she co-founded the Johns Hopkins Science Policy Group, an organization that helps early-career researchers advocate for science-informed decision making in city, state, and federal government. She earned her doctorate in neuroscience from Johns Hopkins University as a National Science Foundation graduate predoctoral research fellow.

Bridget Borel is an administrative assistant and the program coordinator with the Board on Health Sciences Policy at the National Academies of Sciences, Engineering, and Medicine. In addition to providing program support, she helps manage the board's contracts and staff. Ms. Borel has a wide array of writing and research experience. She wrote presidential correspondence for President Clinton on a portfolio including agriculture, science and technology, and military issues. From the White House Executive Office of the President, she joined the National Academies' Board on Life Sciences, where she worked for 3 years before shifting into freelance writing, research, and media analysis. She serves as the communications director for her chapter of Team Red, White, and Blue, a Veteran support organization that aims to support Veterans' mental and physical health by forging positive connections between Veterans and their communities. She earned a B.S. in biology from Tulane University.

Eden Neleman is a senior program assistant with the Forum for Neuroscience and Nervous System Disorders. Prior to joining the National Academies in the summer of 2021, Ms. Neleman volunteered at Hassenfeld Children's Hospital at New York University Langone Health in the art therapy department; was an assistant to family psychologist Dr. Christina Cohen; and worked at WellBe, a company focused on natural health care. Throughout her studies, Ms. Neleman has been passionate about the bridge between mental and physical health and is hoping to further explore this topic at the National Academies. She earned her bachelor's degree in psychology and art history, with a minor in child and adolescent mental studies from the Gallatin School of Individualized Study at New York University.

Andrew M. Pope, Ph.D., is the senior director of the Board on Health Sciences Policy, having been a member of the National Academies of Sciences, Engineering, and Medicine staff since 1982 and the Health and Medicine Division (HMD) staff since 1989. His primary interests are science policy, biomedical ethics, and environmental and occupational influences on human health. During his tenure at the National Academies, Dr. Pope has directed numerous studies on topics that range from injury control, disability prevention, and biologic markers to the protection of human subjects of research, National Institutes of Health priority-setting processes, organ procurement and transplantation policy, and the role of science and technology in countering terrorism. Since 1998, Dr. Pope has served as the director of the Board on Health Sciences Policy, which oversees and guides a program of activities intended to encourage and sustain the continuous vigor of the basic biomedical and clinical research enterprises needed to ensure and improve the health and resilience of the public. Ongoing activities include forums on neuroscience, genomics, drug discovery and development, and medical and public health preparedness for disasters and emergencies. Dr. Pope received HMD's Cecil Award and the National Academy of Sciences President's Special Achievement Award. He has a Ph.D. in physiology and biochemistry from the University of Maryland.

Sharyl Nass, Ph.D., serves as the senior director of the Board on Health Care Services, which undertakes scholarly analysis of the organization, financing, effectiveness, workforce, and delivery of health care, with emphasis on quality, cost, and accessibility. She is also the director of the National Academies' National Cancer Policy Forum, which examines policy issues pertaining to the entire continuum of cancer research and care. For more than two decades, Dr. Nass has worked on a broad range of health and science policy topics that include the quality and safety of health care and clinical trials, developing technologies for precision medicine, and strategies for large-scale biomedical science. She has received the Cecil Medal for Excellence in Health Policy Research, a Distinguished Service Award from the National Academies, the Mentor Award from the Health and Medicine Division, and the Institute of Medicine Staff Team Achievement Award (as team leader). Dr. Nass has a Ph.D. in cell biology from Georgetown University and undertook postdoctoral training at the Johns Hopkins University School of Medicine, as well as a research fellowship at the Max Planck Institute in Germany. She also holds a B.S. and an M.S. from the University of Wisconsin–Madison.

Appendix E

Acronyms and Abbreviations

ACS	American College of Surgeons
AHRQ	Agency for Healthcare Research and Quality
BIPOC	Black, Indigenous, and People of Color
CARE	Concussion Assessment, Research and Education Consortium
CARF	Commission on Accreditation of Rehabilitation Facilities
CCCRP	Combat Casualty Care Research Program
CDC	Centers for Disease Control and Prevention
CDE	Common Data Elements
CDMRP	Congressionally Directed Medical Research Program
CENC	Chronic Effects of Neurotrauma Consortium
CMS	Centers for Medicare & Medicaid Services
CPG	clinical practice guideline
CPP	cerebral perfusion pressure
CT	computed tomography
DALY	disability-adjusted life year
DOC	disorders of consciousness
DoD	Department of Defense
DVBIC	Defense and Veterans Brain Injury Center
ED	emergency department
EHR	electronic health record
EMS	emergency medical services
FDA	Food and Drug Administration
FITBIR	Federal Interagency Traumatic Brain Injury Research (information system)

225

GCS	Glasgow Coma Scale
GFAP	glial fibrillary acidic protein
GOS	Glasgow Outcome Scale
HCBS	home- and community-based services
HCUP	Healthcare Cost and Utilization Project
HHS	Department of Health and Human Services
ICP	intracranial pressure
ICU	intensive care unit
IRF	inpatient rehabilitation facility
JTS	Joint Trauma System
LHS	learning health care system
LIMBIC	Long-Term Impact of Military-Related Brain Injury Consortium
LTACH	long-term acute care hospital
LTSS	long-term services and supports
MRI	magnetic resonance imaging
mTBI	mild traumatic brain injury
NHTSA	National Highway Traffic Safety Administration
NIDILRR	National Institute on Disability, Independent Living, and Rehabilitation Research
NIH	National Institutes of Health
NIMH	National Institute of Mental Health
NINDS	National Institute of Neurological Disorders and Stroke
NRAP	National Research Action Plan
NTDB	National Trauma Data Bank
OEF	Operation Enduring Freedom
OND	Operation New Dawn
OR	operating room
$PbtO_2$	partial brain tissue oxygenation
PM&R	physical medicine and rehabilitation
PST	problem-solving training
PTSD	posttraumatic stress disorder
RCT	randomized controlled trial
RPQ	Rivermead Postconcussion Questionnaire
SIREN	Strategies to Innovate Emergency Care Clinical Trials Network
SNF	skilled nursing facility
TBI	traumatic brain injury
tDCS	transcranial direct-current stimulation
TED	TBI Endpoints Development (project)

TMS	transcranial magnetic stimulation
TRACK-TBI	Transforming Research and Clinical Knowledge in TBI
UCH-L1	ubiquitin carboxy-terminal hydrolase
VA	Department of Veterans Affairs
VIP	Veterans' In-home Program
WHO	World Health Organization
YPLL	years of potential life lost